Incidental Findings in Neuroimaging and Their Management

A Guide for Radiologists, Neurosurgeons, and Neurologists

Kaye D. Westmark, MD
Clinical Assistant Professor of Radiology, Neuroradiology
Department of Diagnostic and Interventional Imaging
The University of Texas Health Science Center at Houston
Houston, Texas

Dong H. Kim, MD
Professor and Chair
Vivian L. Smith Department of Neurosurgery
The University of Texas Health Science Center at Houston;
Director
Mischer Neuroscience Institute
Memorial Hermann–Texas Medical Center
Houston, Texas

Roy F. Riascos, MD
Professor and Chief of Neuroradiology
Department of Diagnostic and Interventional Imaging
McGovern Medical School
The University of Texas Health Science Center at Houston;
Director
Center for Advanced Imaging Processing
Memorial Hermann–Texas Medical Center
Houston, Texas

683 illustrations

Thieme
New York • Stuttgart • Delhi • Rio de Janeiro

Library of Congress Cataloging-in-Publication Data is available from the publisher

© 2020 Thieme. All rights reserved.
Thieme Publishers New York
333 Seventh Avenue, New York, NY 10001 USA
+1 800 782 3488, customerservice@thieme.com

Georg Thieme Verlag KG
Rüdigerstrasse 14, 70469 Stuttgart, Germany
+49 [0]711 8931 421, customerservice@thieme.de

Thieme Publishers Delhi
A-12, Second Floor, Sector-2, Noida-201301
Uttar Pradesh, India
+91 120 45 566 00, customerservice@thieme.in

Thieme Publishers Rio de Janeiro,
Thieme Publicações Ltda.
Edifício Rodolpho de Paoli, 25º andar
Av. Nilo Peçanha, 50 – Sala 2508
Rio de Janeiro 20020-906 Brasil
+55 21 3172 2297

Cover design: Thieme Publishing Group
Cover Image: Laura Ocasio
Typesetting by DiTech Process Solutions, India

Printed in USA by King Printing Company, Inc.   5 4 3 2 1

ISBN 978-1-62623-828-2

Also available as an e book:
eISBN 978-1-62623-829-9

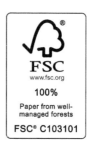

Contents

Section IV Spinal Incidental Findings

Contents

Preface

An incidental finding is a previously undetected imaging finding that is, a priori, unrelated to the purpose of the examination. It may be an artifact, a variant of normal anatomy, or a real abnormality. It may or may not be actionable.

The Prevalence of Incidental Findings

The reported prevalence and types of "incidentalomas" found on MRI examinations range widely from 2.7 to 43%, due to variations in which types of findings are included, MRI resolution, average patient age, and whether a board-certified neuroradiologist has interpreted the exam.[1,2,3,4,5] Whether the studies were looking at the imaging of aging populations or younger research volunteers, a common theme is that although incidental findings are common, only a small percentage are expected to require further clinical or imaging investigation.[4,5,6]

The Impact of Incidental Findings

From 2000 to 2007, health care expenditures (HCE) were skyrocketing, increasing at a rate of 6.6% per year. In the 3 years that followed (2008–2011), the rate of HCE growth decreased markedly, only rising 3.3% per year, with economic factors accounting for the majority of the slowdown.[7] With improvements in the economy, HCE began to rise again and outpaced economic growth for three consecutive years.[8] Imaging utilization trends have also reversed the previous downward trajectory, with increases between 2014 and 2015 of 3.3 and 4.7% for MRI and CT, respectively.[9]

In 2017, 36 million MRI scans were performed in the United States.[10] Recognizing that the "increased utilization of cross-sectional imaging will lead to a marked increase in the number of findings detected that are unrelated to the primary objectives of the examination," the American College of Radiology (ACR) formed committees for incidental findings tasked with the development of evidence-based strategies to guide management decisions. To date, these committees have published a series of white papers on the following topics[11]:

- Incidental findings on abdominal and pelvic CT and MRI, parts 1–4: adnexal, vascular, splenic and nodal, gallbladder, and biliary findings (2013)
- Incidental thyroid findings (2015)
- Incidental liver lesions (2017)
- Incidental adrenal masses (2017)
- Incidental pancreatic cysts (2017)
- Incidental renal mass (2018)
- Incidental thoracic findings (2018)
- Incidental pituitary findings (2018)

With the exception of the pituitary gland "incidentaloma," to date, no management guidelines have been published by the ACR regarding incidental findings in neuroimaging.

The Format and Goals of This Book

Section I presents common variants of normal anatomy that are extremely important to recognize in order to avoid unwarranted additional testing and unnecessary psychological stress for the patient. Section VI concludes this book by outlining CT and MR imaging artifacts that are particularly dangerous in that they may mimic pathology but also degrade imaging quality and obscure real findings.

Extracranial and extraspinal incidental findings in Sections III and V are a source of countless referrals for additional imaging partially due to medical-legal concerns but also due to uncertainty as to which lesions demand further evaluation. Fortunately, many of these findings have been addressed by the ACR's incidental finding committee white papers and diagnostic flow charts, which are presented in this book by body imaging and head and neck radiologists.

The majority of this book is devoted to intracranial and intraspinal "incidentalomas," which are presented in case presentation format in Sections II and IV, respectively. Detailed imaging analysis, the differential diagnosis, and "diagnostic pearls" are given for each case. This book differs from prior neuroimaging textbooks by including management decisions that were made in each case. A clinical Q&A concludes each case and generalizes the discussion by considering the natural history of the disease and its impact on management decisions.

Kaye D. Westmark, MD
Dong H. Kim, MD
Roy F. Riascos, MD

References

1. Morris Z, Whiteley WN, Longstreth WT Jr, et al. Incidental findings on brain magnetic resonance imaging: systematic review and meta-analysis. BMJ 2009;339: b3016

2. Håberg AK, Hammer TA, Kvistad KA, et al. Incidental intracranial findings and their clinical impact; The HUNT MRI Study in a general population of 1006 participants between 50–66 years. PLoS One 2016;11(3): e0151080

3. Vernooij MW, Ikram MA, Tanghe HL, et al. Incidental findings on brain MRI in the general population. N Engl J Med 2007;357(18):1821–1828

4. Orme NM, Fletcher JG, Siddiki HA, et al. Incidental findings in imaging research: evaluating incidence, benefit, and burden. Arch Intern Med 2010;170(17): 1525–1532

5. Katzman GL, Dagher AP, Patronas NJ. Incidental findings on brain magnetic resonance imaging from 1000 asymptomatic volunteers. JAMA 1999;282(1):36–39

6. Reneman L, de Win MM, Booij J, et al. Incidental head and neck findings on MRI in young healthy volunteers: prevalence and clinical implications. AJNR Am J Neuroradiol 2012;33(10):1971–1974

7. Dranove D, Garthwaite C, Ody C. Health spending slowdown is mostly due to economic factors, not structural change in the health care sector. Health Aff (Millwood) 2014;33(8):1399–1406

8. Antos JR, Capretta JC. National health expenditure report shows we have not solved the cost problem. Health Affairs Blog. December 6, 2017. Available at: https://www.healthaffairs.org/do/10.1377/hblog20171205.607294/full/

9. RSNA 2017, David C. Levin of Thomas Jefferson University

10. Organization of Economic Cooperation and Development. Available at: www.oedc.org

11. ACR white papers. Incidental finding committees. Available at: https://www.acr.org/Clinical-Resources/Incidental-Findings

Contributors

Behrang Amini, MD, PhD
Associate Professor
Department of Musculoskeletal Imaging
The University of Texas MD Anderson Cancer Center
Houston, Texas

Octavio Arevalo, MD
Neuroradiology Fellow
Department of Diagnostic and Interventional Imaging
McGovern Medical School
The University of Texas Health Science Center at Houston
Houston, Texas

Spiros L. Blackburn, MD
Associate Professor
Vivian L. Smith Department of Neurosurgery
The University of Texas Health Science Center at Houston
Houston, Texas

Susana Calle, MD
Assistant Professor
Division of Diagnostic Imaging
Department of Neuroradiology
The University of Texas MD Anderson Cancer Center
Houston, Texas

Jeanie M. Choi, MD
Associate Professor of Radiology, Neuroradiology
Department of Diagnostic and Interventional Imaging
The University of Texas Health Science Center at Houston
Houston, Texas

Phillip A. Choi, MD
Neurosurgical Resident
Vivian L. Smith Department of Neurosurgery
The University of Texas Health Science Center at Houston
Houston, Texas

Steven S. Chua, MD, PhD
Assistant Professor
Department of Diagnostic and Interventional Imaging
The University of Texas Health Science Center at Houston
Houston, Texas

Christopher R. Conner, MD, PhD
Neurosurgical Resident
Vivian L. Smith Department of Neurosurgery
The University of Texas Health Science Center at Houston
Houston, Texas

Mark Dannenbaum, MD
Assistant Professor
Vivian L Smith Department of Neurosurgery
The University of Texas Health Science Center at Houston
Houston, Texas

Arthur L. Day, MD
Professor, Co-Chair, and Program Director and Director of
    Cerebrovascular Surgery
Vivian L. Smith Department of Neurosurgery
University of Texas Health Science Center at Houston
Houston, Texas

Mohamed Elgendy, MD
Neuroradiology Department Observership
Department of Diagnostic and Interventional Imaging
The University of Texas Health Science Center at Houston
Houston, Texas

Yoshua Esquenazi, MD
Assistant Professor and Director of Surgical Neuro-Oncology
Vivian L. Smith Department of Neurosurgery
The University of Texas Health Science Center at Houston
Houston, Texas

Anneliese Gonzalez, MD
Associate Professor and Division Director
Division of Oncology
Department of Internal Medicine
McGovern Medical School
The University of Texas Health Science Center
    at Houston
Houston, Texas

Katie B. Guttenberg, MD
Assistant Professor
Division of Endocrinology, Diabetes and Metabolism
Department of Internal Medicine
McGovern Medical School
The University of Texas Health Science Center
    at Houston
Houston, Texas

Leo Hochhauser, MD
Clinical Associate Professor of Radiology, Neuroradiology
Department of Diagnostic and Interventional Imaging
The University of Texas Health Science Center
    at Houston
Houston, Texas

Wesley H. Jones, MD
Assistant Professor
Vivian L. Smith Department of Neurosurgery
The University of Texas Health Science Center at Houston
Houston, Texas

Ron J. Karni, MD
Chief
Division of Head and Neck Surgical Oncology;
Associate Professor
Division of Medical Oncology
Department of Otorhinolaryngology–Head and Neck Surgery
The University of Texas Health Science Center at Houston
Houston, Texas

Keith Kerr, MD
Neurosurgical Resident
Vivian L. Smith Department of Neurosurgery
The University of Texas Health Science Center at Houston
Houston, Texas

Shekhar D. Khanpara, MD
Neuroradiology Fellow
Department of Diagnostic and Interventional Imaging
The University of Texas Health Science Center at Houston
Houston, Texas

Daniel H. Kim, MD
Professor and Director, Reconstructive Spinal and
  Peripheral Nerve Surgery
Vivian L. Smith Department of Neurosurgery
University of Texas Health Science Center at Houston
Houston, Texas

Dong H. Kim, MD
Professor and Chair
Vivian L. Smith Department of Neurosurgery
The University of Texas Health Science Center at Houston;
Director
Mischer Neuroscience Institute
Memorial Hermann–Texas Medical Center
Houston, Texas

Cole T. Lewis, MD
Neurosurgical Resident
Vivian L. Smith Department of Neurosurgery
The University of Texas Health Science Center
  at Houston
Houston, Texas

John A. Lincoln, MD
Associate Professor of Neurology
Bartels Family Professorship in Neurology;
Director, MRI Analysis Center
Multiple Sclerosis Research Group
McGovern Medical School
The University of Texas Health Science Center at Houston
Houston, Texas

Eduardo J. Matta, MD, CMQ
Associate Professor
Department of Diagnostic and Interventional Imaging
The University of Texas Health Science Center at Houston
Houston, Texas

Daniel R. Monsivais, MD
Neurosurgical Resident
Vivian L. Smith Department of Neurosurgery
The University of Texas Health Science Center at Houston
Houston, Texas

Saint-Aaron L. Morris, MD
Neurosurgical Resident
Vivian L. Smith Department of Neurosurgery
The University of Texas Health Science Center at Houston
Houston, Texas

Laura Ocasio, MD
Coordinator of the Center for Advanced Imaging Processing
Memorial Hermann Health System
Houston, Texas

Rajan P. Patel, MD
Associate Professor of Radiology, Neuroradiology
Department of Diagnostic and Interventional Imaging
The University of Texas Health Science Center at Houston
Houston, Texas

Krina Patel, MD, MSc
Assistant Professor and Center Medical Director
Department of Lymphoma/Myeloma
The University of Texas MD Anderson Cancer Center
Houston, Texas

Maria O. Patino, MD
Assistant Professor of Radiology, Neuroradiology
Department of Diagnostic and Interventional Imaging
The University of Texas Health Science Center at Houston
Houston, Texas

Carlos A. Pérez, MD
Neuroimmunology Fellow
Department of Neurology
McGovern Medical School
The University of Texas Health Science Center at Houston
Houston, Texas

Pejman Rabiei, MD
Radiology Resident
Department of Diagnostic and Interventional Imaging
The University of Texas Health Science Center at Houston
Houston, Texas

Roy F. Riascos, MD
Professor and Chief of Neuroradiology
Department of Diagnostic and Interventional Imaging
McGovern Medical School
The University of Texas Health Science Center at Houston;
Director
Center for Advanced Imaging Processing
Memorial Hermann–Texas Medical Center
Houston, Texas

Seferino Romo, ARRT/MR
MR Lead Educator
Memorial Hermann–Texas Medical Center
Houston, Texas

David I. Sandberg, MD, FAANS, FACS, FAAP
Professor and Director of Pediatric Neurosurgery;
Dr. Marnie Rose Professorship in Pediatric Neurosurgery
Departments of Pediatric Surgery and Neurosurgery
McGovern Medical School
The University of Texas Health Science Center at Houston
Houston, Texas, USA

Karl Schmitt, MD
Assistant Professor
Vivian L. Smith Department of Neurosurgery
The University of Texas Health Science Center at Houston
Houston, Texas

Kaustubh G. Shiralkar, MD
Assistant Professor
Department of Diagnostic and Interventional Imaging
The University of Texas Health Science Center at Houston
Houston, Texas

Alexander B. Simonetta, MD
Assistant Professor of Radiology, Neuroradiology
Department of Diagnostic and Interventional Imaging
The University of Texas Health Science Center at Houston
Houston, Texas

Clark W. Sitton, MD
Associate Professor of Radiology, Neuroradiology, and
   Neuroradiology Fellowship Program Director
Department of Diagnostic and Interventional Imaging
The University of Texas Health Science Center at Houston
Houston, Texas

Emilio P. Supsupin, Jr., MD
Assistant Professor of Radiology, Neuroradiology
Department of Diagnostic and Interventional Imaging
The University of Texas Health Science Center
   at Houston
Houston, Texas

Mumtaz B. Syed, MD, PhD
Neuroradiology Fellow
Department of Diagnostic and Interventional Imaging
The University of Texas Health Science Center
   at Houston
Houston, Texas

Nitin Tandon, MD, FAANS
Professor and Vice Chair
Department of Neurosurgery;
Co-Director
Texas Institute of Restorative Neurotechnology;
Director
Epilepsy Surgery Program
Mischer Neuroscience Institute–Memorial Hermann Hospital
McGovern Medical School
The University of Texas Health Science Center at Houston;
Adjunct Professor
Electrical and Computer Engineering
Rice University
Houston, Texas

Chakradhar R. Thupili, MD
Assistant Professor
Department of Diagnostic & Interventional Imaging
The University of Texas Health Science Center at Houston
Houston, Texas

Raul F. Valenzuela, MD
Assistant Professor
Division of Diagnostic Imaging
Department of Muculoskeletal Imaging
The University of Texas MD Anderson Cancer Center
Houston, Texas

Kaye D. Westmark, MD
Clinical Assistant Professor of Radiology, Neuroradiology
Department of Diagnostic and Interventional Imaging
The University of Texas Health Science Center at Houston
Houston, Texas

Richard M. Westmark, MD, FAANS
Assistant Clinical Professor
Department of Neurosurgery
University of Texas Medical School
Houston, Texas

Hussein A. Zeineddine, MD
Neurosurgical Resident
Vivian L. Smith Department of Neurosurgery
McGovern Medical School
The University of Texas Health Science Center at Houston
Houston, Texas

Section I

Normal Variants

Introduction

Normal anatomical variants are frequently encountered in routine clinical imaging. In some cases, they may mimic real anomalies, which could result in unnecessary additional testing and unwarranted intervention. In this section, we will review some commonly encountered normal variants and discuss characteristics of their imaging appearance that may assist in differentiating them from pathologic entities.

1 Persistent Primitive Trigeminal Artery

Kaye D. Westmark, Laura Ocasio, and Roy F. Riascos

1.1 Case Presentation

1.1.1 History and Physical Examination

A 45-year-old man presented with a history of migraine headaches which had recently worsened in severity.

His neurological examination was normal. Specifically, cranial nerves II to XII were intact. An axial T2-weighted image from his brain MRI is shown in ▶ Fig. 1.1.

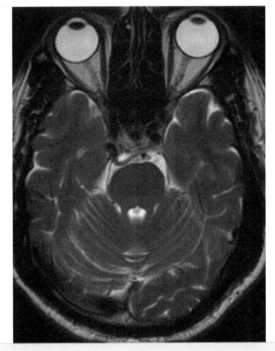

Fig. 1.1

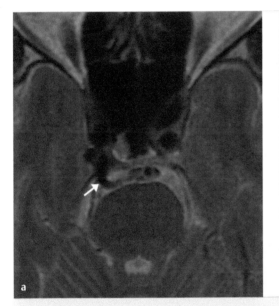
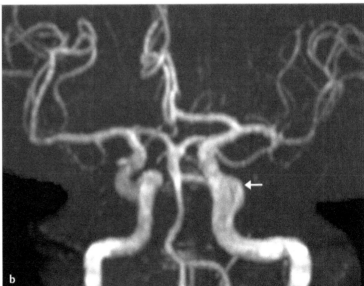

Fig. 1.2 **(a)** The axial FSE T2-weighted image reveals a vascular-appearing flow void (*arrow*), extending from the right cavernous sinus into the prepontine cistern. **(b)** This abnormal vessel is confirmed on the COW MRA, where the proximal basilar artery appears small and the anomalous vessel, arising from the cavernous portion of the right internal carotid artery (*arrow*), can be seen contributing to the distal basilar artery, which it joins immediately proximal to the origin of the superior cerebellar arteries. The P-com arteries were hypoplastic bilaterally. These findings are consistent with a persistent primitive trigeminal artery. COW, circle of Willis; FSE, fast spin echo; MRA, magnetic resonance angiography; P-com, posterior communicating.

1.2 Differential Diagnosis

- Flow void associated with an arterial venous malformation:
  - Typically, numerous enlarged flow voids and a prominent central nidus.
- Flow void associated with a dural arteriovenous fistula:
  - Often occurs in the posterior fossa but in association with a thrombosed dural venous sinus and mastoid air cell opacification.

1.3 Diagnostic Pearls and Pitfalls

Persistent primitive trigeminal artery:
- Classic location of this persistent fetal anastomosis connecting the cavernous carotid artery (anterior circulation) with the basilar artery (posterior circulation) is diagnostic.
- It is very important to recognize this anomalous circulation before doing a Wada test, as the anterior circulation is directly supplying the brainstem.
- The characteristic appearance of this artery on parasellar sagittal images has the shape of the Greek letter "tau" (see ▶ Fig. 1.3a,b).
- The MRA should be closely examined for aneurysm once a trigeminal artery is identified. An increased incidence of aneurysm, typically in the anterior circulation, has been reported due to altered hemodynamics.

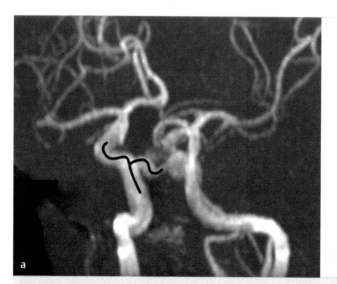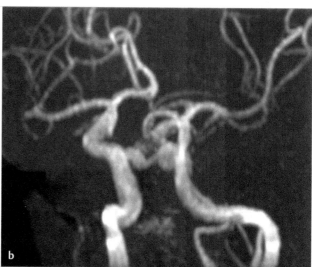

Fig. 1.3 (a, b)

1.4 Essential Information about Persistent Primitive Trigeminal Arteries

- The posterior communicating artery (P-com) is a normal finding, and the most common anterior to posterior circulation anastomosis in the adult.
- In utero, the trigeminal artery supplies the basilar artery before development of the P-com and vertebral arteries.
- Fetal anastomoses may fail to involute and be seen as incidental findings or, more rarely, cause symptoms (i.e., trigeminal neuralgia may be associated with a persistent trigeminal artery).
  - Four types (from inferior to superior):
    - Proatlantal–cervical internal carotid artery (ICA) to vertebral artery (VA).
    - Hypoglossal–distal cervical or petrous ICA to VA. It traverses the hypoglossal canal.
    - Otic–petrous ICA to basilar artery. It traverses the internal auditory canal.
    - Trigeminal:
      - The most common and largest of the persistent fetal anastomoses.
      - May course through the sella or exit the cavernous sinus and accompany the trigeminal nerve.

- Angiographic types:
  - Saltzman I—P-coms are hypoplastic and the persistent trigeminal artery supplies the distal posterior circulation.
  - Saltzman II—The P-coms supply the posterior cerebral arteries. The persistent trigeminal artery supplies the superior cerebellar artery territory. The distal basilar artery is poorly visualized angiographically.
  - Saltzman III—The persistent trigeminal artery terminates into the superior cerebellar artery and does not join the basilar artery.

Suggested Readings

Alcalá-Cerra G, Tubbs RS, Niño-Hernández LM. Anatomical features and clinical relevance of a persistent trigeminal artery. Surg Neurol Int. 2012; 3:111

de Bondt BJ, Stokroos R, Casselman J. Persistent trigeminal artery associated with trigeminal neuralgia: hypothesis of neurovascular compression. Neuroradiology. 2007; 49(1):23–26

Goyal M. The tau sign. Radiology. 2001; 220(3):618–619

Tyagi G, Sadashiva N, Konar S, et al. Persistent trigeminal artery: neuroanatomic and clinical relevance. World Neurosurg 2020;134:e214–e223

2 Arachnoid Granulations

Susana Calle, Pejman Rabiei, Shekhar D. Khanpara, and Roy F. Riascos

2.1 Case Presentation

2.1.1 History and Physical Examination

A 17-year-old girl with a past medical history of migraine headaches since the age of 14 years presents with a severe headache.

On neurological examination, CNs II–XII were intact. There was no evidence of papilledema on fundoscopy examination.

2.1.2 Imaging Findings and Impression

MRI of the brain with contrast shows an oval lesion (*white arrows*; ▶ Fig. 2.1a,b) in the distal left transverse sinus, which is isointense to cortex on T2-weighted imaging (T2WI) and on fluid-attenuated inversion recovery (FLAIR; ▶ Fig. 2.1c) and hypointense on T1-weighted imaging (T1WI). The lesion is seen as a filling defect on postcontrast T1WI (▶ Fig. 2.1d) and does not show any susceptibility on susceptibility weighted imaging (SWI; ▶ Fig. 2.1e) to suggest a venous clot. An intralesional vein (*black arrow*) is seen draining the area. All these features are consistent with an arachnoid granulation.

2.2 Differential Diagnosis

- **Arachnoid granulation:**
  - Represent enlarged arachnoid villi and are seen as nonenhancing filling defects within venous sinuses causing scalloping of the inner table when large.

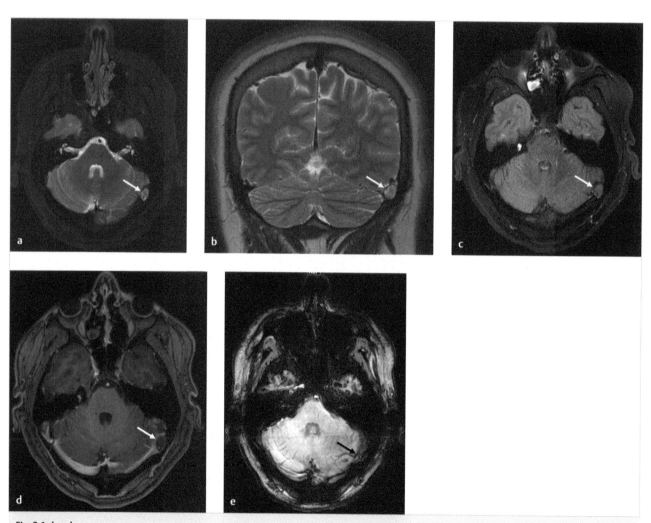

Fig. 2.1 (a–e)

- Often seen is a superficial cortical vein draining into the arachnoid granulation.
  - Absence of susceptibility on gradient echo (GRE) images.
- Venous thrombosis:
  - Usually involves an entire segment of one sinus or multiple sinuses.
  - May be associated with mastoid inflammation.
  - Can extend into cortical veins and may involve the distal sigmoid sinus and jugular vein, which does NOT occur with arachnoid granulations.
  - Unlike arachnoid granulations, acute thrombus is hyperdense to the brain on CT, hyperintense on T1WI, and hypointense on FLAIR sequences and shows susceptibility artifact on GRE/SWI.
- Intrasinusal tumor:
  - Enhances with gadolinium administration.

2.3 Diagnostic Pearls and Pitfalls

- CT:
  - Nonenhancing, hypo- to isodense to the brain, frondlike filling defects within venous sinuses.[1]
  - The density measures around 20 HU.
  - They tend to cause scalloping of the inner table of skull if large, likely due to cerebrospinal fluid (CSF) pulsations.
- MRI:
  - Hyperintense to the brain on T2WI and hypointense on T1WI. Partial or no suppression on FLAIR sequences.
  - No enhancement on postcontrast images.
  - Visualization of superficial cortical veins draining into the granulation is a specific sign for arachnoid granulation.
- Since arachnoid granulations protrude into the dural venous sinuses, they may mimic venous thrombosis or a dural-based

tumor. Careful analysis of the density on CT, MRI signal characteristics, and the finding of intralesional flow voids are important in making the distinction.
- In the chronic phases, sinus thrombosis can enhance.

2.4 Essential Information about Arachnoid Granulations

- Arachnoid granulations represent enlarged arachnoid villi and are fluid-filled extensions of arachnoid membrane into dural venous sinuses whose function is to drain CSF.[2]
- They are present in all superficial venous sinuses but are most common in the transverse sinus, followed by the superior sagittal sinus.
- If large, they may obstruct the venous flow, leading to venous hypertension and may predispose to venous thrombosis.
- They are called giant granulations when larger than 1 cm.

2.5 Companion Case

2.5.1 History and Physical Examination

A 56-year-old woman presents with a history of weakness in the right upper extremity.

Patient is conscious and oriented to time, place, and person. Strength in the right upper extremity appears decreased compared to the opposite side.

Noncontrast CT brain (▶ Fig. 2.2a) and bone (▶ Fig. 2.2b) windows show a prominent sagittal sinus with scalloping (*asterisk*) of the inner table of the skull.

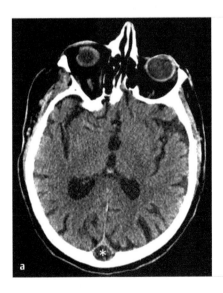 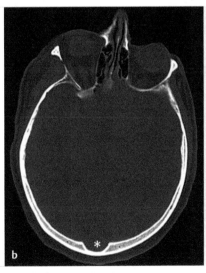

Fig. 2.2 (a, b)

MRI of the brain including axial T2WI (▶ Fig. 2.3a), axial T1WI without contrast (▶ Fig. 2.3b), and axial FLAIR (▶ Fig. 2.3c) shows a round filling defect (*white arrow*) in the posterior aspect of the superior sagittal sinus with flow voids within it. The lesion is centrally hyperintense to the cortex on T2WI, hypointense on T1WI and FLAIR, and shows no restriction on diffusion weighted imaging (DWI; ▶ Fig. 2.3d). Axial postcontrast T1WI (▶ Fig. 2.3e) demonstrates enhancement of only the vessels. All findings are consistent with the diagnosis of a prominent arachnoid granulation.

Some incidental periventricular white matter changes are noted secondary to small vessel ischemia with prominence of Virchow–Robin spaces in the bilateral basal ganglia.

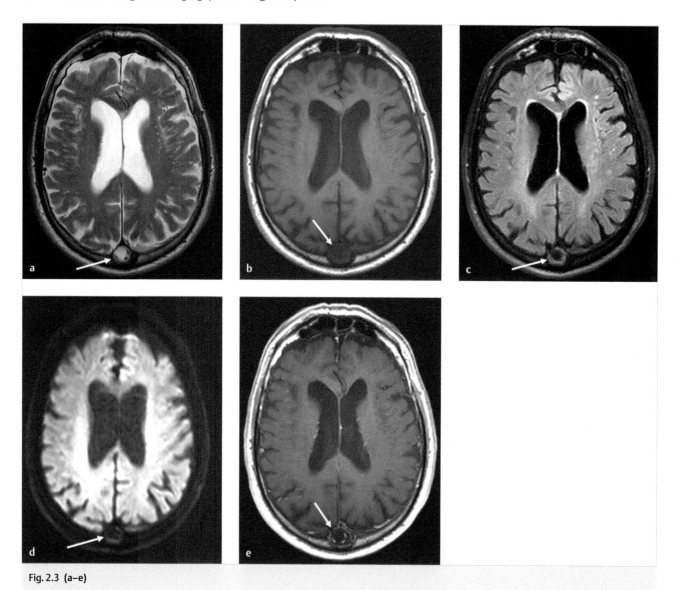

Fig. 2.3 (a–e)

References

[1] De Keyzer B, Bamps S, Van Calenbergh F, Demaerel P, Wilms G. Giant arachnoid granulations mimicking pathology. A report of three cases. Neuroradiol J. 2014; 27(3):316–321

[2] Brunori A, Vagnozzi R, Giuffrè R. Antonio Pacchioni (1665–1726): early studies of the dura mater. J Neurosurg. 1993; 78(3):515–518

3 Asymmetry of the Lateral Ventricles

Susana Calle, Pejman Rabiei, Shekhar D. Khanpara, and Roy F. Riascos

3.1 Case Presentation

3.1.1 History and Physical Examination

A 59-year-old male presented with headaches.
The neurological examination was unremarkable.

3.1.2 Imaging Findings and Impression

Axial (▶ Fig. 3.1a) and coronal (▶ Fig. 3.1b) images from a noncontrast head CT show asymmetry of the frontal horns (*white arrows*) of the lateral ventricles. There was no dilatation of the temporal horns (not shown).

Axial T2-weighted imaging (T2WI; ▶ Fig. 3.2a) and fluid-attenuated inversion recovery (FLAIR) weighted imaging (▶ Fig. 3.2b) of the brain without contrast show asymmetrical prominence of the right lateral ventricle as compared to the opposite side (*black arrows*). The temporal horns were normal in size and there is no evidence of transependymal flow of cerebrospinal fluid (CSF) to suggest hydrocephalus (▶ Fig. 3.2c).

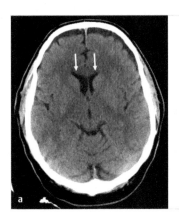 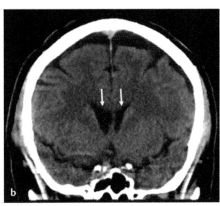

Fig. 3.1 (a, b)

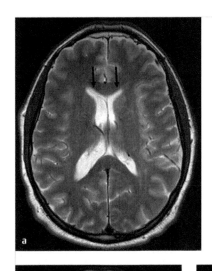 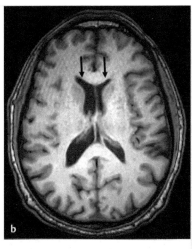
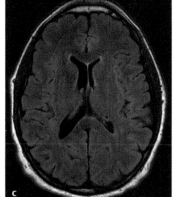 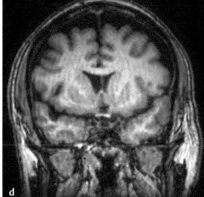

Fig. 3.2 (a–d)

3.2 Differential Diagnosis

- **Asymmetric lateral ventricles:**
  - Minimal asymmetry of the lateral ventricles, involving the frontal horns without signs of transependymal flow or mass involving the foramen of Monro.
- Unilateral obstructive hydrocephalus:
  - The degree of asymmetry is typically more severe.
  - Associated with periventricular edema or transependymal flow of CSF.
  - An intraventricular or periventricular lesion may be causing obstruction of one foramen of Monro.
  - Causes may include the following:
    - Adhesion/synechiae post infectious ventriculitis or hemorrhage.
    - Congenital atresia.
    - Choroid plexus lesion.
    - Cysts: colloid cysts, neurocysticercosis, ependymal cysts, etc.
    - Tumor: subependymal giant cell astrocytoma (SEGA).
    - Vascular malformations.
  - High-resolution, multiplanar 3D sequences and heavily T2WI that are immune to CSF flow artifact have better specificity as they are able to directly visualize the foramina and look to see if there is a mass causing obstruction.
  - When questions remain, CSF flow studies can be performed to see if there is evidence of normal flow through the foramen of Monro, thus supporting the diagnosis of a normal variant, lateral ventricular asymmetry.
- Ipsilateral atrophy due to encephalomalacia (Dyke–Davidoff–Masson syndrome):
  - Ipsilateral dilatation of ventricle secondary to atrophy of the brain.
  - Associated hypertrophy of calvarium and sinuses on the ipsilateral side.
- Ipsilateral hemimegalencephaly:
  - Congenital malformation with defective cellular organization/migration.
  - Presence of polymicrogyria/lissencephaly/pachygyria ipsilateral to dilatation of ventricle.
  - Ipsilateral thickened calvarium.
- Contralateral extrinsic mass effect.
- Herniation syndromes leading to compression of the foramen of Monro, post shunting.

3.3 Diagnostic Pearls

- Asymmetric lateral ventricles:
  - Minimal asymmetry of ventricles.
  - Lack of mass effect or periventricular interstitial edema (transependymal flow of CSF).
  - Symmetry of the hemispheres.
- Severe degrees of asymmetry, diffuse nonfocal ventricular enlargement, and evidence of transependymal CSF migration should prompt a search for possible obstruction.

3.4 Essential Information about Asymmetric Lateral Ventricles

- Asymmetry of the frontal horns of the lateral ventricles is a fairly common phenomenon[1]. Shapiro et al examined 300 patients, out of which 10.3% of patients had an asymmetric frontal horn.[2]
- Bowing, deviation, or displacement of the septi pellucidi across the midline.
- It may be a normal finding but should prompt closer evaluation of the foramen of Monro.

3.5 Companion Case

3.5.1 History and Physical Examination

A 44-year-old man presents with complain of ataxia.
The neurological examination was normal.

3.5.2 Imaging Findings and Impression

Axial (▶ Fig. 3.3a) and coronal (▶ Fig. 3.3b) images from a noncontrast head CT scan show asymmetric prominence of the right lateral ventricle (*white asterisk*) as compared to the opposite side. A 5-mm hyperdense colloid cyst is noted within the foramen of Monro (*white arrow*), possibly causing unilateral obstruction of right lateral ventricle. Axial and coronal FLAIR images (▶ Fig. 3.3c,d) confirms the presence of FLAIR hyperintense colloid cyst and unilateral prominence of the right lateral ventricle. In this case, the patient had a history of new onset, progressively worsening headaches and, therefore, electively underwent resection of the colloid cyst. Postresection, the lateral ventricles were symmetric.

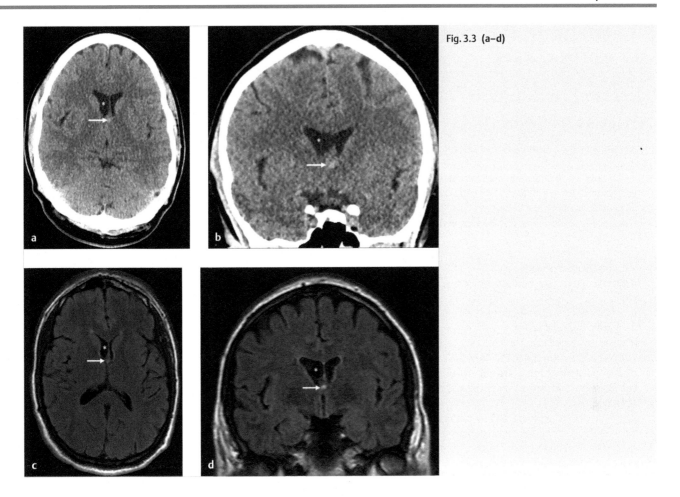

Fig. 3.3 (a–d)

References

[1] Grosman H, Stein M, Perrin RC, Gray R, St Louis EL. Computed tomography and lateral ventricular asymmetry: clinical and brain structural correlates. Can Assoc Radiol J. 1990; 41(6):342–346

[2] Shapiro R, Galloway SJ, Shapiro MD. Minimal asymmetry of the brain: a normal variant. AJR Am J Roentgenol. 1986; 147(4):753–756

4 Basal Ganglia/Dentate Nuclei Mineralization

Susana Calle, Pejman Rabiei, Shekhar D. Khanpara, and Roy F. Riascos

4.1 Case Presentation

4.1.1 History and Physical Examination

A 62-year-old woman with past medical history of type 2 diabetes mellitus (DM) presents with right lower extremity edema, pain, fever and confusion. The patient was admitted to the emergency room for cellulitis of the right lower extremity and altered mental status.

The patient is febrile. Her cranial nerves II–XII were intact with no focal neurologic deficit.

4.1.2 Imaging Findings and Impression

Axial CT scans of the head without contrast (▶ Fig. 4.1a,b) show hyperdensities (HU of 110) involving the bilateral basal ganglia and the bilateral dentate nuclei (*black arrows*). Axial gradient-echo images (▶ Fig. 4.1c,d) show susceptibility artifact in the corresponding areas consistent with calcification (*white arrows*). The calcifications are symmetric without associated edema or mass effect.

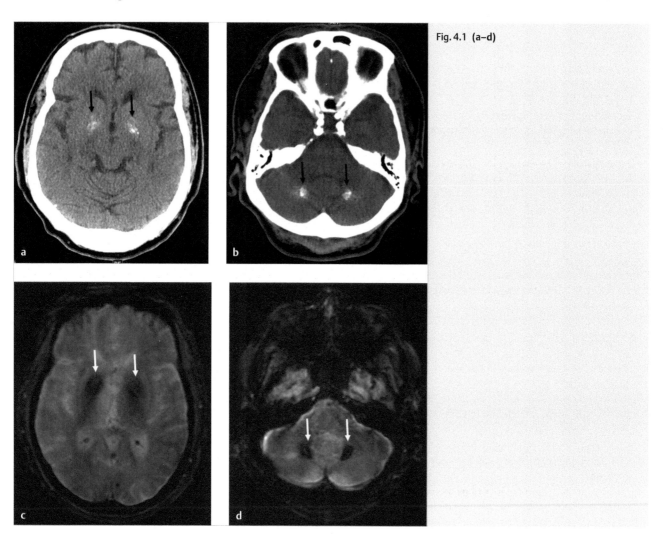

Fig. 4.1 (a–d)

4.2 Differential Diagnosis[1]

- **Basal ganglia calcification:**
  - Bilateral calcification involving the basal ganglia with a predominance for globus pallidus interna seen as hyperdensity on CT and presence of susceptibility on gradient-echo images.
- Fahr's syndrome:
  - Rare genetic disorder of abnormal vascular calcium deposition.
  - Presents as symmetrical calcifications of the bilateral globus pallidus, caudate, lentiform nucleus, thalamus, and dentate nucleus.
  - MR images may be normal or have hyperintense signal on the T1-weighted images.
  - PET scan may show degrees of fluorodeoxyglucose (FDG) uptake.
  - Should be differentiated from underlying metabolic causes such as hyperparathyroidism and hypoparathyroidism by measuring serum calcium, phosphorus, and alkaline phosphatase levels.
- Mineralizing microangiopathy:
  - Usually seen in children receiving chemotherapy or radiotherapy.
  - Areas typically involved are the gray–white matter interface, lentiform nucleus, and dentate nucleus of the cerebellum.
- Mitochondrial encephalomyopathy, lactic acidemia, and stroke-like symptoms (MELAS):
  - MELAS is a mitochondrial disease with maternal inheritance.
  - Presents in younger adults with multiple strokes in different stages of development, not confining to a specific vascular territory.
  - May show symmetric basal ganglia calcification.[2,3]
- CNS tuberculosis:
  - Multiple punctate calcified and noncalcified lesions involving bilateral cerebral hemispheres, including the basal ganglia.
  - Since the noncalcified lesions are active granulomas, they tend to enhance with gadolinium administration.
- Cockayne's syndrome:
  - Rare genetic dysmyelinating disorder. Patients are children with neurodevelopmental delay and hearing and skin problems.
  - On brain MR images, there is atrophy of cerebellum, corpus callosum, brain stem, and supratentorial white matter.
- TORCH (toxoplasmosis, other [syphilis, varicella-zoster, parvovirus B19], rubella, cytomegalovirus, and herpes) infection.

- Congenital HIV infection and HIV encephalopathy may have basal ganglia calcifications which are NOT seen when the virus infection occurs later in life.

4.3 Diagnostic Pearls

- Normal physiologic calcifications that occur more frequently in older patients are considered an incidental finding but should be considered pathological when present in the pediatric and young adult populations.
- Normal basal ganglia calcifications tend to involve the globus pallidus interna.
- Noncontrast CT: faint or course hyperdense areas. It is sometimes difficult to differentiate from hemorrhage, but bilaterality, symmetry, and complete lack of mass effect and surrounding edema suggest basal ganglia calcifications.
- MR: appear as hypointense to the brain on T2-weighted images and hyperintense on T1-weighted images involving the bilateral basal ganglia with susceptibility artifact on T2*-weighted images.

4.4 Essential Information about Basal Ganglia Mineralization

- It is frequently seen in the elderly population and represents deposition of minerals within the basal ganglia and dentate nuclei.
- It is fairly common in the general population with an incidence of about 1%.

4.5 Companion Case

4.5.1 History and Physical Examination

A 42-year-old man presented with complaint of intermittent headaches.

The neurological examination was normal.

4.5.2 Imaging Findings and Impression

Axial CT head (▶ Fig. 4.2a) demonstrates calcification within bilateral caudate and lentiform nuclei (*arrows*) with faint curvilinear calcification in subcortical white matter of bilateral frontal lobes (*arrowheads*).

Corresponding axial T1 image (▶ Fig. 4.2b) illustrates hyperintensity in bilateral caudate and lentiform nuclei (*arrows*). An underlying subclinical hypoparathyroidism was identified on laboratory studies. The diagnosis was Fahr's syndrome.

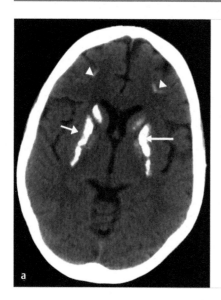 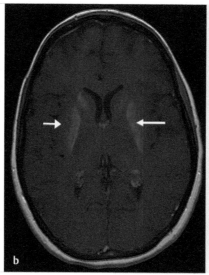

Fig. 4.2 (a, b)

References

[1] Hegde AN, Mohan S, Lath N, Lim CCT. Differential diagnosis for bilateral abnormalities of the basal ganglia and thalamus. Radiographics. 2011; 31(1):5–30

[2] Pauli W, Zarzycki A, Krzyształowski A, Walecka A. CT and MRI imaging of the brain in MELAS syndrome. Pol J Radiol. 2013; 78(3):61–65

[3] Sue CM, Crimmins DS, Soo YS, et al. Neuroradiological features of six kindreds with MELAS tRNA(Leu) A2343G point mutation: implications for pathogenesis. J Neurol Neurosurg Psychiatry. 1998; 65(2):233–240

5 Cavum Septum Pellucidum

Susana Calle, Pejman Rabiei, Shekhar D. Khanpara, and Roy F. Riascos

5.1 Case Presentation

5.1.1 History and Physical Examination

An 18-year-old man with no significant past medical history presents with an episode of seizure-like activity.

On physical examination, the patient is alert and oriented with no focal neurologic deficit.

5.1.2 Imaging Findings and Impression

Coronal CT scan of the head without contrast (▶ Fig. 5.1a) and brain MR images without contrast including axial T2-weighted (▶ Fig. 5.1b), axial T1-weighted (▶ Fig. 5.1c), and coronal fluid-attenuated inversion recovery (FLAIR; ▶ Fig. 5.1d)

images show persistence of a fluid-filled cavity (*white arrows*) in between leaflets of the septum pellucidum extending posteriorly to the foramina of Monro, consistent with a cavum septum pellucidum. There is an incidental curvilinear pericallosal lipoma (*white arrowhead*) along the splenium.

5.2 Differential Diagnosis

- **Cavum septum pellucidum (CSP):**
  - It is a fluid-filled cavity within the leaflets of septum pellucidum, which follows the cerebrospinal fluid (CSF) signal intensity on all sequences located anterior to columns of fornix.

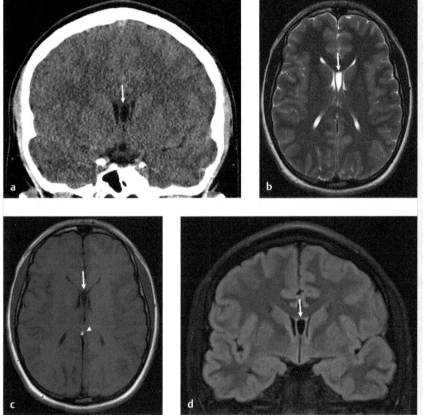

Fig. 5.1 (a–d)

- Cavum septum vergae (CSV):
  - Posterior extension of CSP beyond the columns of the fornix and foramen of Monro.
  - CSV is located posterior to the CSP and posterior and superior to the columns of fornix.[1]
  - It is hypodense with CSF density on head CT scans without contrast. It follows CSF signal intensity on MR images of the brain and will be suppressed on FLAIR sequences.
  - Although the CSP and CSV are believed to represent anatomic variations, investigators have shown an increased prevalence of them in traumatic brain injury patients.[2,3]
  - A large CSP in patients with schizophrenia can also be associated with more severe symptoms.[4]
- Cavum velum interpositum:
  - It is an enlarged potential space in between infolded layers of the velum interpositum.
  - Anatomically, it is triangle shaped and lies between the internal cerebral veins.
  - It is located below the column of the fornix and the splenium of corpus callosum and posterior to the foramen of Monro.
  - It has CSF-like density on head CT scans with a triangular configuration pointing forward and not extending anterior to the foramen of Monro.[5]
  - Isointense to CSF on all MR sequences with a hypointense membrane surrounding it.

5.3 Diagnostic Pearls

- It is a fluid-filled cavity within the leaflets of septum pellucidum located anterior to columns of fornix.
- It follows CSF signal on all sequences.

5.4 Essential Information about Cavum Septum Pellucidum

- It is a fluid-filled cavity between the frontal horns of the lateral ventricles.

- It occurs due to persistence of fluid in between the leaflets of the septum pellucidum during fetal life.
- It is commonly seen in around 85% of infants at age 3 to 6 months. However, the incidence tends to decrease with increasing age.
- It is lined with ependyma on ventricular sides.[6]
- It is bounded on all sides: anteriorly by the genu of the corpus callosum, superiorly by the body of the corpus callosum, posteriorly by the anterior limb and pillars of the fornix, inferiorly by the anterior commissure and the rostrum of the corpus callosum, and laterally by the leaflets of the septum pellucidum.[1]
- It does not communicate with the subarachnoid space and can occur in isolation or along with a CSV.

5.5 Companion Cases

5.5.1 Companion Case 1

History and Physical Examination

A 62-year-old woman with past medical history of stroke was admitted because of severe headache.

Physical examination failed to reveal any neurologic deficit.

Imaging Findings and Impression

Axial CT scan of the head without contrast (▶ Fig. 5.2a, *white arrow*) and noncontrast MR images of the brain including axial T1-weighted (▶ Fig. 5.2b) and coronal T2-weighted (▶ Fig. 5.2c) images demonstrate persistence of a fluid-filled cavity (*asterisks*) in between leaflets of the septum pellucidum extending posteriorly beyond the foramen of Monro, consistent with a CSP and vergae.

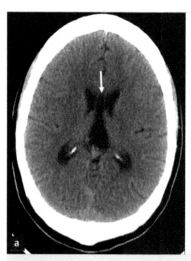
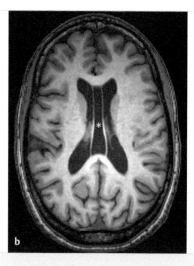
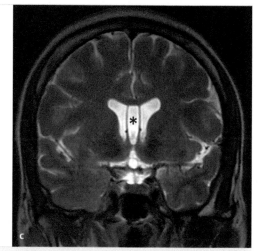

Fig. 5.2 (a–c)

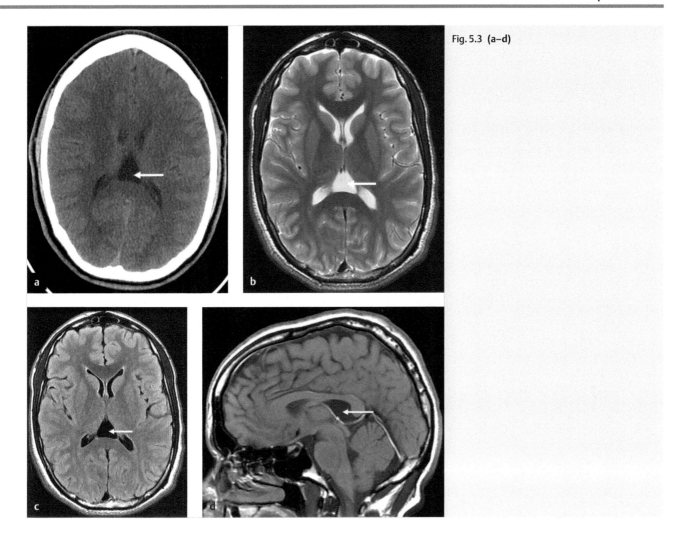

Fig. 5.3 (a–d)

5.5.2 Companion Case 2

History and Physical Examination

A 19-year-old woman with past medical history of right-sided craniotomy presents with severe nausea and vomiting.

Physical examination revealed that cranial nerves II to XII are grossly intact without any neurologic deficit.

Imaging Findings and Impression

Axial CT of the head (▶ Fig. 5.3a) demonstrates a triangular fluid-filled cavity within the lateral ventricle just anterior to splenium of corpus callosum.

MRI of the brain (▶ Fig. 5.3b,c) in the same patient re-illustrates the triangular fluid-filled cavity (*white arrow*; follows CSF signal on all sequences) in between the leaflets of the septum pellucidum extending from the foramen of Monro anteriorly to the splenium of the corpus callosum posteriorly consistent with a cavum velum interpositum. The sagittal T1 image (▶ Fig. 5.3d) demonstrates the location of cavum veli interpositum (*white arrow*) below the splenium and above the internal cerebral veins (*white asterisk*).

References

[1] Tubbs RS, Krishnamurthy S, Verma K, et al. Cavum velum interpositum, cavum septum pellucidum, and cavum vergae: a review. Childs Nerv Syst. 2011; 27(11):1927–1930

[2] Bonfante E, Riascos R, Arevalo O. Imaging of chronic concussion. Neuroimaging Clin N Am. 2018; 28(1):127–135

[3] Spillane JD. Five boxers. BMJ. 1962; 2(5314):1205–1210

[4] Flashman LA, Roth RM, Pixley HS, et al. Cavum septum pellucidum in schizophrenia: clinical and neuropsychological correlates. Psychiatry Res. 2007; 154(2):147–155

[5] Glastonbury CM, Osborn AG, Salzman KL. Masses and malformations of the third ventricle: normal anatomic relationships and differential diagnoses. Radiographics. 2011; 31(7):1889–1905

[6] Sarwar M. The septum pellucidum: normal and abnormal. AJNR Am J Neuroradiol. 1989; 10(5):989–1005

6 Choroid Fissure Cyst

Susana Calle, Pejman Rabiei, Shekhar D. Khanpara, and Roy F. Riascos

6.1 Case Presentation

6.1.1 History and Physical Examination

A 5-year-old girl with a 1-year history of occasional mild occipital headache admitted to the ER (emergency room) because of a facial laceration from a fall.

The patient had a small facial laceration but was otherwise normal with no neurological deficits.

6.1.2 Imaging Findings and Impression

Axial (▶ Fig. 6.1a) and coronal (▶ Fig. 6.1b) CT scans of the head without contrast demonstrate a well-circumscribed cerebrospinal fluid (CSF) density lesion (*white arrows*) measuring approximately 10 × 10 mm in the choroidal fissure. The lesion has an imperceptible wall with no evidence of a solid component within the cyst.

However, MR was performed to exclude the less likely possibility of a small cystic lesion. The cyst follows CSF signal

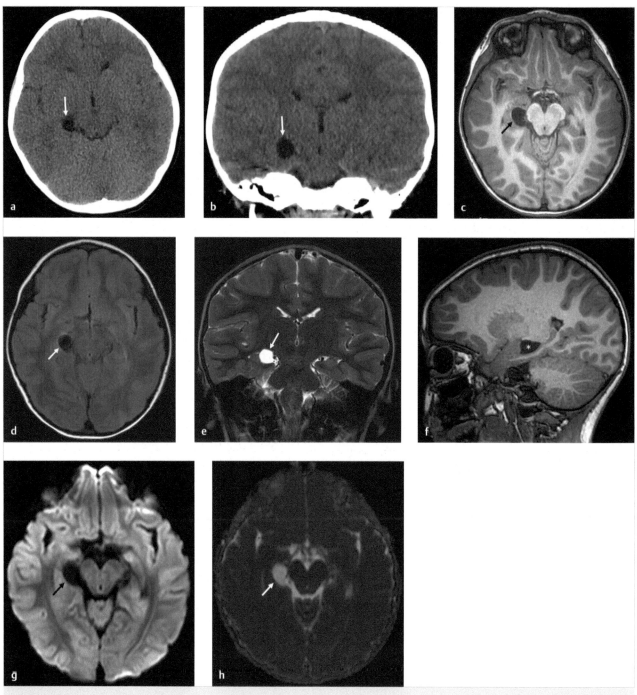

Fig. 6.1 (a–h)

intensity on axial T1-weighted (*black arrow* on ► Fig. 6.1c), axial fluid-attenuated inversion recovery (FLAIR; ► Fig. 6.1d), and coronal high-resolution fast spin-echo (FSE) T2-weighted (► Fig. 6.1e) images (*white arrows*). Coronal image (► Fig. 6.1e) clearly shows that the 10-mm cyst lies within the choroidal fissure. The distinctive spindle shape of the lesion is best seen in the T1-weighted sagittal plane (*asterisk* on ► Fig. 6.1f). The lesion does not show restriction on diffusion-weighted and ADC (apparent diffusion coefficient) map images (*arrows* on ► Fig. 6.1g,h).

6.2 Differential Diagnosis .

- **Choroid fissure cysts:**
  - Choroid fissure cysts are a normal variant occurring in the choroidal fissure and follow the CSF signal intensity on all sequences, with the absence of nodular enhancement.
- Mesial temporal sclerosis:
  - This is rarely an incidental finding but rather a common cause of epilepsy.
  - The hippocampus (uni- or bilateral) is atrophic with abnormal signal intensity on FLAIR images and with loss of normal internal architecture on T2-weighted images.
  - The ipsilateral fornix is also often noted to be small.
  - This atrophy may result in ipsilateral widening of the temporal horn and choroidal fissure.
  - The primary abnormality of the hippocampus and secondary widening of adjacent CSF spaces should distinguish this from a choroid fissure cyst in which the adjacent brain is displaced due to mass effect but is otherwise normal.[1]
- Epidermoid cysts:
  - They are more commonly found in the CPA (cerebellopontine angle) cistern.
  - Epidermoid cysts do not suppress on FLAIR images completely and are bright on diffusion-weighted images, unlike choroid fissure cysts.
- Parasitic cysts (neurocysticercosis):
  - They are more common in tropical countries.
  - Typically, they are parenchymal but can be present in the subarachnoid space.
  - The vesicular stage of neurocysticercosis (tapeworm infection) can look similar, but the cysts are most often multiple.
  - Nonenhancing T2 hypointense/T1 hyperintense scolex can be identified within the cysts.
  - They evolve into colloidal vesicular, granular nodular, and nodular calcified stages over time.
- Hippocampal sulcus remnants:
  - They are multiple tiny cysts within the hippocampus itself and are therefore seen just medial to the temporal horn of the lateral ventricle but between the dentate gyrus and subiculum.
  - They are incidental findings and follow the CSF signal intensity on all sequences.

- DNETs (dysembryoplastic neuroepithelial tumors):
  - Intra-axial mass/masslike abnormalities as opposed to a choroid fissure cyst that may compress adjacent brain but is extra-axial in location.
  - They often occur in the temporal lobes and have a pseudo-cystic/bubbly appearance.
  - They do not suppress on FLAIR sequences and often have a bright rim, which should help distinguish them.
  - Calcification and cortical remodeling may be seen.
  - Contrast enhancement is unusual.[2]

6.3 Diagnostic Pearls

- It occurs in a typical location (choroidal fissure).
- CT: well-delineated, extra-axial homogeneous CSF density cystic lesion with an imperceptible wall.
- MRI: follows CSF signal with complete suppression of signal on FLAIR sequences and no perceptible wall.
- No edema in the adjacent brain.
- Associated linear areas of enhancement may be present due to enhancing choroid plexus or choroidal vessels; however, nodular enhancement in the walls of the cyst should not be present.

6.4 Essential Information about Choroid Fissure Cyst

- A choroid fissure cyst is a CSF-containing embryological remnant occurring in a thin **C**-shaped cleft along the medial aspect of the lateral ventricle called the choroidal fissure. During development, tela choroidea invaginates through the choroidal fissure to reach the lateral ventricles and any anomalous development may lead to choroidal cyst formation.[3]
- They are commonly are incidental findings and are often considered to be clinically benign, although some have been reported in association with epilepsy, migraine, gait disturbance, tremor, paresthesia, and hemiparesis.
- They are usually small and range from around 1 to 2 cm in diameter. Larger cysts may also be seen occasionally.
- Often they are quite round on axial and coronal scans, with a characteristic spindle or ovoid shape paralleling the long axis of the temporal lobe and choroid fissure on sagittal images. Rarely they may enlarge and cause mass effect on the temporal lobe or may hemorrhage internally.[4]

References

[1] Karatas A, Gelal F, Gurkan G, Feran H. Growing hemorrhagic choroidal fissure cyst. J Korean Neurosurg Soc. 2016; 59(2):168–171

[2] Osborn AG. Osborn's Brain, Imaging, Pathology, and Anatomy. 2nd ed. Philadelphia, PA: Elsevier; 2017

[3] de Jong L, Thewissen L, van Loon J, Van Calenbergh F. Choroidal fissure cerebrospinal fluid-containing cysts: case series, anatomical consideration, and review of the literature. World Neurosurg. 2011; 75(5–6):704–708

[4] Morioka T, Nishio S, Suzuki S, Fukui M, Nishiyama T. Choroidal fissure cyst in the temporal horn associated with complex partial seizure. Clin Neurol Neurosurg. 1994; 96(2):164–167

7 Empty Sella Configuration

Susana Calle, Pejman Rabiei, Shekhar D. Khanpara, and Roy F. Riascos

7.1 Case Presentation

7.1.1 History and Physical Examination

A 70-year-old man with past medical history of hypertension complains of an episode of weakness and tingling in the left upper extremity. MRI was performed to rule out stroke.

The neurological examination was normal.

7.1.2 Imaging Findings and Impression

Sagittal (*white arrow* on ▸ Fig. 7.1a) and axial (*asterisk* on ▸ Fig. 7.1b) CT scans of the head without contrast show an empty sella configuration filled with cerebrospinal fluid (CSF) and no visualization of the pituitary gland.

Brain MR images without contrast including axial T2-weighted (▸ Fig. 7.2a), sagittal T1-weighted (▸ Fig. 7.2b), and coronal fluid-attenuated inversion recovery (FLAIR; ▸ Fig. 7.2c) sequences demonstrate an empty sella (*white arrows*) filled with CSF with nonvisualization of the pituitary gland. However, the pituitary stalk can be visualized (*arrow head*).

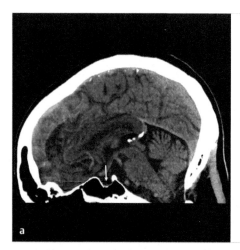
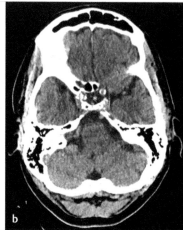

Fig. 7.1 (a, b)

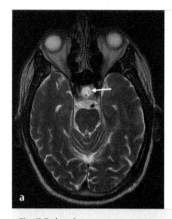
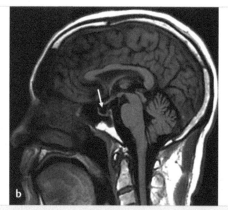
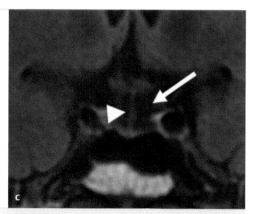

Fig. 7.2 (a–c)

7.2 Differential Diagnosis

- **Empty sella configuration:**
  - It is seen due to partial or complete absence of the pituitary gland in the sella turcica.
  - It is a normal-appearing sella filled with CSF with the infundibular stalk traversing it and absence of mass effect or remodeling of sella.
- Rathke's cleft cyst:
  - It often does not follow the CSF signal intensity on MR images as 50% are of high signal on T1-weighted images.
  - A small hypointense intracystic nodule may be seen on T2-weighted images and is considered virtually pathognomonic of a Rathke cleft cyst. Small T2 hypointense intracystic nodules may also be present.
- Cystic pituitary macroadenoma:
  - It usually has solid components and septation and does not follow the CSF signal intensity on MR images.
- Arachnoid cyst:
  - Although the signal intensity is very similar to an empty sella, mass effect on the infundibulum will be seen.
  - In addition, the margins of the cyst may be visible on high-resolution MR images.
- Epidermoid cyst:
  - This tumor is more commonly located in the CP (cerebellopontine) angle, but it can exist in the suprasellar region and can appear very similar to a cyst on T1- and T2-weighted sequences.
  - It frequently engulfs the adjacent vasculature rather than displacing vessels.
  - Most importantly, epidermoid cysts are bright on diffusion-weighted images with corresponding dark signal on ADC (apparent diffusion coefficient) due to the presence of keratin.
  - Incomplete suppression ("dirty CSF") is seen on FLAIR images.
- Craniopharyngioma:
  - This suprasellar tumor most commonly presents as a multiloculated cystic and solid mass that frequently calcifies and does not follow the CSF signal intensity.

7.3 Diagnostic Pearls

- The sella is empty with complete/partial absence of pituitary tissue.
- There is no associated mass lesion.

- The bony sella otherwise most often appears normal.
- On MR images, the infundibulum will be seen traversing the sella filled with CSF, which excludes the presence of a cystic lesion ("infundibulum sign").[1]

7.4 Essential Information about Empty Sella

- It was first described as an empty sella by Busch in 1951, after performing an autopsy study on cadavers.[2]
- It is a relatively common incidental finding on brain imaging with an overall incidence of 12%[3] and is often asymptomatic.
- It may be partial, in which some pituitary tissue is still visualized or complete, in which the sella appears entirely empty.
- The pituitary fossa can be normal in size or enlarged.
- The empty sella syndrome (ESS) may be primary or secondary:
  - Primary ESS:
    - It is believed to be secondary to intrasellar herniation of suprasellar arachnoid and subarachnoid space through the diaphragma sellae into the sella turcica, resulting in flattening of the pituitary gland.[4,5]
  - Secondary ESS:
    - It occurs when there has been prior injury to the pituitary gland.
    - Possible causes include prior surgery, postpartum infarction of the pituitary gland (Sheehan's syndrome), or the sequelae of hemorrhage and subsequent involution of an adenoma or lymphocytic hypophysitis.

References

[1] Haughton VM, Rosenbaum AE, Williams AL, Drayer B. Recognizing the empty sella by CT: the infundibulum sign. AJR Am J Roentgenol 1981;136 (2): 293–295

[2] Busch W. Die Morphologie der Sella turcica und ihre Beziehungen zur Hypophyse. Virchows Arch Pathol Anat Physiol Klin Med. 1951; 320(5):437–458

[3] Foresti M, Guidali A, Susanna P. Primary empty sella. Incidence in 500 asymptomatic subjects examined with magnetic resonance. Radiol Med (Torino). 1991; 81(6):803–807

[4] Sage MR, Blumbergs PC. Primary empty sella turcica: a radiological-anatomical correlation. Australas Radiol. 2000; 44(3):341–348

[5] Saindane AM, Lim PP, Aiken A, Chen Z, Hudgins PA. Factors determining the clinical significance of an "empty" sella turcica. AJR Am J Roentgenol. 2013; 200(5):1125–1131

8 High-Riding Jugular Bulb

Susana Calle, Pejman Rabiei, Shekhar D. Khanpara, and Roy F. Riascos

8.1 Case Presentation

8.1.1 History and Physical Examination

A 26-year-old woman presents for a CT status-post penetrating trauma to her neck. A "mass" was seen in right external auditory canal on otoscopic examination. Her neurologic examination was normal.

8.1.2 Imaging Findings and Impression

Axial and coronal images (▶ Fig. 8.1a,b) of a contrast CT of the head and neck show the jugular bulb (*white arrow*) extending superior to the floor of the external auditory canal. An axial contrast MR image (▶ Fig. 8.1c) of the same patient re-illustrates the findings. The left-sided internal jugular vein and jugular bulb are hypoplastic.

In this case, the thin bony septum separating the jugular bulb from the external auditory canal was be dehiscent. Special care should be taken during examination of the ear to avoid puncturing the jugular bulb.

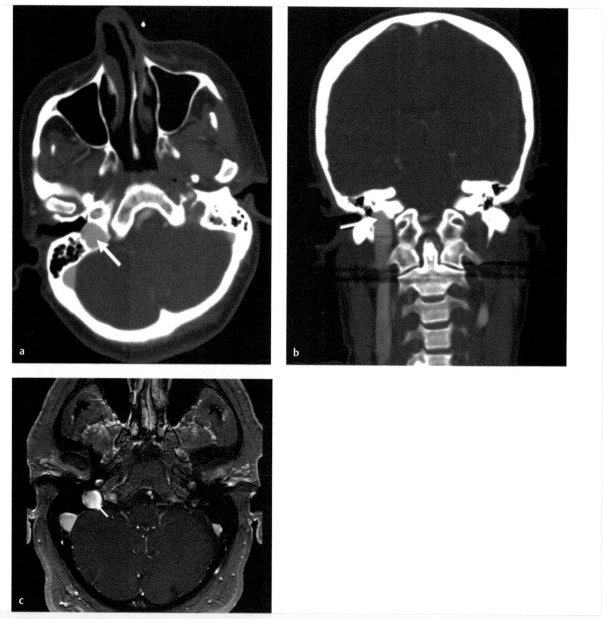

Fig. 8.1 (a c)

8.2 Differential Diagnosis

- **High-riding jugular bulb:**
  - A high-riding jugular bulb is defined as a jugular bulb reaching above the floor of the middle ear cavity. In this case, the sigmoid plate which is normally present between a high riding jugular bulb and middle ear cavity, is absent which defines this as a focal dihiscence. In this case, the patient was asymptomatic. In other cases, this may be a cause of pulsatile tinnitus or even conductive hearing loss if the bulb extends into the middle ear cavity.
- Asymmetrical large jugular bulb:
  - It is a normal variation and usually asymptomatic.
  - It has been shown that the right-sided jugular bulb in two-thirds of the population is larger compared to the left side.
- Glomus jugulare:
  - It is a paraganglioma confined to the jugular fossa, which may arise from the jugular bulb, the tympanic branch of CN IX, or the auricular branch of CN X.
  - Patients usually present with tinnitus and hearing loss and commonly show some patterns of cranial nerve palsies (Vernet's syndrome, Horner's syndrome and Collet–Sicard syndrome).
  - It should be fully assessed on CT as it usually manifests with irregularly moth-eaten bony margins and an eroded jugular spine.
  - It enhances on postcontrast MR images and shows low signal intensity on T1-weighted images and high signal intensity on T2-weighted images.

8.3 Diagnostic Pearls

- It should be recognized when the jugular bulb extends superiorly to the floor of the middle ear cavity.
- There is no associated mass effect or erosion of the adjacent bone.

8.4 Pitfalls

- Signal on MR images of a large high-riding jugular bulb can be confusing to radiologists because of the presence of turbulent flow in the bulb and should not be mistaken for a tumor.

- Evaluation of a high-riding jugular bulb with thin-slice CT scans of the petrous bone may be helpful in differentiating it from other pathologies.

8.5 Essential Information about High-Riding Jugular Bulb

- This condition is recognized when the dome of an asymmetrical large jugular bulb extends above the floor of the middle ear cavity.
- A thin plate of bone (sigmoid plate) should separate the middle ear cavity from the jugular bulb; if absent, this is known as a dehiscent jugular bulb. When the bulb protrudes into the middle ear cavity, it is known as a jugular bulb diverticulum. Both dehiscent jugular bulbs and jugular bulb diverticulums may be incidental findings but are often associated with pulsatile tinnitus and conductive hearing loss.
- The sigmoid plate is appreciable on thin-slice petrous bone CT and is not visible on MR images.
- Most cases of high-riding jugular bulb are asymptomatic, while symptomatic cases have also been reported[1] as it can mimic Meniere's disease.

8.6 Companion Case

8.6.1 History and Physical Examination

An 18-year-old woman presents with complaint of right sided tinnitus.

The neurological examination was normal. There was no hearing loss on audiometry.

8.6.2 Imaging Findings and Impression

Coronal bone window temporal bone CT (▶ Fig. 8.2a) shows a prominent high-riding jugular bulb with wedge-shaped protrusion. Contrast T1 axial MRI (▶ Fig. 8.2b) confirms the presence of a right-sided high-riding jugular bulb and a hypoplastic jugular bulb on the left side. Contrast T1 coronal and sagittal MR images (▶ Fig. 8.2c,d) demonstrate a protrusion of the superior aspect of the right jugular bulb.

Diagnosis: High-riding jugular bulb with diverticulum.

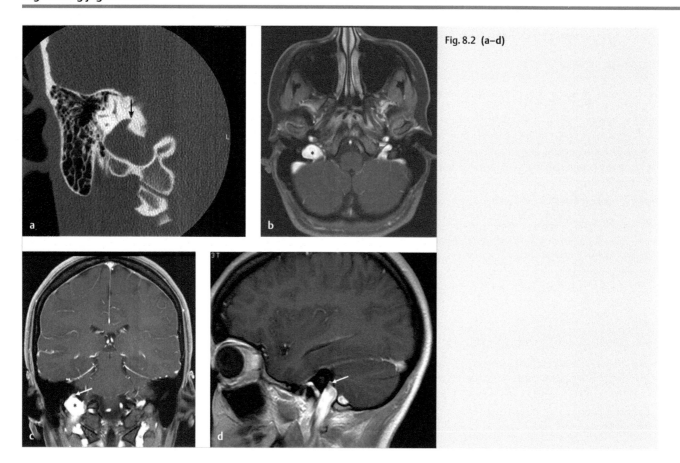

Fig. 8.2 (a–d)

Reference

[1]   Wadin K, Thomander L, Wilbrand H. Effects of a high jugular fossa and jugular bulb diverticulum on the inner ear. A clinical and radiologic investigation. Acta Radiol Diagn (Stockh). 1986; 27(6):629–636

9 Hyperostosis Frontalis Interna

Susana Calle, Pejman Rabiei, Shekhar D. Khanpara, and Roy F. Riascos

9.1 Case Presentation

9.1.1 History and Physical Examination

A 45-year-old woman presents with headache and nausea. Physical examination was normal with no neurologic deficit.

9.1.2 Imaging Findings and Impression

Axial (▶ Fig. 9.1a), sagittal (▶ Fig. 9.1b), and coronal (▶ Fig. 9.1c) CT scans of the head without contrast show symmetric thickening (*white arrow*) of the inner table of the frontal bone.

9.2 Differential Diagnosis

- **Hyperostosis frontalis interna:**
  - Symmetrical thickening involving the inner table of the frontal bones with no enhancement. It is frequently seen in middle-aged women.
- Acromegaly:
  - Diffuse calvarial thickening associated with enlargement of the sinuses, enlargement of the sella turcica, frontal bossing, and prominence of the mandible.
  - Other skeletal features are also present involving the spine and joints.

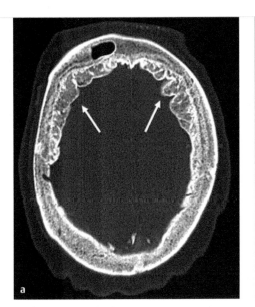
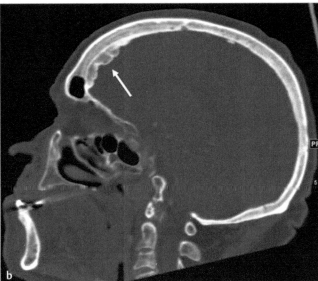
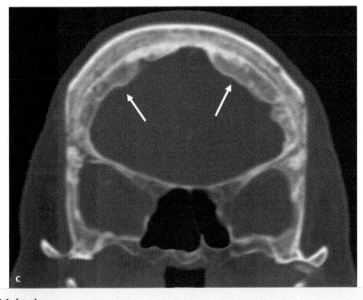

Fig. 9.1 (a–c)

- Fibrous dysplasia:
  - A non-neoplastic condition involving the bones and commonly occurring in children and young adults.
  - Normal bone is replaced with fibrous stroma and immature woven bone. The skull is involved in the polyostotic form.
  - It is characterized by focal or diffuse ground glass thickening of the skull.
  - The ethmoid bone is the most common involved area of the skull base.
  - The inner table is more frequently involved.
- Paget's disease of the bone:
  - A chronic bone disorder characterized by excessive bone remodeling with replacement of normal bone architecture with a coarsened trabecular pattern.
  - Commonly involved sites include the skull, spine, pelvis, and long bones.
  - It is more common in individuals older than 40 years with a slight male predilection.
  - Involvement of the skull is characterized by diffuse thickening of the inner and outer tables as opposed to fibrous dysplasia, which predominantly affects the inner table.
  - Other findings in the skull are widening of the diploic space, mixed lytic and sclerotic lesions (cotton wool appearance), or large well-defined lytic lesions (osteoporosis circumscripta).
  - Enhancement of the lesions is seen in active disease.
- Meningioma:
  - An extra-axial tumor arising from the arachnoid cap cells of the meninges.
  - Classically, it presents as a homogeneously enhancing dural-based lesion with a characteristic dural tail sign.
  - It is often associated with hyperostosis of the overlying skull that has been shown to be due to either hypervascularity or direct infiltration of tumor cells.
- Sclerotic metastasis:
  - It can arise from a variety of primary malignancies including prostate carcinoma, breast carcinoma, transitional cell carcinoma of urothelial origin, medulloblastoma, neuroblastoma, and lymphoma, among others.
  - It is characterized by single or multiple focal areas of increased density as compared to the normal skull.
  - It tends to enhance.

9.3 Diagnostic Pearls

- The thickening of the inner table is symmetric and can extend to involve parietal bones.[1]
- The thickening can be focal, flat, or nodular in appearance.
- It does not enhance.

9.4 Essential Information about Hyperostosis Frontalis Interna

- It is characterized by thickening of the inner table of the frontal bone.[2]
- It has predominant female predilection, especially among postmenopausal women.
- It is primarily considered an incidental finding and not associated with any symptoms.
- Its exact cause is not known. It is associated with multiple conditions, namely, seizures, headaches, obesity, and sexual disturbances. It is believed to be hereditary in nature.
- It can also be associated with seizures (or antiepileptic medicine), headaches, obesity, excessive hair growth, and sexual disturbances.

9.5 Companion Case

9.5.1 History and Physical Examination

A 60-year-old woman presents with sensorineural hearing loss and headaches.

Neurological examination was normal, except for the presence of bilateral sensorineural hearing loss.

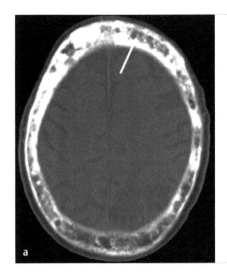 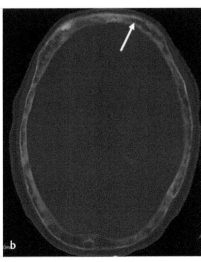

Fig. 9.2 (a, b)

9.5.2 Imaging Findings and Impression

Axial CT head (▶ Fig. 9.2a,b) demonstrates multiple lytic and sclerotic lesions diffusely involving the skull with widening of diploic space and involvement of inner and outer tables of the skull. Diagnosis: Paget's disease.

References

[1] Akashi T. MRI findings of hyperostosis frontalis interna: a case of Morgagni syndrome. No To Shinkei. 1996; 48(7):667–670

[2] She R, Szakacs J. Hyperostosis frontalis interna: case report and review of literature. Ann Clin Lab Sci. 2004; 34(2):206–208

10 Prominent Perivascular Space

Susana Calle, Pejman Rabiei, Shekhar D. Khanpara, and Roy F. Riascos

10.1 Case Presentation

10.1.1 History and Physical Examination

A 40-year-old man with no major past medical history complains of headache following a minor head trauma.

The patient is alert and oriented and his cranial nerves II–XII are grossly intact.

10.1.2 Imaging Findings and Impression

Brain MR images including axial T2-weighted (*white arrow* in ▶ Fig. 10.1a), axial noncontrast T1-weighted (*white arrow* in ▶ Fig. 10.1b), and fluid-attenuated inversion recovery (FLAIR; *black arrow* in ▶ Fig. 10.1c) demonstrate a small fluid-filled cystlike lesion measuring 3 × 6 mm involving the left thalamus. It follows cerebrospinal fluid (CSF) signal intensity on all the sequences. Axial diffusion-weighted image (▶ Fig. 10.1d) and apparent diffusion coefficient (ADC) map (▶ Fig. 10.1e) show no restriction. The fluid-filled lesion is nonenhancing on the axial postcontrast T1-weighted image (▶ Fig. 10.1f), consistent with a prominent perivascular space (PVS).

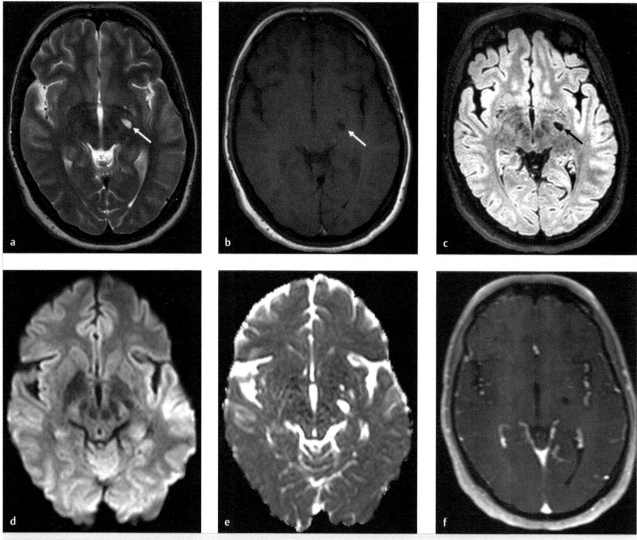

Fig. 10.1 (a–f)

10.2 Differential Diagnosis

- **Prominent PVS:**
  - It represents enlarged PVSs that follow cerebrospinal fluid (CSF) signal intensity on all MRI sequences.
- Neurocysticercosis:
  - May mimic a PVS in the initial vesicular stage. Endemic area and additional lesions in regions of the brain that are atypical for PVSs is helpful. Additional calcified lesions, representing the nodular calcified stage of neurocysticercosis, are helpful in making this diagnosis.
  - A "dot sign" may be seen inside the cyst, representing the parasite scolex.
- Cryptococcosis:
  - It spreads along the PVSs and becomes distended with mucoid, gelatinous material.
  - When multiple, they should be differentiated from prominent PVSs.
  - If the patient is immunocompromised, cryptococcus should be considered highly in the differential diagnosis!
  - Cryptococcomas can manifest with low signal intensity on T1-weighted images, high signal intensity on T2-weighted images and fluid-attenuated inversion recovery (FLAIR) images, and variable enhancement on postcontrast images.
- Arachnoid cyst:
  - CSF-containing cysts that are most commonly found in the middle cranial fossa, the parasellar region, and the subarachnoid space over the convexities.
  - It follows CSF signal intensity on all sequences.
- Lacunar infarctions:
  - They show abnormal increased FLAIR signal intensity along the rim and more commonly happen in the upper two-thirds of the basal ganglia.
  - Acute lacunar infarcts show restricted diffusion.
- Cystic neoplasm:
  - They have solid components, may enhance, and commonly show surrounding edema.
  - Diffusion-weighted images and the FLAIR sequence should be evaluated for better differentiating cystic neoplasms from prominent PVSs.
- Dysembryoplastic neuroepithelial tumor (DNET) and multinodular and vacuolating neuronal tumor (MVNT):
  - These are similar-appearing cystic bubbly lesions most frequently located in the temporal lobe.
  - DNETs are cortical lesions, while MVNTs are subcortical in location.
  - MVNT is a recently introduced entity in WHO 2016 classification.
  - The cystic component does not suppress completely on the FLAIR sequence and often has a hyperintense rim.
  - Lack of enhancement is most common.
- Non-neoplastic neuroepithelial cyst:
  - It is spherical to ovoid and measures up to several centimeters.
  - It may involve the lateral ventricles or the fourth ventricle with which they do not communicate.
  - CSF-like signal on MR images with no enhancement on postcontrast images.[1]

10.3 Diagnostic Pearls

- It follows CSF signal on all sequences with complete suppression on FLAIR.
- The surrounding brain parenchyma is usually normal with classic locations described as: along the lenticulostriate arteries in the basal ganglia, along the high convexities associated with perforating medullary arteries, and around the midbrain associated with collicular and accessory collicular arteries.
- It does not restrict on diffusion-weighted images.
- It never enhances.

10.4 Pitfalls

- In patients with multiple enlarged PVSs, clinicians have to rule out underlying diseases such as mucopolysaccharidosis (Hunter's, Hurler's, and Sanfilippo's syndromes), which might result in accumulation of undegraded mucopolysaccharides within enlarged PVSs.[2]
- Tumefactive PVSs may mimic tumors and may have surrounding abnormal signal on FLAIR due to reactive gliosis in the surrounding white matter. Lack of contrast enhancement and stabilty on follow-up imaging is helpful in excluding tumor.

10.5 Essential Information about Prominent Perivascular Space

- PVSs are also known as Virchow–Robin spaces.
- PVSs are pia-lined spaces and follow the penetrating arteries and arterioles into the brain parenchyma.
- They do not communicate directly with the subarachnoid spaces.[3]
- They are filled with interstitial fluid (ISF) and are a pathway for ISF and cerebral metabolites to exit the brain.
- They can become enlarged in some circumstances, which is known as tumefactive PVSs.
- They are found most frequently in the basal ganglia.

10.6 Companion Case

10.6.1 Imaging Findings and Impression

Brain MR images demonstrate a cystic bubbly lesion (*white arrow*) involving the left mesial temporal lobe. The lesion is hyperintense on T2 and hypointense on T1 with incomplete suppression of contents of the cysts on FLAIR (► Fig. 10.2a–d). A hyperintense rim is also noted surrounding the lesion on FLAIR (► Fig. 10.2d). The lesion does not restrict on diffusion-weighted images (► Fig. 10.2e) with no enhancement postgadolinium administration (► Fig. 10.2f).

Diagnosis: dysembryoplastic neuroepithelial tumor.

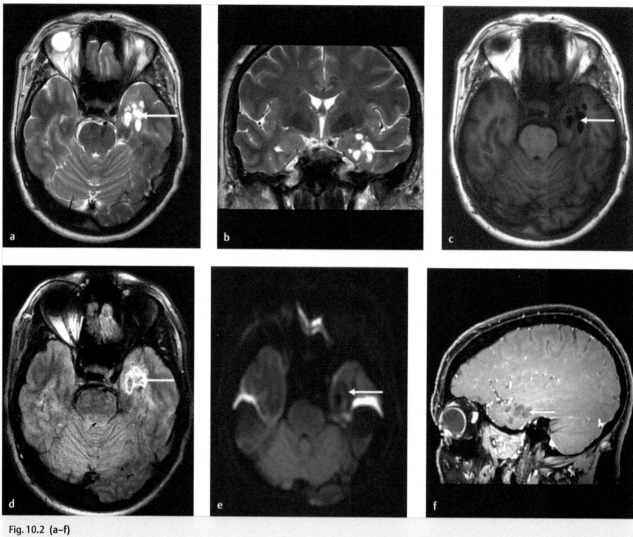

Fig. 10.2 (a–f)

References

[1] Kwee RM, Kwee TC. Virchow-Robin spaces at MR imaging. Radiographics. 2007; 27(4):1071–1086

[2] Reichert R, Campos LG, Vairo F, et al. Neuroimaging findings in patients with mucopolysaccharidosis: what you really need to know. Radiographics. 2016; 36(5):1448–1462

[3] Osborn AG. Osborn's Brain, Imaging, Pathology, and Anatomy. 2nd ed. Amsterdam: Elsevier; 2017

11 Simple Pineal Cyst

Susana Calle, Pejman Rabiei, Shekhar D. Khanpara, and Roy F. Riascos

11.1 Case Presentation

11.1.1 History and Physical Examination

A 32-year-old woman presents to ER with head trauma.

The patient is alert and oriented. Cranial nerves II–XII are grossly intact with no focal neurologic deficit.

11.1.2 Imaging Findings and Impression

Axial CT scan of the head without contrast show a well-defined and rounded cystic lesion (*white arrows*) measures 5 × 6 mm in the pineal region with focal calcification along with anterior wall (▶ Fig. 11.1).

MR images of the brain with and without contrast show a well-defined and rounded cystic lesion in the pineal region. The lesion is hyperintense on the axial T2-weighted image (▶ Fig. 11.2a) and hypointense on noncontrast T1-weighted image (▶ Fig. 11.2b) with incomplete suppression on the axial fluid-attenuated

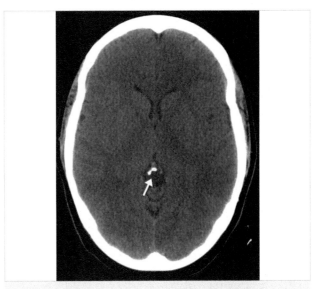

Fig. 11.1

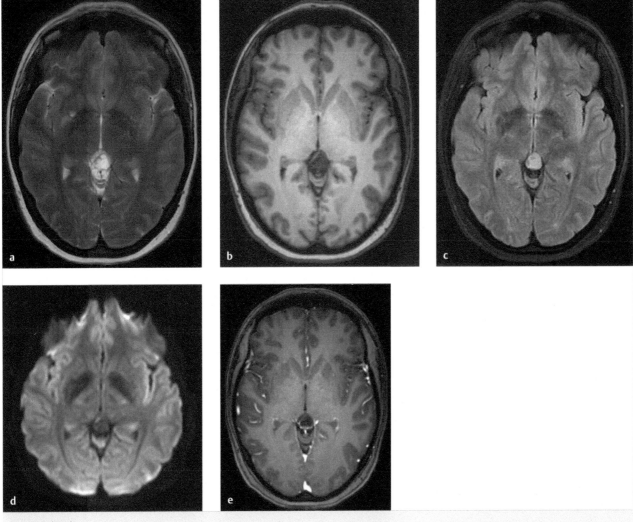

Fig. 11.2 (a–e)

inversion recovery (FLAIR) image (▶ Fig. 11.2c). Diffusion-weighted image shows no evidence of restricted diffusion (▶ Fig. 11.2d). Axial (▶ Fig. 11.2e) postcontrast T1-weighted images demonstrate minimal, linear enhancement of the wall of the cyst. No solid component can be identified. Importantly, there is no evidence of enlargement of the ventricles to suggest obstruction.

11.2 Differential Diagnosis

- **Simple pineal cyst:**
  - It is a benign cyst involving the pineal gland usually measuring less than 1 cm with no enhancing nodular, solid component. It usually follows the cerebrospinal fluid (CSF) signal intensity on all MRI sequences but may not completely suppress on T2-weighted FLAIR sequences. It often has concentric calcification involving the wall of the cyst.
  - It does not result in obstruction of CSF flow nor symptomatic compression of the tectal plate, which could result in upgaze paralysis.
- Pineocytoma:
  - Pineocytomas are benign pineal parenchymal tumors frequently seen in females.
  - They are round or oval well-demarcated tumors measuring less than 3 cm in diameter.
  - CT: hypodense to intermediate-density lesion arising from the pineal gland with peripheral calcifications.
  - MRI: hypo- to isointense on T1-weighted images and isointense to the brain parenchyma on the T2-weighted images.[1]
  - Larger tumors can demonstrate cystic degeneration within them.
  - Solid component shows vivid enhancement on MR after gadolinium administration.
- Pineoblastoma[2]:
  - Pineoblastomas are malignant pineal parenchyma tumors typically seen in children with a slight female predilection.
  - They are ill-defined heterogeneous tumors usually larger than 3 cm with an aggressive growth pattern.
  - CT: A large heterogeneous, irregularly marginated tumor that is hyperdense as compared to the normal brain parenchyma attributed to the high cellularity. Calcification is often seen peripherally dispersed within the tumor.
  - MRI: Isointense on T1- and T2-weighted images with marked heterogeneous enhancement following gadolinium administration. As this tumor has high cellularity, it appears dark on apparent diffusion coefficient (ADC) maps.
  - Imaging of the entire neuraxis is recommended as approximately 40 to 50% of these tumors can develop leptomeningeal spread.
- Germinoma:
  - Germinoma is the most common intracranial germ cell tumor common in children and young adults with higher predilection in males.
  - CT: hyperdense due to high cellularity. It tends to engulf pineal calcifications centrally within the mass.
  - MRI: isointense to hyperintense on the T2-weighted and isointense on T1 weighted-images and demonstrate homogeneous enhancement following contrast administration.
    - They can have a cystic component and appear darker on ADC maps. They are associated with elevated levels of placental alkaline phosphatase and beta-human chorionic gonadotropin (beta-hCG) in blood.
- Arachnoid cyst:
  - Arachnoid cysts are benign cystic lesions filled with CSF with an imperceptible wall and presumed to be arising from arachnoid cells of the meninges.
  - They are extra-axial lesions that commonly occur in the subarachnoid space.
  - They are most commonly found in the region of the anterior temporal pole, but can be seen in the pineal region in some cases.
  - CT: well-circumscribed cystic lesions with an imperceptible wall.
  - MRI: cyst follows CSF signal intensity on all sequences.
- Epidermoid cyst:
  - Epidermoid cysts are benign cystic lesions arising from inclusion of ectodermal elements during neural tube closure.
  - They are extra-axial lesions most commonly occurring in the cerebellopontine cisterns.
  - They are nonenhancing, well-circumscribed lobulated slow-growing tumors.
  - CT: The density of the epidermoid cysts approximates 0 HU and can seem identical to CSF. Calcification is seen in 10 to 20% of cases.
  - MRI: Isointense to CSF on T2- and T1-weighted images with incomplete suppression (dirty signal) on FLAIR images:
    - On diffusion-weighted images, it appears bright with corresponding hypointensity on ADC images due to keratin.

11.3 Diagnostic Pearls

- It is a well-demarcated cystic lesion.
- It is usually less than 1 cm in diameter.
- It is isointense to CSF on T2- and T1-weighted images with complete or incomplete suppression on FLAIR images depending on the composition of the fluid.
- There is no restriction on diffusion-weighted images.
- Gradient recalled echo (GRE) images may demonstrate peripheral susceptibility artifact along the wall of the cyst.
- On postcontrast images, a thin rim of enhancement may be noted along the wall.
- Nodular enhancement should raise the suspicion of other diagnosis, for example, pineocytoma.
- It may be impossible to differentiate a pineal cyst from a cystic pineocytoma on imaging alone. Clinical correlation by neurosurgery and follow-up imaging may be required especially with larger, more complex cystic lesions.

11.4 Essential Information about Simple Pineal Cyst

- It is a benign cyst involving the pineal gland, seen in all age groups. It is more common in young adults and less frequent in the pediatric and geriatric population suggesting a "life-cycle".

- It presents as a unilocular cyst within the pineal gland with a very thin wall.
- The finding of lateral and third ventricular enlargement due to aqueduct of Sylvius compression should be noted and results called to the referring physician as this is an indication for emergent neurosurgical evaluation.
- The cyst contains fluid similar to CSF or slightly hyperdense.
- It is seen in around 5% MRI scans and 20 to 40% of autopsies.[4]
- Most of them are smaller than 1 cm and asymptomatic.
- It may increase or decrease in size gradually over the years.
- Rapid enlargement with internal hemorrhage has rarely been reported.

11.5 Companion Case

11.5.1 History and Physical Examination

A 5-year-old boy presents with headache, nausea, and difficulty in walking.

Neurological examination was notable for the presence of papilledema and up-gaze paralysis.

11.5.2 Imaging Findings and Impression

Axial and sagittal (▶ Fig. 11.3a,b) CT scans of the head without contrast shows a 3 × 2 cm hyperdense mass lesion involving the pineal gland with central speckled calcification. The mass is causing compression of the aqueduct with resultant obstructive hydrocephalus. T2, FLAIR, and GRE axial MR images (▶ Fig. 11.3c–e) demonstrate T2 and FLAIR hyperintense mass lesion involving the pineal region with a central hypointensity that corresponds to increased susceptibility representing calcification. Contrast T1 sagittal image (▶ Fig. 11.3f) shows heterogeneous enhancement following gadolinium administration. Diagnosis: pineal germinoma.

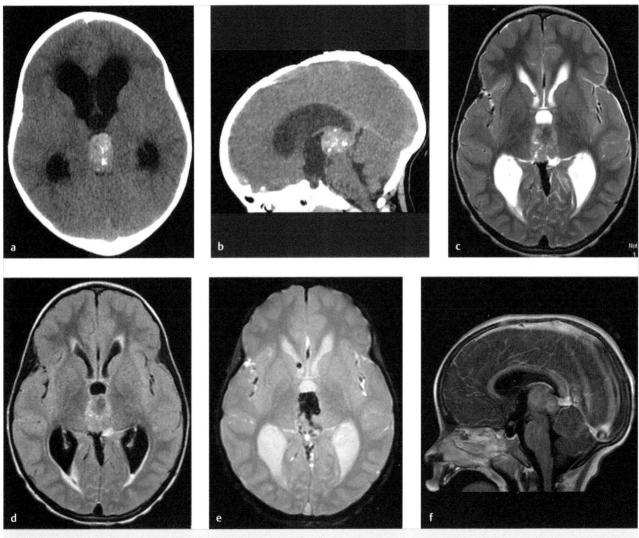

Fig. 11.3 (a–f)

References

[1] Fakhran S, Escott EJ. Pineocytoma mimicking a pineal cyst on imaging: true diagnostic dilemma or a case of incomplete imaging? AJNR Am J Neuroradiol. 2008; 29(1):159–163

[2] Fang AS, Meyers SP. Magnetic resonance imaging of pineal region tumours. Insights Imaging. 2013; 4(3):369–382

[3] Karthik DK, Khardenavis V, Kulkarni S, et al. "Pineal gland apoplexy mimicking as migraine-like headache". Case Reports 2018;2018:bcr-2018-225187

[4] Pu Y, Mahankali S, Hou J, et al. High prevalence of pineal cysts in healthy adults demonstrated by high-resolution, noncontrast brain MR imaging. AJNR Am J Neuroradiol. 2007; 28(9):1706–1709

Section II

Intracranial Incidental Findings

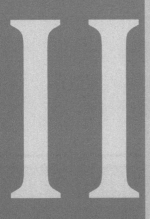

12 Diffuse White Matter Hyperintensities

Carlos A. Pérez and John A. Lincoln

12.1 Introduction

Diffuse white matter hyperintensities on brain MRIs are a common finding with an extensive differential diagnosis. In this chapter, we describe a case in which a diagnosis of CNS demyelination was highly suggested based on the appearance of white matter lesions identified on MRI. The necessary imaging, clinical evaluation, and laboratory testing that led to a diagnosis of radiologically isolated syndrome (RIS) are outlined. In addition, companion cases of diffuse white matter signal abnormalities secondary to small vessel ischemic disease are presented to highlight key differences in imaging appearance and clinical presentation between these conditions. The differential diagnosis of diffuse white matter hyperintensities and imaging "red flags" that should suggest a diagnosis other than CNS demyelination are also discussed.

12.2 Case Presentation

12.2.1 History

A 26-year-old woman who presents to the hospital for evaluation of syncope and collapse. A brain MR was performed. ▶ Fig. 12.1 shows the axial T2-weighted images (T2WIs; **a**) and axial fluid-attenuated inversion recovery (FLAIR) image (**b**).

12.3 Imaging Analysis

12.3.1 Imaging Findings and impression

▶ Fig. 12.2a,b shows large, discrete ovoid lesions that are hyperintense on T2WIs and FLAIR (*arrows*) MRI sequences. Many of

these lesions measure greater than 6 mm in diameter and are located adjacent to the ventricles, and involve the deep white matter. The orientation of many lesions is perpendicular to the lateral ventricles (*arrows* in ▶ Fig. 12.2b,d). ▶ Fig. 12.2c shows infratentorial lesions, which are also hyperintense on T2WIs (*arrow* indicating largest infratentorial lesion). ▶ Fig. 12.2d shows the lesions are hypointense on T1WIs with the "Dawson's fingers" appearance (*white arrows*).

The multifocal periventricular and posterior fossa white matter lesions have an appearance typical of demyelinating disease. (See Section 12.5, "Differential Diagnosis of White Matter Lesions.")

12.3.2 Additional Imaging Recommended

- Postcontrast MRI of the brain should be obtained if gadolinium was not administered for the initial brain MRI. Ideally, a high-quality MRI at 1.5 or 3T should be obtained.
- MRI of the cervical spine is recommended with and without gadolinium given the suspicious nature of the brain MR findings. Although the vast majority of cervical spinal cord lesions would not be clinically "silent," if present, they would impact management decisions and provide additional prognostic information in patients with multiple sclerosis

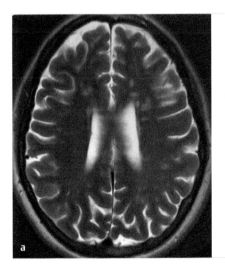
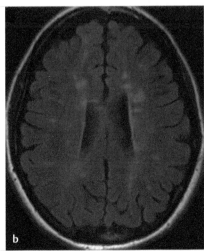

Fig. 12.1 (a, b)

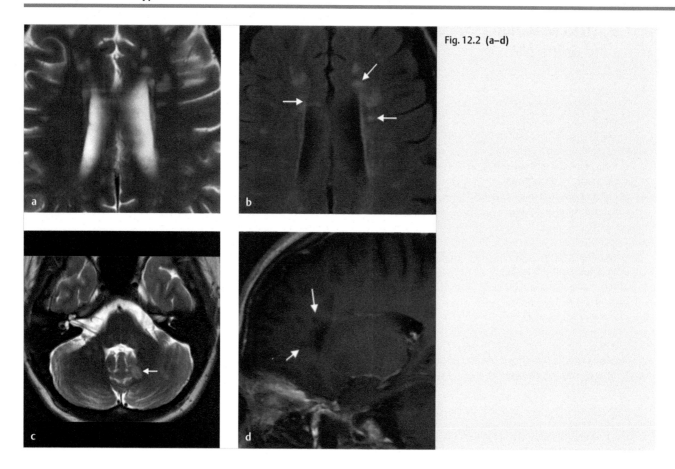

Fig. 12.2 (a–d)

12.4 Clinical Evaluation

12.4.1 Neurologist History and Physical Examination

The patient is a 26-year-old, right-handed, Caucasian woman with a history of type 1 diabetes mellitus, depression, and anxiety with anxiety who presented to the hospital after a possible "syncopal" episode that occurred while she was having an argument with a family member. She denied any prior symptoms other than the single fainting episode.

A complete neurological examination was performed. The patient was awake, alert, and oriented. Her speech was fluent and she answered all questions appropriately. Visual acuity was 20/20 bilaterally as tested by the Snellen chart with intact peripheral visual fields. Her face was symmetric bilaterally with intact facial expressions. Facial sensation was intact to light touch, pinprick, and temperature. Her tongue was midline and palate elevated equally bilaterally. A motor examination was normal in both proximal and distal upper and lower extremities. Sensation was intact in all extremities to light touch, pinprick, temperature, position, and vibration. Deep tendon reflexes were normal in all extremities and no pathologic

reflexes were elicited. Gait and station were normal with full arm swing. Finger-to-nose and heel-to-shin tests were also normal bilaterally.

12.4.2 Recommended Additional Testing

- MRI of the brain should be of high quality, preferably 1.5 or 3 T (see (Magnetic Resonance Imaging in multiple sclerosis [MAGNIMS] protocol).
- MRI of the cervical spine with and without gadolinium.
- Peripheral blood/serum studies: complete blood cell count (CBC), erythrocyte sedimentation rate (ESR), antinuclear antibody (ANA), rheumatoid factor, vitamin B12, homocysteine, methylmalonic acid, antiphospholipid antibody, thyroid function tests, angiotensin-converting enzyme (ACE), anticardiolipin antibody screen and Lyme disease antibody titers.[2]
- Routine cerebrospinal fluid (CSF) analysis should be performed to exclude other diagnoses—particularly infection.[1]
- Visual evoked potential (VEP) testing can also be obtained to look for signs of subclinical demyelination.[1]

12.4.3 2015 MAGNIMS Standardized Brain and Spine MRI Protocol[3,4]

- Brain:
  - Mandatory:
    - Axial: proton-density and/or T2 FLAIR/T2-weighted.
    - Sagittal: 2D or 3D T2 FLAIR.
    - 2D or 3D contrast-enhanced T1-weighted imaging.
  - Optional:
    - Unenhanced 2D or high-resolution isotropic 3D T1-weighted imaging.
    - 2D and/or 3D dual inversion recovery.
    - Axial diffusion-weighted imaging.
- Spinal cord:
  - Mandatory
    - Dual echo (proton density and T2 weighted) conventional and/or fast spin echo (FSE).
    - Short tau inversion recovery (STIR; as an alternative to proton-density-weighted images).
    - Contrast-enhanced T1-weighted spin echo (if lesions that are hyperintense on T2-weighted imaging are present).
  - Optional:
    - Phase-sensitive inversion recovery (as an alternative to STIR at the cervical segment).

12.4.4 Results of Additional Testing

Cerebrospinal fluid (CSF) studies showed an immunoglobulin index of 1.0 (normal < 0.7) and three oligoclonal bands (OCBs) that were not observed in the serum. All other serum labs were unremarkable. Additional testing performed in this patient included VEP and optical coherence tomography (OCT), both of which were normal.

The cervical spine MR failed to reveal any additional lesions.

There were no enhancing lesions in the brain or in the cervical spine.

12.4.5 Clinical Impression

Radiologically isolated syndrome (RIS).

12.4.6 Management Decision in This Case

VEPs can be performed on a case-by-case basis as they can add an additional risk factor for progression to symptomatic MS when positive. In this case, they would have offered information about prior optic nerve inflammation had they been positive.

There is currently no consensus as to routine use of disease-modifying therapies (DMTs) in patients presenting with RIS, even for those with abnormal cervical and/or thoracic spinal cord findings. A randomized clinical trial to determine the utility of early intervention in RIS patients is currently in progress.

In this case, a decision was made to pursue active monitoring with periodical clinical and radiological follow-up every 6 to 12 months.

12.5 Differential Diagnosis of White Matter Lesions

- Inflammatory:
  - Multiple sclerosis (MS), radiologically isolated syndrome (RIS), vasculitis (systemic lupus erythematosus [SLE], Sjögren's syndrome, Behçet's syndrome, primary CNS vasculitis), neurosarcoidosis.
- Hypoxic/ischemic:
  - Atherosclerosis, stroke, hypertension, migraine, amyloid angiopathy, vasculopathy (CADASIL, Susac's syndrome).
- Infectious:
  - HIV, syphilis, Lyme disease, TB, progressive multifocal leukoencephalopathy (PML).
- Toxic/metabolic.
- Traumatic:
  - Posttraumatic, radiotherapy.
- Metabolic:
  - Leukodystrophies.
- Neoplastic:
  - Metastatic or primary disease.
- Normal:
  - Age-related or Virchow–Robin spaces.

12.6 Diagnostic Imaging Pearls

Imaging findings suggestive of a demyelinating process[1]:
- Lesion size: usually greater than 5 mm.
- Asymmetric.
- Location: cortical/juxtacortical, periventricular (Dawson's fingers), infratentorial, spinal cord, corpus callosum.
- Gadolinium-enhancing lesions (incomplete rim enhancement in larger lesions).
- Most typically, all lesions do NOT enhance simultaneously at onset.
- "Central vein sign."[1]
- New lesions on repeat imaging are common with possible regression of older lesions.
- Nonconfluent except in very advanced cases.

12.7 Clinical and Diagnostic Imaging Pitfalls

"Red flag" clinical and imaging findings that are atypical for MS (RIS) and should suggest an alternative diagnosis (see ▶ Table 12.1).

Table 12.1 Clinical and imaging red flags in the differential diagnosis of white matter lesions

Clinical or imaging finding	Alternative diagnosis
• Bone lesions	• Sarcoidosis; histiocytosis
• Lung involvement	• Sarcoidosis; lymphoid granulomatosis
• Multiple cranial nerve involvement	• Sarcoidosis
• Cerebral sinus thrombosis	• Vasculitis; antiphospholipid antibody syndrome
• Cardiac disease	• Embolic infarctions
• Myopathy	• MELAS; Sjogren's syndrome
• Renal involvement	• SLE; vasculitis; Fabry's disease
• Hemorrhage	• Amyloid angiopathy; CADASIL; vasculitis
• Meningeal enhancement	• Sarcoidosis; lymphoma; TB; CNS vasculitis
• Retinopathy	• Susac's syndrome
• Calcifications on CT brain	• Cysticercosis; toxoplasmosis; mitochondrial disorders
• Diabetes insipidus	• Sarcoidosis; histiocytosis
• Anterior temporal lobe involvement	• CADASIL
• Lacunar infarctions	• CADASIL; Susac's syndrome; hypertensive small-vessel disease
• Persistent lesion enhancement	• Lymphoma; glioma; vasculitis; sarcoidosis
• Mucosal ulcers	• Behcet's disease
• Simultaneous enhancement of all lesions	• Vasculitis; lymphoma; sarcoidosis
• Hyperintense basal ganglia on T1WI	• Fabry's disease; hepatic disease; manganese toxicity
• Predominantly cortical/subcortical lesions	• Embolic infarctions; vasculitis; PML
• Symmetric, confluent white matter lesions	• Seen in MS only when advanced; toxic exposure; post hypoxic leukoencephalopathy; HIV-related white matter disease; and the leukodystrophies (adrenoleukodystrophy, metachromatic leukodystrophy, and Krabbe's disease are the most common to have an atypical, "MS-like" presentation in an adult).

Abbreviations: CADASIL, cerebral autosomal dominant arteriopathy with subcortical infarcts and leukoencephalopathy; CNS, central nervous system; CT, computed tomography; DI, diabetes insipidus; MELAS, mitochondrial myopathy, encephalopathy, lactic acidosis, and stroke-like episodes; HIV, human immunodeficiency disease; MS, multiple sclerosis; PML, progressive multifocal leukoencephalopathy; SLE, systemic lupus erythematosus; TB, tuberculosis; T1WI, T1-weighted image.
Source: Adapted from Miller DH, Weinshenker BG, Filippi M, et al. Differential diagnosis of suspected multiple sclerosis: a consensus approach. Mult Scler 2008;14(9):1157–1174.

12.8 Companion Cases

12.8.1 Companion Case 1

History

A 45-year-old woman presents with episodes of painless blurred vision that lasts for several days without an associated headache.

Imaging Analysis

Imaging Findings and Impression

Multifocal round and punctate white matter lesions that are hyperintense on FLAIR (▶ Fig. 12.3a) and FSE T2WIs (▶ Fig. 12.3b) are seen in this case and do not involve the corpus callosum or the callosal–septal interface. They are not oval, nor do they have a perpendicular orientation to the ventricles and are therefore not

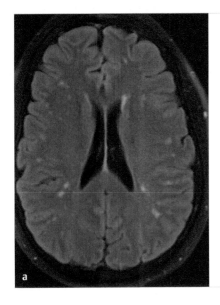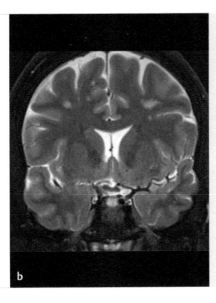

Fig. 12.3 Companion case 1. Axial fluid attenuated inversion recovery (FLAIR) **(a)** and coronal T2WI **(b)** are shown.

typical for neither MS nor Susac's syndrome. These nonspecific lesions are seen more commonly in patients who suffer from migraines or they could be vascular, secondary to small-vessel ischemic disease. The differential diagnosis is broad as in the lead case presentation in this chapter. See Section 12.5, "Differential Diagnosis of White Matter Lesions." Clinical correlation is needed before any additional imaging testing is recommended.

Clinical Evaluation

Neurologist History and Physical Examination

The patient is a 45-year-old, right-handed, Caucasian woman with history of uncontrolled hypertension, migraine during pregnancy, and fibromyalgia presented with episodic painless bilateral blurred vision without color desaturation. Episodes generally persisted for several days and were not associated with headache.

She was referred to an ophthalmologist who found 20/20 visual acuity bilaterally with intact peripheral visual fields, normal VEPs, and normal retinal nerve fiber layer thickness on optical coherence tomography. As part of her workup, she had brain MRI that showed the multifocal T2 hyperintensities shown above.

A complete neurological examination was performed. The patient was awake, alert, and oriented. Her speech was fluent and she answered all questions appropriately. Her face was symmetric bilaterally with intact facial expressions. Facial sensation was intact to light touch, pinprick, and temperature. Her tongue was midline and palate elevated equally bilaterally. A motor examination was normal in both proximal and distal upper and lower extremities. Sensation was intact in all extremities to light touch, pinprick, temperature, position, and vibration. Deep tendon reflexes were normal in all extremities and no pathologic reflexes were elicited. Gait and station were normal with full arm swing. Finger-to-nose and heel-to-shin tests were also normal bilaterally.

Recommended Additional Testing

The brain MRI showed nonspecific T2 hyperintensities that can be seen in the setting of chronic migraine and prior uncontrolled hypertension. In addition, an increased incidence of peripartum migraine and stroke risk has been reported. Given the abnormal brain MRI, an MRI of the cervical spine with and without gadolinium as well as serum and CSF studies were obtained. Finally, given the pattern, the patient was evaluated for intermediate and small-vessel vasculitis.

Results

CSF showed an immunoglobulin index of 0.5 (normal < 0.7) and no OCBs. Erythrocyte sedimentation rate was normal and serum studies for large vessel vasculitides (Sjogren's syndrome, antineutrophil cytoplasmic antibodies, antiphospholipid antibodies) were negative.

Clinical Impression and Management in Companion Case 1

Abnormal brain MRI without clear etiology. The patient does not have clinical or radiologic findings to suggest CNS demyelination, and CSF and serum studies did not support the diagnosis of vasculitis.

Clinical management included stricter control of hypertension and routine clinical and imaging follow-up.

12.8.2 Companion Case 2

History

A 40-year-old African-American male patient with poorly controlled hypertension and headache.

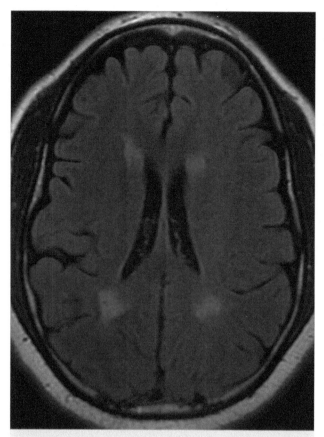

Fig. 12.4 Companion case 2. Axial FLAIR image is shown.

Imaging Analysis, Clinical Correlation, and Management in Companion Case 2

Axial FLAIR image of the brain reveals prominent, confluent areas of increased signal in the periventricular white matter (▶ Fig. 12.4). There is lack of involvement of the corpus callosum and the lesions are confluent without discrete oval-shaped lesions perpendicular to the ventricles.

This white matter change is consistent with the patient's history of poorly controlled hypertension rather than demyelinating disease. Other than recommend increased follow-up with the patient's primary care physician to promote better blood pressure medication compliance, no further work-up was recommended.

12.8.3 Companion Case 3

History

A 70-year-old man with chronic hypertension and a headache.

Imaging Analysis, Clinical Correlation, and Management in Companion Case 3

FLAIR image (▶ Fig. 12.5a) of the brain reveals extensive white matter signal abnormality, which is confluent in the periventricular and deep white matter. Ventricles and sulci are prominent as expected in this 70-year-old man with chronic hypertension. A gradient recalled echo (GRE) T2WI (▶ Fig. 12.5b) shows punctate areas of very low signal in the left thalamus that were not detected on T1WI or FSE T2WI. These are felt to represent small

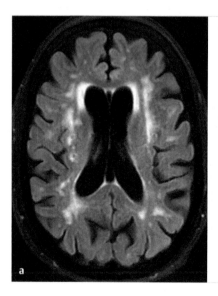
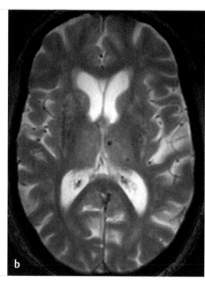

Fig. 12.5 Companion case 3. Axial FLAIR **(a)** and GRE T2WI **(b)** are shown.

areas of microhemorrhage due to chronic hypertensive, small-vessel ischemic disease. These areas of microhemorrhage are found in the same distribution as the typical location of lobar hemorrhages associated with chronic hypertensive encephalopathy, that is, the basal ganglia, pons, and cerebellum. Similar punctate areas of signal loss that are best seen "blooming" on susceptibility-weighted imaging (SWI) or GRE images can also be seen in amyloid angiopathy but are more peripheral at the gray-white junction where amyloid-associated lobar hemorrhages occur. Multiple familial cavernous malformations would appear similar but be more randomly distributed in a younger patient and not be as uniform in size. Hemorrhagic metastatic disease tends to be larger with associated edema and are more peripheral. Lesions due to neurocysticercosis may appear similar on MR but are most often more peripheral and calcified on CT scan.

If there had been a history of longstanding, prior demyelinating disease, it could appear in this manner. However, due to this patient's advanced age, male sex, and underlying hypertension, it is much more likely that this represents small vessel ischemic disease, white matter leukoaraiosis. Follow-up with the patient's primary care physician was recommended in hopes of achieving better blood pressure control.

12.9 Clinical and Diagnostic Imaging Pearls: "MS-Like lesions" versus Hypoxic–Ischemic Lesions (i.e., Small-Vessel Ischemic Disease)

- Periventricular white matter hyperintensities (WMHs) are often nonspecific and have a broad differential diagnosis. Clinical correlation taking into account the age of the patient and any associated medical conditions, like hypertension and diabetes, is important.
- Small-vessel ischemic disease affecting the white matter is far more common than demyelinating lesions due to MS.
- The presence of basal ganglia lacunes, microhemorrhages, and cortical infarctions increases the probability that the WMHs are secondary to small-vessel ischemic disease.
- The corpus callosum and juxtacortical (U-fiber) white matter are typically involved in MS and spared in small-vessel ischemic disease.
- Perivenular, ovoid configuration is typical for MS. Typical Dawson's fingers are not seen in small-vessel ischemic disease.
- Posterior fossa lesions in MS typically involve the surface of the pons, base of the fourth ventricle and trigeminal track rather than the central region of the pons diffusely, which is typical of small-vessel ischemia.
- Chronic ischemic white matter changes in the periventricular white matter do not typically enhance, whereas enhancement of an acute demyelinating MS plaque is common.
- Lesions typically associated with migraines are punctate and round, located in the periventricular and deep white matter, spare the corpus callosum and do not enhance.

12.10 Essential Information about Leukoaraiosis ("Age-Related" White Matter Changes and Small-Vessel Ischemic Disease)

- The Fazekas scale is the most commonly used metric to quantify WMHs[5]:
  - 0 = no abnormal white matter signal intensities.
  - 1 = punctate foci.
  - 2 = lesions becoming confluent.
  - 3 = large confluent areas of abnormal signal.
- Periventricular–ependymal "caps," mild atrophy, and incidental WMHs (Fazekas 1 and 2) are normal "age-related" findings with over 90% prevalence in those older than 80 years.
- When extensive small-vessel ischemic change is identified, hypertension is the most common risk factor.
- Extensive small vessel disease–related WMH is an important prognosticator. The LADIS study found that severe WMHs (Fazekas 3) independently predict disability in older adults with a more than double risk of transition from autonomous to dependent status or death within 3 years.[6]

12.11 Clinical Questions and Answers with a Neurologist about Radiologically Isolated Syndrome

1. **What is the definition of radiologically isolated syndrome (RIS)?**
   The term radiologically isolated syndrome (RIS) refers to the incidental detection of radiological findings highly suggestive of MS in the absence of clinical signs and symptoms of CNS demyelination.[1] Diagnostic criteria for this nosological entity were first described by Okuda et al in 2009 (▶ Table 12.2).[7] These criteria imply the exclusion of an alternative diagnosis in addition to the presence of CNS lesions meeting the criteria for dissemination in space (DIS).[1]

2. **What is the role of MRI in the diagnosis of RIS?**
   The MRI in multiple sclerosis (MAGNIMS) collaborative research network published new recommendations in 2016 to upgrade the imaging diagnostic criteria for MS in an effort to improve the previous 2010 McDonald criteria for MS.[8] These recommendations were partially incorporated into the revised 2017 McDonald criteria (▶ Table 12.3)[9], which should be applied for the establishment of dissemination in time (DIT) and DIS in patients with RIS.[8] Although the use of 3.0-T MRI scanners is not likely to result in an earlier diagnosis compared to 1.5-T scanner, the use of high-field scanners might help enhance differentiation of MS lesions.[3] Typical MS lesions are typically greater than 3 mm in diameter, ovoid in shape, well circumscribed, and with a homogeneous signal within the lesions that are commonly in the juxtacortical, periventricular, infratentorial regions of the brain, or spinal cord.[10] In addition, the use of SWI can help discriminate MS lesions from other related disorders by its ability to detect small veins ("central vein sign"), which is

Table 12.2 Proposed diagnostic criteria for radiologically isolated syndrome

A. The presence of incidentally identified CNS white matter anomalies meeting the following MRI criteria

1. Ovoid, well-circumscribed, and homogeneous foci observed with or without involvement of the corpus callosum.
2. T2 hyperintensities measuring ≥ 3 mm and fulfilling the Barkhof criteria (at least three out of four) for dissemination in space.
3. Anomalies not following a clear vascular pattern.
4. Structural neuroimaging abnormalities identified not explained by another disease process.

B. No historical accounts of remitting clinical symptoms consistent with neurological dysfunction.

C. The MRI anomalies do not account for clinically apparent impairments in social, occupational, or generalized area of functioning.

D. The MRI anomalies are not due to the direct physiological effects of substances (recreational drug use, toxic exposure) or a medical condition.

E. Exclusion of individuals with MRI phenotypes suggestive of leukoaraiosis or extensive white matter changes lacking clear involvement of the corpus callosum.

F. The MRI anomalies are not better accounted for by another disease process.

Source: Okuda et al.[2]

Table 12.4 The Barkhof criteria for prediction of CIS conversion to clinically definite MS

- ≥ 1 gadolinium-enhancing lesion or ≥ 9 T2-hyperintense lesions
- ≥ 1 infratentorial lesion
- ≥ 1 juxtacortical lesion
- ≥ 3 periventricular lesions

Source: Barkhof et al.[17]

commonly seen in MS-related white matter lesions.[1] Cortical lesions are present in up to 97% of patients with MS but are not easily detected on conventional MRI.[11] Double inversion recovery (DIR) allows for better detection of cortical lesions by using two sequential 180-degree inversion pulses to null the signal from the CSF and white matter.[12] Although cortical lesions have been identified in up to 40% of patients with RIS,[13] whether the occurrence of these lesions can be used as an indicator of possible clinical evolution to MS cannot be established at this time and additional studies are warranted to determine the clinical utility of this entity in patients with RIS.

3. **What is the prevalence of RIS in the general population?**
   A large population-based study in Sweden reported an incidence of 0.8 cases of RIS per 100,000 person-years compared to 10.2 cases of MS per 100,000 person-years.[14] These results suggest that RIS is relatively uncommon even in high-incidence regions. However, the prevalence of RIS seems to be higher (2.9–10.3%) in healthy relatives of patients with MS compared to nonrelatives (2.4–3.7%)[15].

Table 12.3 The 2017 McDonald criteria for demonstration of dissemination in space and time by MRI

Dissemination in space

- ≥ 1 T2-hyperintense lesions in two or more areas of the CNS: periventricular, cortical or juxtacortical, infratentorial, and spinal cord.

Dissemination in time

- Simultaneous presence of gadolinium-enhancing and nonenhancing lesions at any time or by a new T2-hyperintense or gadolinium-enhancing lesion on follow-up MRI, irrespective of the timing of the baseline MRI.

Source: Thompson et al.[9]

4. **How often does RIS progress to MS?**
   Approximately one-third of individuals with RIS will be diagnosed with MS and the remaining two-thirds will develop new lesions within 5 years of presentation.[16] The Barkhof criteria (▶ Table 12.4),[17] which were the basis of the Okuda criteria, were designed to predict conversion of clinically isolated syndrome (CIS) to MS. This may be of particular importance in the case of headache, which is by far the most common reason why RIS patients obtain a brain MRI scan and where multifocal white matter lesions are oftentimes identified in a significant proportion of individuals.[1]

5. **What are the most significant predictive factors for clinical conversion of RIS to CIS or MS?**
   According to a recent large, multicenter, retrospective study performed by the RIS Consortium (RISC), age (< 37 years), sex (male), and the presence of demyelinating lesions in the spinal cord are significant predictors for a first clinical event.[2] Specifically, around 58% of patients older than 37 years with spinal cord lesions are predicted to become symptomatic within 5 years, and up to 90% if male gender is added as an additional risk factor.[18] Other risk factors include high cerebral lesion load, gadolinium-enhancing lesions, abnormal VEPs, and CSF-specific OCBs.[9] In a recent study of 75 patients with RIS, the presence of more than two OCBs was an independent predictor of conversion to CIS with a hazard ratio of 14.7.[19]

6. **What is the recommended clinical management of RIS?**
   There are no official consensus guidelines regarding the management of patents with RIS and current evidence does not support treatment initiation in these patients, even when the radiographic findings suggest subclinical MS.[1] The use of DMT is not routinely recommended outside of clinical trials.

7. **How should patients with RIS be followed over time?**
   The approach to the patient with RIS should focus on obtaining further evidence that supports CNS demyelination or an alternative diagnosis. Attempts to determine if involvement is present in other regions, such as the spinal cord, and to better characterize the radiologic features through the use of SWI or other imaging techniques, may assist with refining the overall impression. Active monitoring of patients with periodical clinical and radiological follow-up every 6 to 12 months is currently recommended though this might change based upon the results of the clinical trial currently in progress.[1,18]

12.12 Key Point Summary

- Radiologically isolated syndrome (RIS) refers to the incidental detection of radiological findings highly suggestive of multiple sclerosis (MS) in the absence of clinical signs and symptoms of CNS demyelination.
- About one-third of individuals with RIS will be diagnosed with MS. The remaining two-thirds will develop new lesions within 5 years of presentation.
- The approach to the patient with RIS should focus on obtaining further evidence that supports CNS demyelination or an alternative diagnosis.
- Active monitoring of patients with periodical clinical and radiological follow-up every 6 to 12 months is currently recommended.

References

[1] De Stefano N, Giorgio A, Tintoré M, et al. MAGNIMS study group. Radiologically isolated syndrome or subclinical multiple sclerosis: MAGNIMS consensus recommendations. Mult Scler. 2018; 24(2):214–221

[2] Okuda DT, Siva A, Kantarci O, et al. Radiologically Isolated Syndrome Consortium (RISC), Club Francophone de la Sclérose en Plaques (CFSEP). Radiologically isolated syndrome: 5-year risk for an initial clinical event. PLoS One. 2014; 9(3):e90509

[3] Rovira À, Wattjes MP, Tintoré M, et al. MAGNIMS study group. Evidence-based guidelines: MAGNIMS consensus guidelines on the use of MRI in multiple sclerosis-clinical implementation in the diagnostic process. Nat Rev Neurol. 2015; 11(8):471–482

[4] Arevalo O, Riascos R, Rabiei P, Kamali A, Nelson F. Standardizing Magnetic Resonanace Imaging Protocols, Requisitions, and Reports in Multiple Sclerosis: an update for radiologist based on 2017 Magnetic Resonance Imaging in Multiple Sclerosis and 2018 Consortium of Multiple Sclerosis Centers Consensus Guidelines. J Comput Assist Tomogr. 2019; 43(1):1–12

[5] Fazekas F, Chawluk JB, Alavi A, Hurtig HI, Zimmerman RA. MR signal abnormalities at 1.5 T in Alzheimer's dementia and normal aging. AJR Am J Roentgenol. 1987; 149(2):351–356

[6] The LADIS Study Group. 2001–2011: a decade of the LADIS study: what have we learned about white matter changes and small-vessel disease? Cerebrovasc Dis. 2011; 32(6):577–588

[7] Okuda DT, Mowry EM, Beheshtian A, et al. Incidental MRI anomalies suggestive of multiple sclerosis: the radiologically isolated syndrome. Neurology. 2009; 72(9):800–805

[8] Filippi M, Rocca MA, Ciccarelli O, et al. MAGNIMS Study Group. MRI criteria for the diagnosis of multiple sclerosis: MAGNIMS consensus guidelines. Lancet Neurol. 2016; 15(3):292–303

[9] Thompson AJ, Banwell BL, Barkhof F, et al. Diagnosis of multiple sclerosis: 2017 revisions of the McDonald criteria. Lancet Neurol. 2018; 17(2):162–173

[10] Okuda DT. Radiologically isolated syndrome: MR imaging features suggestive of multiple sclerosis prior to first symptom onset. Neuroimaging Clin N Am. 2017; 27(2):267–275

[11] Balashov K. Imaging of central nervous system demyelinating disorders. Continuum (Minneap Minn). 2016; 22 5, Neuroimaging:1613–1635

[12] Kolber P, Montag S, Fleischer V, et al. Identification of cortical lesions using DIR and FLAIR in early stages of multiple sclerosis. J Neurol. 2015; 262(6):1473–1482

[13] Giorgio A, Stromillo ML, Rossi F, et al. Cortical lesions in radiologically isolated syndrome. Neurology. 2011; 77(21):1896–1899

[14] Forslin Y, Granberg T, Jumah AA, et al. Incidence of radiologically isolated syndrome: a population-based study. AJNR Am J Neuroradiol. 2016; 37(6):1017–1022

[15] Gabelic T, Ramasamy DP, Weinstock-Guttman B, et al. Prevalence of radiologically isolated syndrome and white matter signal abnormalities in healthy relatives of patients with multiple sclerosis. AJNR Am J Neuroradiol. 2014; 35(1):106–112

[16] Lebrun C. Radiologically isolated syndrome should be treated with disease-modifying therapy: commentary. Mult Scler. 2017; 23(14):1821–1823

[17] Barkhof F, Filippi M, Miller DH, et al. Comparison of MRI criteria at first presentation to predict conversion to clinically definite multiple sclerosis. Brain. 1997; 120(Pt 11):2059–2069

[18] Yamout B, Al Khawajah M. Radiologically isolated syndrome and multiple sclerosis. Mult Scler Relat Disord. 2017; 17(July):234–237

[19] Matute-Blanch C, Villar LM, Álvarez-Cermeño JC, et al. Neurofilament light chain and oligoclonal bands are prognostic biomarkers in radiologically isolated syndrome. Brain. 2018; 141(4):1085–1093

13 Brain Capillary Telangiectasias

Emilio P. Supsupin Jr.

13.1 Introduction

Brain capillary telangiectasias (BCTs) are rare findings often found incidentally on imaging workup of unrelated symptoms. Because of their benign nature, it is important not to mistake BCTs from more serious conditions (such as neoplasm, demyelination, or infarct) that have worse prognoses. Familiarity with the imaging findings of BCTs is crucial, not only to avoid unwarranted and potentially hazardous biopsies, but also to allay patient's fears and concerns arising from a "wrong diagnosis." The epidemiology, pathology, characteristic imaging features, and pertinent clinical issues, including the management of BCTs, are discussed.

13.2 Case Presentation

An otherwise healthy 56-year-old man was referred to our outpatient imaging facility for behavioral changes. The patient had no other symptoms or neurologic complaints. On examination, he was neurologically intact.

13.3 Imaging Analysis

13.3.1 Imaging Findings

Axial T1 precontrast MRI (▶ Fig. 13.1a) showed no abnormality. Axial T1 postcontrast study revealed an enhancing lesion in the left paramedian pons. The lesion shows **brush-like or stippled pattern of enhancement**. The brain MRI examination is otherwise unremarkable.

Impression: The imaging findings are consistent with capillary telangiectasia. This is an incidental finding and the patient's history and clinical presentation are noncontributory.

13.4 Clinical Evaluation and Management

No follow-up imaging is recommended for an asymptomatic capillary telangiectasia with no evidence of cavernous malformation.

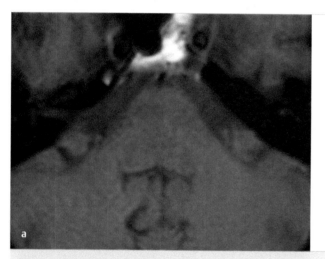
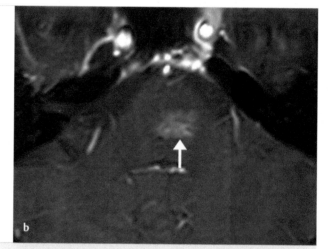

Fig. 13.1 Axial T1 **(a)** precontrast and **(b)** postcontrast MRI are shown.

13.5 Differential Diagnosis

- **Capillary telangiectasia** (see Companion Case 5, ► Fig. 13.6):
  - Lack of any abnormality on the precontrast T1-weighted and fast spin-echo (FSE) T2-weighted images is characteristic.
  - It is most commonly found in the pons, although it may occur in other locations within the brain parenchyma
  - Gradient recalled echo (GRE) and susceptibility-weighted imaging (SWI) shows low signal.
  - Enhancement is brushlike or stippled.
- Neoplasm (see Companion Case 1, ► Fig. 13.2):
  - Enhancement is almost always more nodular and solid.
  - Abnormality on the T2-weighted images is frequent but not always present.
  - Multiple lesions favor metastatic disease.
- Subacute infarction (see Companion Case 2, ► Fig. 13.3):
  - It follows a vascular territory and respects the midline.
  - It restricts on diffusion-weighed imaging (DWI).
  - It may also show decreased signal on GRE and SWI, but only if hemorrhagic.
  - It may have patchy enhancement in the subacute phase.
- Active demyelination (see Companion Case 3, ► Fig. 13.4):
  - Abnormal signal is present on fluid-attenuated inversion recovery (FLAIR) and T2-weighted images.
  - Supratentorial callososeptal lesion (Dawson fingers) is usually present if due to multiple sclerosis.
- Inflammatory processes, that is, chronic lymphocytic inflammation with pontine perivascular enhancement responsive to steroids (CLIPPERS; see Companion Case 4, ► Fig. 13.5):
  - CLIPPERS is a pontine centric condition with variable involvement of adjacent structures.[1] Lesions are typically less numerous and smaller as distance from the pons increases.[1]
  - Nodular and curvilinear enhancement "peppering" the pons is the MRI signature of CLIPPERS,[1] which appears different from the "brushlike" enhancement of a capillary telangiectasia.
  - Patchy, nonspecific T2 signal elevation in the areas of enhancement is seen,[1] whereas no abnormality is evident on the T2-weighted images with capillary telangiectasia.
  - All patients are symptomatic with cranial sensory abnormalities, diplopia, ataxia, and dysarthria.[1]
- Behcet's disease:
  - This is a chronic, idiopathic, relapsing-remitting, multisystem inflammatory vascular disease characterized mainly by skin lesions and CNS involvement in 20 to 25% of patients[2] (neuro-Behcet's disease).
  - Mucocutaneous recurrent oral and genital ulcers, aphthous stomatitis, ophthalmologic lesions such as uveitis and iridocyclitis, and multiple arthralgias are the major clinical features of Behcet's disease.[2]
  - Brainstem involvement is typical, although any part of the central nervous system may be affected.[2]
  - Typical MRI findings are small circular, linear, crescent-shaped, or irregular T2/FLAIR hyperintensity in the brainstem, usually with minimal mass effect [2] unlike capillary telangiectasia.
  - Mild to moderate patchy enhancement is common; strong uniform enhancement is rare.[2]

13.6 Diagnostic Imaging Pearls

- The combination of signal-intensity loss on SWI and focal enhancement in a lesion that is otherwise unremarkable on conventional MR images is virtually diagnostic for BCT[3] (► Fig. 13.6).
- Classic capillary telangiectasia can be distinguished from cavernous malformation.[4] The latter shows a hypointense hemosiderin ring and marked signal loss (termed "blooming") on GRE.[4]
- BCTs are typically small with a stippled or brushlike pattern of enhancement on postcontrast MRI[2] (► Fig. 13.1). They lack edema and the hemosiderin halo of cavernous malformations.[2,4]
- BCTs show low signal intensity (susceptibility) on GRE sequence.[5] The presence of susceptibility makes the diagnosis of demyelination, neoplasm, or subacute infarction unlikely[5] (► Fig. 13.7).
- SWI is a better technique than GRE in the diagnosis of BCT[3,6] (► Fig. 13.8).
- BCTs are angiographically occult.[2,7]
- A small draining vein sometimes associated with BCT[5] may serve as a useful clue to the diagnosis (► Fig. 13.8).

13.7 Essential Facts about BCTs

- It is important to recognize the MRI features of BCTs in order to avoid unnecessary biopsies, which may be potentially dangerous.[8] The implications of an erroneous diagnosis are profound because of the different prognoses of these other lesions, including their potentially devastating psychological impact to patients and their families.[5]
- BCTs are typically asymptomatic and incidentally found.[2,9] They are considered "leave-me-alone" lesions.
- SWI is superior to GRE (► Fig. 13.8)[3,6] in confirming the diagnosis and differentiating BCT from more serious lesions. This serves to discard serious differential diagnoses with high specificity, reassuring patients and referring physicians.[3]
- SWI is particularly helpful for BCT in atypical locations and may replace T2*-GRE.[3] SWI is extremely sensitive to susceptibility effects and offers high spatial resolution and excellent contrast.[3]
- Diffusion-weighted imaging (DWI) may also help differentiate BCTs from other lesions such as infarct. They have a consistently low signal on DWI, contrary to elevated DWI signal for recent infarcts.[10]
- A draining vein from the lesion is frequently found on postcontrast T1-weighted MRI as an enhancing structure. This may serve as a useful clue to the diagnosis of BCTs.[11]
- The presence of a small draining vein may also help differentiate BCTs from other lesions.[5] Infarct, neoplasm, or demyelination typically do not harbor such draining vein.
- Because they are composed of sacs of stagnant blood that has presumably partially converted to deoxyhemoglobin, they exhibit susceptibility dephasing, which is evident only on GRE (T2*-weighted) images.[5] This dephasing is probably due to the BOLD effect.[5]

13.8 Companion Cases

13.8.1 Companion Case 1: Breast Cancer Metastases

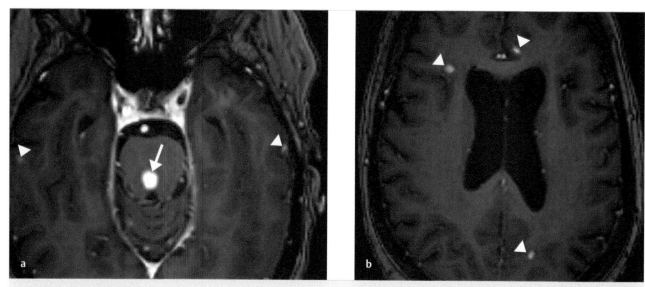

Fig. 13.2 (a, b) Companion case 1. Nodular enhancing pontine lesion (*long arrow*) in this patient with known breast cancer metastases. Note multiple other metastatic deposits in the supratentorial brain (*arrowheads*).

13.8.2 Companion Case 2: Recent (Subacute) Pontine Infarct

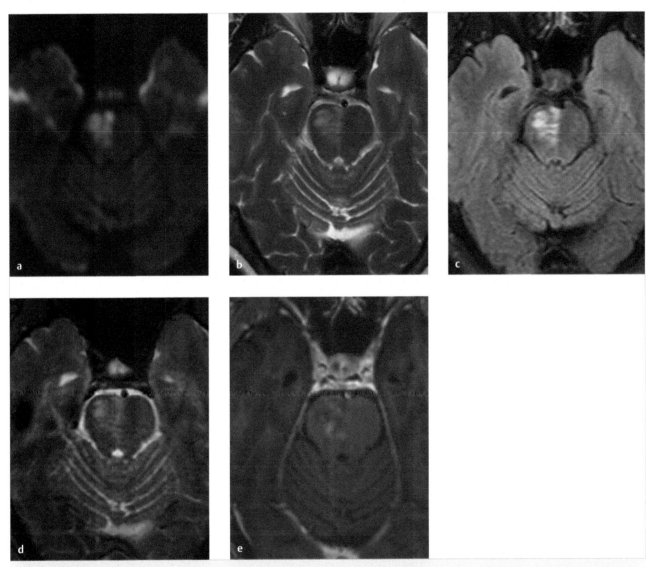

Fig. 13.3 Companion case 2. Recent (subacute) pontine infarct showing diffusion restriction (a) and elevated signal on T2-weighted (b) and FLAIR (c) sequences. Unlike capillary telangiectasias, nonhemorrhagic pontine infarcts do not exhibit susceptibility or low signal on GRE (d) or SWI sequences. A subacute pontine infarct may show patchy enhancement (e).

13.8.3 Companion Case 3: Active Pontine Demyelination

13.8.4 Companion Case 4: CLIPPERS (Chronic Lymphocytic Inflammation with Pontine Perivascular Enhancement Responsive to Steroids)

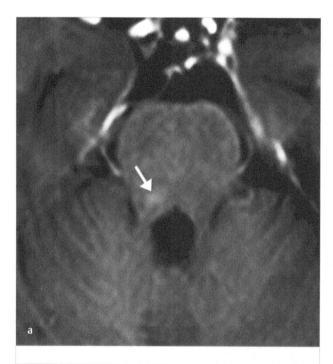

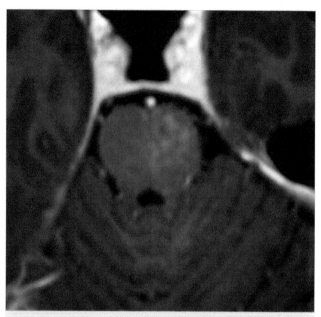

Fig. 13.5 Companion case 4. Typical pattern of nodular and curvilinear enhancement peppering the pons in chronic lymphocytic inflammation with pontine perivascular enhancement responsive to steroids (CLIPPERS). CLIPPERS is a definable, chronic inflammatory central nervous system disorder amenable to immunosuppressive treatment.[1]

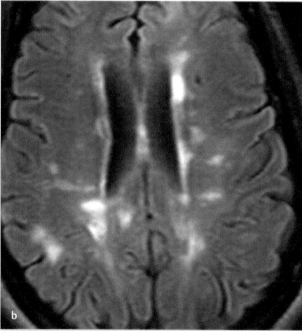

Fig. 13.4 (a, b) Companion case 3. Focal enhancement in the right superior cerebellar peduncle reflecting active demyelination. Same patient with multiple sclerosis showing multiple T2-hyperintense lesions in the supratentorial white matter in a callososeptal distribution.

13.8.5 Companion Case 5: Capillary Telangiectasia

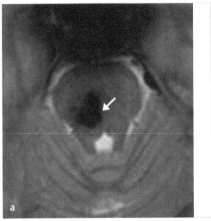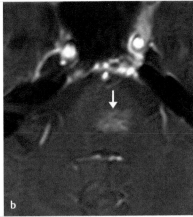

Fig. 13.6 Companion case 5. Susceptibility (*arrow* in **a**) and brushlike enhancement (*arrow* in **b**) in a pontine lesion are characteristic features of capillary telangiectasia on MRI.

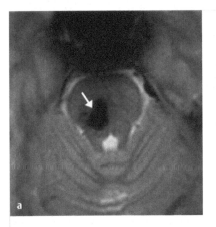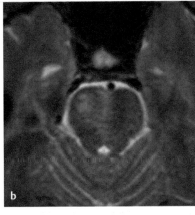

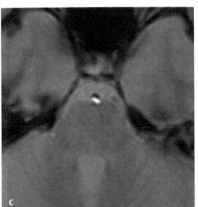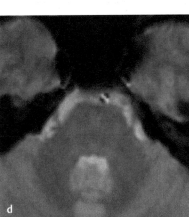

Fig. 13.7 Companion case 5. Diagnostic value of GRE in BCTs. **(a)** Susceptibility effect (low signal) is invariably seen in BCTs (*arrow*). The lack of susceptibility in other pontine lesions including **(b)** nonhemorrhagic infarct, **(c)** demyelination, and **(d)** inflammatory process (CLIPPERS) helps distinguish them from BCTs.

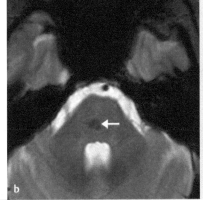

Fig. 13.8 Companion case 5. SWI versus GRE in the diagnosis of BCT. Susceptibility focus representing BCT more conspicuously depicted on SWI (*arrow* in **a**) as compared to GRE (*arrow* in **b**). The associated small draining vein (*arrowhead* in **a**) is clearly displayed on SWI but is barely visible on GRE. This associated small draining vein may serve as a useful clue to the diagnosis and differentiate BCT from other pontine lesions. Infarct, neoplasm, or demyelination typically do not harbor such a draining vein.

13.9 Questions and Answers

1. **What are capillary telangiectasias?**

   Capillary telangiectasias are a type of vascular malformation. They are considered the most benign among the vascular malformations in the brain.[12] The lesions are a collection of enlarged, thin-walled blood vessels resembling capillaries that are separated and surrounded by normal brain parenchyma.[2]

2. **What other terms are used to describe BCTs?**

   Capillary angiomas or capillary malformations. These lesions consist of small collections of dilated capillaries occupying an area measuring several millimeters to 2 to 3 cm in diameter, and may be seen as a pink or pink-gray circular lesion that is sometimes mistaken for a cluster of petechiae.[13]

3. **What causes BCTs?**

   The exact pathogenesis of BCTs is unknown. BCTs were originally thought to be congenital, forming as a result of failure of blood vessel involution.[14,15] However, more recent literature suggests that both BCTs and cavernous malformations are acquired lesions that may share the same pathophysiology.[16,17,18]

   De novo formation of BCT and cerebral cavernous malformation in association with developmental venous anomaly have been reported.[15,17,18,19] The coexistence of pontine capillary telangiectasia and multiple classic-appearing cavernomas support the hypothesis that these lesions may represent two ends of a spectrum of angiographically occult vascular malformations.[5] The presence of a small draining vein in association with BCT suggests a possible spectrum between BCT and venous angioma (developmental venous anomaly).[5]

4. **How common are BCTs?**

   BCTs are rare. Most are discovered as incidental findings on autopsy or imaging. Their incidence ranges from 0.1 to 0.7% in five population-based post mortem examinations.[13] BCTs represent 12% of pontine lesions discovered on MRI.[10,16] BCTs account for up to 20% of all brain vascular malformations[2,13] and 56% of pontine vascular malformations.[10,16] BCTs may occur at any age without gender predilection.[2] Peak presentation is at 30 to 40 years.[2]

5. **Where are BCTs located?**

   The most common location is the pontine basis near the raphe nuclei,[2,5,11,13,20,21] less often the subcortical or deep white matter of the cerebellar hemispheres,[11,13,21] the cortex and basal ganglia,[13,21] spinal meninges, or spinal cord.[2,11,13,21]

6. **What symptoms are associated with BCTs? How do these lesions come to light?**

   These lesions are quiescent and discovered incidentally.[2,5,9] They rarely cause mass effect or hemorrhage.[20,22,23] Other symptoms rarely reported include tinnitus,[4,24] headache,[5,8] vertigo,[5,8] upper extremity numbness,[8] drowsiness,[4] lip smacking,[24] mild facial weakness,[5] transient Bell's palsy,[24] and basilar-type migraine.[25]

   The pathophysiology of transient or intermittent symptoms in patients harboring BCTs is not established. In one case report of tinnitus, the vascular anomaly involved the acoustic pathway.[24]

7. **Which imaging modality is best in diagnosing BCTs? Describe the imaging appearance of BCTs.**

   MRI is the modality of choice in the diagnosis of BCTs. The lesions lack edema and have a low signal on GRE sequence or SWI.[2] SWI is superior to GRE in detecting BCTs[3] (▶ Fig. 13.8). The combination of signal-intensity loss on SWI and focal enhancement in a lesion that is otherwise unremarkable on conventional MR images is virtually diagnostic for BCT.[3]

   BCTs exhibit contrast enhancement with a "brushlike" or "stippled" pattern.[2,5] BCTs are typically inconspicuous on conventional MRI pulse sequences.[2,5] Unless unusually large, the lesions are invisible on CT scans.[2]

8. **Describe the pathology of BCTs?**

   BCTs consist of small vascular spaces lined by a single layer of endothelium and normal intervening neural tissue.[13,22,23] Microscopically, they are composed of thin-walled capillaries that are devoid of smooth muscle or elastic fibers.[22] The capillaries may vary greatly in size and may resemble cavernous spaces in some areas.[22] The presence of normal intervening brain tissue distinguishes BCTs from cerebral cavernous malformations.[22] BCTs typically do not hemorrhage or calcify.[2] Hemosiderin deposition and gliosis are absent.[2]

9. **Are there other vascular lesions associated with BCTs?**

   Associations between BCTs and other vascular anomalies such cavernous malformation,[16,17,18,26] developmental venous anomaly,[15,16,18,27] or arteriovenous malformation[15] have been rarely reported. BCTs are the most common vascular malformation in hereditary hemorrhagic telangiectasia (HHT), occurring in 60% of patients.[2]

10. **How are BCTs managed clinically?**

    BCTs are clinically benign,[16] and isolated lesions **do not** usually require treatment.[2] Given the exceedingly low risk of progression or hemorrhage from these lesions, asymptomatic patients can be treated conservatively.[16] Persistently symptomatic patients can be managed surgically if the lesion is located in a noneloquent part of the brain.[16] Because of their predilection to the pons, however, symptomatic lesions in this locale should be managed nonoperatively and symptomatically.[16] In the case of a mixed lesion, treatment is dictated by the lesion associated with the BCT.[2]

13.10 Key Point Summary

- BCTs are the most benign among the vascular malformations in the brain. They are considered "leave-me-alone" lesions.
- MRI is the imaging modality of choice, with SWI being particularly useful in the diagnosis of BCTs.
- Brushlike or stippled enhancement on the postcontrast images, no perceptible abnormality on the FSE T2-weighted images, and susceptibility (low signal) on GRE or SWI are the signature MRI features of BCTs.

References

[1] Pittock SJ, Debruyne J, Krecke KN, et al. Chronic lymphocytic inflammation with pontine perivascular enhancement responsive to steroids (CLIPPERS). Brain. 2010; 133(9):2626–2634

[2] Osborn AG, Hedlund GL, Salzman KL. Osborn's Brain: Imaging, Pathology, and Anatomy. 2nd ed. Philadelphia, PA: Elsevier; 2018

[3] El-Koussy M, Schroth G, Gralla J, et al. Susceptibility-weighted MR imaging for diagnosis of capillary telangiectasia of the brain. AJNR Am J Neuroradiol. 2012; 33(4):715–720

[4] Heremans B, Wilms G, Marchal G. Symptomatic brain capillary telangiectasia. JBR-BTR. 2010; 93(3):138–139

[5] Lee RR, Becher MW, Benson ML, Rigamonti D. Brain capillary telangiectasia: MR imaging appearance and clinicohistopathologic findings. Radiology. 1997; 205(3):797–805

[6] Chaudhry US, De Bruin DE, Policeni BA. Susceptibility-weighted MR imaging: a better technique in the detection of capillary telangiectasia compared with T2* gradient-echo. AJNR Am J Neuroradiol. 2014; 35(12):2302–2305

[7] Dillon WP. Cryptic vascular malformations: controversies in terminology, diagnosis, pathophysiology, and treatment. AJNR Am J Neuroradiol. 1997; 18 (10):1839–1846

[8] Tan LA, Munoz LF. Giant Pontine Capillary Telangiectasia. Br J Neurosurg. 2015; 29(4):574–575

[9] Milan, dre L, Pellissier JF, Boudouresques G, Bonnefoi B, Ali Cherif A, Khalil R. Non-hereditary multiple telangiectasias of the central nervous system. Report of two clinicopathological cases. J Neurol Sci. 1987; 82(1–3):291–304

[10] Finkenzeller T, Fellner FA, Trenkler J, Schreyer A, Fellner C. Capillary telangiectasias of the pons. Does diffusion-weighted MR increase diagnostic accuracy? Eur J Radiol. 2010; 74(3):e112–e116

[11] Yoshida Y, Terae S, Kudo K, Tha KK, Imamura M, Miyasaka K. Capillary telangiectasia of the brain stem diagnosed by susceptibility-weighted imaging. J Comput Assist Tomogr. 2006; 30(6):980–982

[12] Nussbaum ES. Vascular malformations of the brain. Minn Med. 2013; 96(5):40–43

[13] Jellinger K. Vascular malformations of the central nervous system: a morphological overview. Neurosurg Rev. 1986; 9(3):177–216

[14] Mullan S, Mojtahedi S, Johnson DL, Macdonald RL. Embryological basis of some aspects of cerebral vascular fistulas and malformations. J Neurosurg. 1996; 85(1):1–8

[15] Awad IA, Robinson JR, Jr, Mohanty S, Estes ML. Mixed vascular malformations of the brain: clinical and pathogenetic considerations. Neurosurgery. 1993; 33(2):179–188, discussion 188

[16] Gross BA, Puri AS, Popp AJ, Du R. Cerebral capillary telangiectasias: a meta-analysis and review of the literature. Neurosurg Rev. 2013; 36(2):187–193, discussion 194

[17] Gross BA, Lin N, Du R, Day AL. The natural history of intracranial cavernous malformations. Neurosurg Focus. 2011; 30(6):E24

[18] Abla A, Wait SD, Uschold T, Lekovic GP, Spetzler RF. Developmental venous anomaly, cavernous malformation, and capillary telangiectasia: spectrum of a single disease. Acta Neurochir (Wien). 2008; 150(5):487–489, discussion 489

[19] Barr RM, Dillon WP, Wilson CB. Slow-flow vascular malformations of the pons: capillary telangiectasias? AJNR Am J Neuroradiol. 1996; 17(1):71–78

[20] McCormick WF, Hardman JM, Boulter TR. Vascular malformations ("angiomas") of the brain, with special reference to those occurring in the posterior fossa. J Neurosurg. 1968; 28(3):241–251

[21] Castillo M, Morrison T, Shaw JA, Bouldin TW. MR imaging and histologic features of capillary telangiectasia of the basal ganglia. AJNR Am J Neuroradiol. 2001; 22(8):1553–1555

[22] McCormick WF. The pathology of vascular ("arteriovenous") malformations. J Neurosurg. 1966; 24(4):807–816

[23] Sarwar M, McCormick WF. Intracerebral venous angioma. Case report and review. Arch Neurol. 1978; 35(5):323–325

[24] Scaglione C, Salvi F, Riguzzi P, Vergelli M, Tassinari CA, Mascalchi M. Symptomatic unruptured capillary telangiectasia of the brain stem: report of three cases and review of the literature. J Neurol Neurosurg Psychiatry. 2001; 71(3):390–393

[25] Beukers RJ, Roos YB. Pontine capillary telangiectasia as visualized on MR imaging causing a clinical picture resembling basilar-type migraine: a case report. J Neurol. 2009; 256(10):1775–1777

[26] Roberson GH, Kase CS, Wolpow ER. Telangiectases and cavernous angiomas of the brainstem: "cryptic" vascular malformations. Report of a case. Neuroradiology. 1974; 8(2):83–89

[27] De Gennaro A, Manzo G, Serino A, Fenza G, Manto A. Large capillary telangiectasia and developmental venous anomaly of the basal ganglia: an unusual finding. Neuroradiol J. 2012; 25(6):744–749

14 Developmental Venous Anomaly

Emilio P. Supsupin Jr.

14.1 Introduction

Developmental venous anomalies (DVAs) are the most common vascular anomalies of the brain. They are most often discovered incidentally given the widespread use of MRI. Although they are rarely symptomatic, hemorrhage may occur, which was erroneously attributed to the DVA prior to the advent of MRI. It is now known that an associated cavernous malformation is the likely culprit for cerebral hemorrhage. Therefore, when hemorrhagic complications are encountered in the context of a known DVA, a thorough search for an associated cerebral cavernous malformation must be undertaken. The epidemiology, pathology, characteristic imaging features, and pertinent clinical issues including workup and management of DVAs are addressed.

14.2 Case Presentation

A 29-year-old Hispanic woman presented to a primary care clinic complaining of burning sensation to the right side of her head. The patient had no associated symptoms such as headaches, vision changes, or other neurologic complaints. On examination, she was neurologically intact. The patient was referred to our outpatient imaging facility.

14.3 Imaging Analysis

14.3.1 Imaging Findings

Initial postcontrast CT showed linear enhancing structures in the right frontal lobe (▶ Fig. 14.1). The smaller enhancing structures represented by dilated small veins are radially arranged and converge centripetally and drain into a larger venous structure (the "collector vein"; see ▶ Fig. 14.2). This pattern, described as the "caput medusae," is the characteristic appearance of a DVA.

No additional imaging was recommended in this case.

14.3.2 Impression

Typical developmental venous anomaly, also known as venous angioma.

14.4 Clinical Evaluation

No follow-up is recommended for an incidental, asymptomatic DVA without associated cavernous malformation.

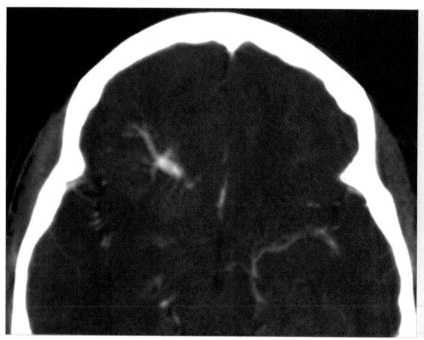

Fig. 14.1 Axial contrast-enhanced CT.

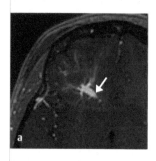
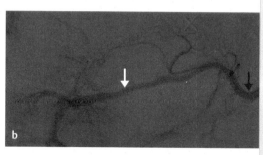

Fig. 14.2 (a) Postcontrast MRI depicting enhancing linear and curvilinear structures (i.e., dilated medullary venous radicles) converging into the collector vein (*white arrow*). There is normal intervening brain parenchyma between the dilated medullary veins. **(b)** Catheter angiogram demonstrating the caput medusae and collector vein (*white arrow*) with deep venous drainage into the Galenic system (*black arrow*). Medullary veins depend on the collector vein as they have lost their normal connections to the brain surface or ependyma.[1]

14.5 Differential Diagnosis

None. The classic caput medusae pattern is diagnostic of a DVA.[2]

14.5.1 Diagnostic Imaging and Clinical Pearls

- The caput medusae pattern is virtually diagnostic of a DVA.[2]

- DVAs are frequently incidental findings that are asymptomatic and follow a benign clinical course.[3]
- Prior to the advent of MRI, hemorrhage may have been wrongly attributed to DVAs. An associated vascular anomaly, most commonly a cavernous malformation, must be sought when hemorrhagic complications are seen.
- Susceptibility-weighted imaging (SWI) allows better visualization of DVAs without requiring contrast media[4,5] (▶ Fig. 14.3).

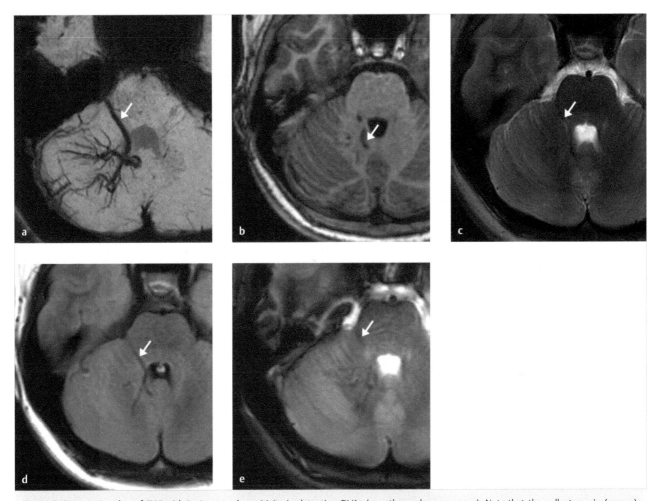

Fig. 14.3 Diagnostic value of SWI with its increased sensitivity in detecting DVAs (vs. other pulse sequences). Note that the collector vein (*arrows*) and draining venous radicles are much better visualized on SWI **(a)**. These structures are barely visible on T1- and T2-weighted images **(b, c)**, fluid-attenuated inversion recovery (FLAIR) **(d)**, and Gradient recalled echo (GRE) sequences **(e)**. Although contrast-enhanced CT or MRI has been traditionally used as the gold standard in diagnosis, the increased sensitivity of SWI in detecting DVAs practically obviates the need for intravenous contrast.

14.6 Essential Imaging Facts about DVAs

- Perfusion imaging and pathophysiology:
  - Perfusion imaging allows qualitative and quantitative assessment of the flow characteristics throughout DVAs.[6]
  - Venous congestion pattern is seen in larger DVAs with increased cerebral blood flow, cerebral blood volume, and mean transit time.[1,6,7]
  - Abnormal perfusion parameters in some DVAs may indicate that they have less robust venous drainage capacity in comparison to normal brain.[7,8]
  - DVAs may remain completely asymptomatic, suggesting that the diminished venous capacity is still sufficient to accommodate the physiologic needs of the territory drained.[8]
  - Most importantly, the DVA drains normal brain and large venous infarctions often result from their surgical disruption.[7] Therefore, careful planning is needed when surgical intervention involves the territory of a DVA (i.e., cavernous malformation resection).[7]
  - The term cerebral "developmental venous anomaly" was coined by Lasjaunias et al,[9] and it is recognized as a distinct clinical, radiological, and pathological entity.[10,11]
  - DVA is a specific type of malformation of intracranial blood vessels that is composed exclusively of venous structures.[2,10,12]
- Conventional catheter angiography:
  - The diagnosis of DVAs has been historically based on their classic appearance on cerebral angiography.[1,13,14] "Caput medusae" describes a drainage pattern in which a myriad of small veins arising at the periphery converge into a larger central vein (the "collector vein").[2] The collector vein follows a transcerebral course to reach a cortical surface, where it ascends to empty into larger cortical veins or a dural sinus.[2,14] Alternatively, the collector vein may drain into a subependymal vein in the wall of a lateral ventricle.[2]
  - On angiogram, the dilated veins appear on the venous phase, and the collector vein persistently opacifies until the late venous phase.[11,14,15] DVA shows a normal circulation time and a normal arterial phase.[16]
  - The majority of DVAs drain into the superficial venous system (70%), followed by deep drainage (20%), and less commonly a combination of both superficial and deep drainage.[9,11,17] They drain normal cerebral tissue within a functionally normal arterial territory.[9,16]
  - Most importantly, DVAs are associated with absence of a venous pathway that would normally drain the territory.[9,16,18]
- On contrast-enhanced CT or MRI, DVAs appear as numerous linear and/or punctate enhancing foci converging on a well-delineated tubular collector.[1,7,11]

14.7 Companion Cases

14.7.1 Companion Case 1

A 37-year-old man presented to the emergency center (EC) with headaches. On examination, the patient was neurologically intact with no focal deficits.

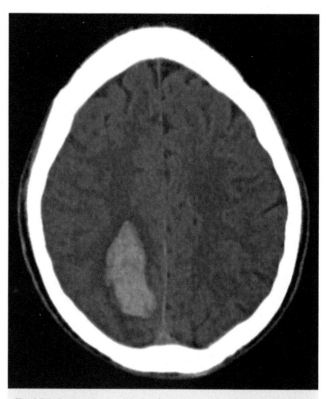

Fig. 14.4 Companion case 1. Axial noncontrast head CT shows right parietal hemorrhage.

Imaging Findings

Initial noncontrast head CT in the EC revealed an acute parenchymal hematoma in the right parietal lobe with localized surrounding edema.

Additional Imaging in Companion Case 1

Further workup was undertaken to elucidate any underlying vascular etiology for the right parietal lobe hematoma. CT angiogram (CTA; ▶ Fig. 14.5a), MRI (▶ Fig. 14.5b), and catheter angiogram (▶ Fig. 14.6 and ▶ Fig. 14.7) were negative. However, an incidental DVA was found in the left frontal lobe, which did not have any associated parenchymal abnormality.

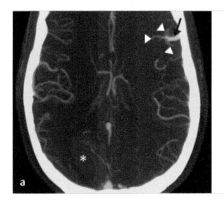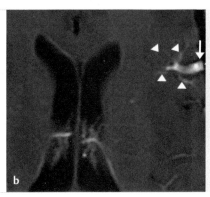

Fig. 14.5 Companion case 1. CTA **(a)** and post-contrast T1-weighted image from the brain MRI **(b)** show the classic "caput medusae" appearance of a DVA. There are multiple, radially arranged dilated small veins (*arrowheads*) that converge centripetally into the collector vein (*arrows*). Parenchymal hematoma is indicated by the asterisk.

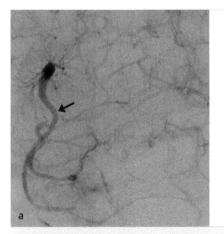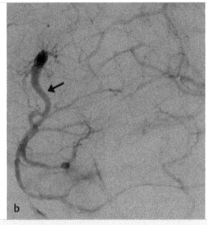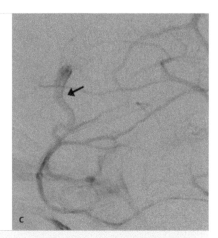

Fig. 14.6 **(a–c)** Catheter angiogram from companion case 1 (lateral view of left internal carotid artery injection) showing opacification of the collector vein (*arrows*) during the early, mid, and late venous phases of injection. The collector vein appears in the early venous phase and is persistently opacified until the late venous phase. There are no enlarged feeding arteries. Circulation time is normal with no evidence of arteriovenous shunting.

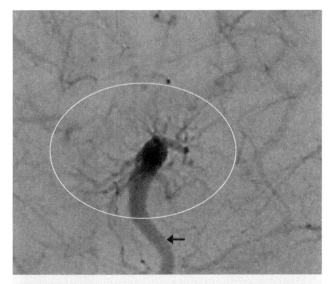

Fig. 14.7 Companion case 1. Venous phase angiogram shows classic caput medusae pattern in a DVA with multiple small dilated veins (*circle*) converging centripetally into the collector vein (*arrow*).

Follow-up Imaging in Companion Case 1

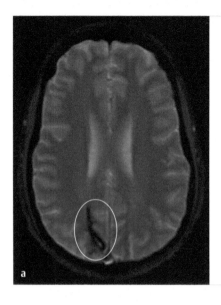
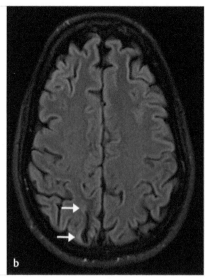

Fig. 14.8 Companion case 1. Follow-up MRI was performed to ensure normal evolution of the hematoma. GRE sequence (a) depicting hypointense signal (*circle*) in the previous hemorrhage bed, reflecting hemosiderin staining. There is surrounding gliosis represented by T2 signal hyperintensities on FLAIR sequence (*arrows* in **b**). In this case, DVA was incidentally found and was unrelated to the patient's clinical presentation. In this fairly young patient without prior neurologic symptoms and no history of coagulopathy, drug abuse, or evidence of vasculitis on angiogram, the most likely cause of symptomatic hemorrhage in the right parietal lobe was believed to be either a cavernous malformation or small arteriovenous malformation (AVM) that bled and was subsequently obliterated.

14.7.2 Companion Case 2

A 66-year-old woman presented to the EC with episodes of ataxia. Workup for stroke was negative. An incidental DVA was found on CTA and CT perfusion. (▶ Fig. 14.9 and ▶ Fig. 14.10)

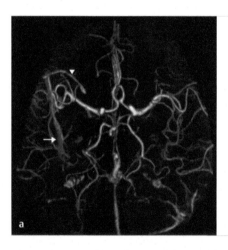
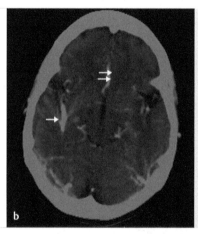

Fig. 14.9 (a, b) Companion case 2. CTA and CT perfusion showing dilated, radially oriented veins converging into the collector vein (*arrows*). The venous collector empties into the sphenoparietal sinus (*arrowhead*).

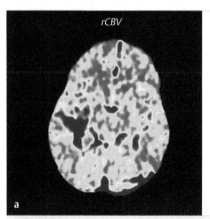
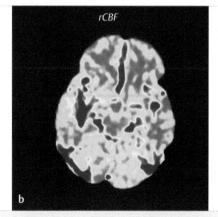
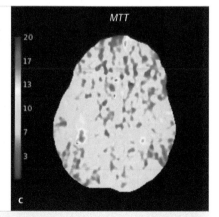

Fig. 14.10 (a–c) Companion case 2. DVAs may show a venous congestion pattern with increased cerebral blood volume, increased cerebral blood flow, and delayed mean transit time on CT perfusion.[1,6,7]

14.8 Questions and Answers

1. **What other terms (or synonyms) are used to describe DVAs?**

   Various terminologies have been used to describe the unique aspect of the same clinical entity.[13] For example, the description "caput medusae"[2] emphasizes its classic imaging appearance.[13] Other terms such as medullary venous malformation, venous angioma, and venous malformation stress on anatomy and pathology/pathogenesis of the lesion.[13]

2. **How common are DVAs?**

   DVAs are the most frequently encountered among all vascular malformations on autopsy and imaging. The prevalence of DVAs in an autopsy study four decades ago of 4,069 consecutive brains is approximately 2.6%.[19] With today's use of modern imaging, the estimated prevalence of DVAs is much higher (i.e., up to 6.4%).[20]

3. **Where are DVAs located?**

   DVAs are most commonly located in the frontal lobe, followed by the cerebellum.[11] DVAs localize less commonly in the parietal lobe, temporal lobe, basal ganglia and thalamus, occipital lobe, and pons.[21,22]

4. **How do these lesions typically come to the clinician's attention?**

   DVAs are not associated with a specific clinical presentation.[23] With the widespread use of MRI, DVAs have been increasingly diagnosed as an incidental finding on imaging workup of nonspecific symptoms.[13,24]

5. **What symptoms are most commonly associated with DVAs?**

   Most patients harboring a DVA have no symptoms. The finding is incidentally discovered during an imaging investigation. Typically, the diagnosis is made in a young adult presenting with symptoms that are often unrelated to the DVA itself. Headaches and seizures are common presentations that lead to imaging workup in this subset of patients. In a systematic review and prospective, population-based study, the clinical presentation and clinical course of DVAs were described.[3] This review included fifteen studies, and 8 of the 15 studies also described the clinical course of DVAs. In the 15 studies of 714 people first presenting with a DVA, 61% were incidental findings, the mode of presentation was unclear in 23%, 6% presented with nonhemorrhagic focal neurological deficit, 6% had caused symptomatic hemorrhage, 3.7% were associated with epileptic seizure, and 0.3% were associated with infarction. In the population-based study of 93 adults with DVAs, 98% were incidental, 1% presented with symptomatic hemorrhage, and 1% presented with an infarct, but there were no symptomatic hemorrhages or infarcts in 492 person-years of follow-up.[3]

6. **How may DVAs produce symptoms?**

   DVAs are rarely symptomatic. The major mechanisms explaining the symptoms produced by DVAs are divided into two: mechanical and flow related.[18]

   When a component of the DVA (typically the draining collector vein) compresses an intracranial structure (such as brain parenchyma, ventricle, cranial nerve) and produces compressive symptoms that could be documented by imaging, mechanical complications were considered.[18] Obstructive hydrocephalus[18,25] and neurovascular nerve compression syndromes, being trigeminal neuralgia,[18,26,27,28] hemifacial spasm,[18,29] and tinnitus,[18,30] were the most common findings.[18]

   A misbalance between the inflow and outflow of blood in the DVA system raising the pressure in the DVA either due to an increased flow or restricted outflow characterize the flow-related complications.[18] Examples of symptoms attributed to flow-related complications include focal neurological deficits, headaches, seizures, and altered mental status or altered level of consciousness.[18] Venous outflow restriction such as stenosis or occlusion of the collector vein may lead to venous[18,31,32,33] or hemorrhagic infarction.[18,34,35,36] The term "idiopathic" was used when no clear mechanism for the underlying symptoms could be identified.[18]

7. **Are DVAs associated with other brain abnormalities? How can this be explained?**

   One theory regarding the association of DVAs with various abnormalities such as regional atrophy, parenchymal signal abnormalities, and cavernous malformations is that hemodynamic changes occur in the adjacent brain. The application of advanced physiological imaging techniques may elucidate the underlying pathophysiology of DVA and its effects on the brain parenchymal abnormalities.[7]

8. **What imaging modality is mainly used to diagnose DVAs?**

   Conventional MRI is typically diagnostic of a DVA, which limits the role of conventional angiography only for cases with a symptomatic presentation.

   On brain MRI scans, DVAs usually demonstrate a flow void on both T1- and T2-weighted sequences with homogeneous enhancement following gadolinium contrast administration.[7] Postcontrast T1 MRI shows a stellate collection of linear enhancing structures converging on the transparenchymal or subependymal vein collector.[1] The collector vein may show variable high-velocity signal loss.[1] Gradient echo or SWI is useful in detecting DVAs and associated cavernous malformations.[7] These techniques are sensitive to blood products typically seen in these lesions that produce magnetic field inhomogeneity producing a characteristic imaging appearance.[7] Lack of contrast enhancement should raise the possibility of DVA thrombosis.[7]

   Describe the pathology of DVAs.

   Grossly, DVAs consist of a cluster of variably sized prominent medullary veins (so-called "caput medusae") converging on an enlarged "collector" vein.[1] The medullary veins have lost their normal connections to the brain surface and depend on the collector vein.[1] DVAs are embedded within a grossly normal-appearing brain parenchyma, serving as its primary or sole venous drainage pathway.[1] Histologically, DVAs are malformations that are composed entirely of veins interspersed in normal brain parenchyma.[10] The walls of the vessels are devoid of large quantities of smooth muscles and elastic tissue.[10] Hyalinization and thickening of the walls are common.[10]

9. **What other vascular anomalies are associated with DVAs?**

DVAs are frequently associated with cavernous malformations.[37,38,39,40,41,42] DVAs associated with capillary telangiectasia,[43] true AVM,[44] and varix[45] have been rarely described. DVAs may coexist with sinus pericranii.[1,9,46] Typically, sinus pericranii is the cutaneous sign of an underlying venous anomaly.[1] Sinus pericranii is a rare benign venous anomaly that consists of an emissary intradiploic vein that connects an intracranial dural venous sinus with an extracranial venous varix.[1] DVAs are also associated with hereditary hemorrhagic telangiectasia,[1] blue rubber bleb nevus syndrome,[46] and periorbital lymphatic/lymphaticovenous malformations.[1] Other reported associations include malformations of cortical development.[1]

10. **Do DVAs have a role in the evolution or existence of other vascular anomalies?**

The role of DVAs in the de novo formation of cavernous malformations has been well documented.[23,47,48,49] Most cavernous malformations form at a distal radicle of a venous malformation.[40] It was shown that DVAs communicate freely with the venous circulation.[50,51] It was postulated that venous outflow obstruction and increased venous pressure induce a cascade of events including ischemia, petechial hemorrhage, and release of angiogenic factors that stimulate growth of new blood vessels and a new cavernous malformation.[40,52,53]

11. **How do DVAs form?**

The exact etiology of DVAs is unclear. DVAs are considered congenital abnormalities of the venous system of the brain.[7] DVAs are considered an extreme variation of venous architecture and venous drainage.[9,54] It has been proposed that it is related to complete arrest in venous development during intrauterine life causing the development of an aberrant venous architecture.[9,12] DVAs illustrate a transhemispheric anastomotic pathway in response to a hemodynamic "need."[9] Sometimes DVAs obey a dominant pattern of inheritance due to a gene mutation on the short arm of chromosome 9, which is thought to alter early venous development.[17,55,56]

12. **How are DVAs managed clinically?**

DVAs are incidental findings frequently encountered in routine imaging of the brain. Long-term cohort studies have unveiled the benign natural history of DVAs.[3,13] In the vast majority of cases, they follow a benign clinical course[3] and *do not require* imaging follow-up nor specific medical management.[3,54] However, they are frequently associated with cavernous malformations. Morbidity is largely attributed to coexisting cavernous malformations that are thought to be responsible for their clinical presentation (particularly hemorrhage and seizures).[13,54] Therefore, whenever DVAs are encountered, efforts in detecting associated cavernous malformation (or other vascular anomalies) through specific MRI protocols must be undertaken.[54] The

high sensitivity of SWI in detecting DVAs may obviate the need for intravenous contrast[4,5] (as exemplified on ▶ Fig. 14.3).

14.9 Key Point Summary

- DVAs are the most common vascular anomalies of the brain.
- When hemorrhagic complications are encountered, a thorough search for an associated cavernous malformation must be undertaken.
- "Caput medusae" is the characteristic imaging appearance of DVAs.

References

[1] Osborn AG, Hedlund GL, Salzman KL. Osborn's Brain: Imaging, Pathology, and Anatomy. 2nd ed. Philadelphia, PA: Elsevier; 2018

[2] Wendling LR, Moore JS, Jr, Kieffer SA, Goldberg HI, Latchaw RE. Intracerebral venous angioma. Radiology. 1976; 119(1):141–147

[3] Hon JM, Bhattacharya JJ, Counsell CE, et al. SIVMS Collaborators. The presentation and clinical course of intracranial developmental venous anomalies in adults: a systematic review and prospective, population-based study. Stroke. 2009; 40(6):1980–1985

[4] Mittal S, Wu Z, Neelavalli J, Haacke EM. Susceptibility-weighted imaging: technical aspects and clinical applications, part 2. AJNR Am J Neuroradiol. 2009; 30(2):232–252

[5] Young A, Poretti A, Bosemani T, Goel R, Huisman TAGM. Sensitivity of susceptibility-weighted imaging in detecting developmental venous anomalies and associated cavernomas and microhemorrhages in children. Neuroradiology. 2017; 59(8):797–802

[6] Kroll H, Soares BP, Saloner D, Dillon WP, Wintermark M. Perfusion-CT of developmental venous anomalies: typical and atypical hemodynamic patterns. J Neuroradiol. 2010; 37(4):239–242

[7] Nabavizadeh SA, Mamourian AC, Vossough A, Loevner LA, Hurst R. The many faces of cerebral developmental venous anomaly and its mimics: spectrum of imaging findings. J Neuroimaging. 2016; 26(5):463–472

[8] Sharma A, Zipfel GJ, Hildebolt C, Derdeyn CP. Hemodynamic effects of developmental venous anomalies with and without cavernous malformations. AJNR Am J Neuroradiol. 2013; 34(9):1746–1751

[9] Lasjaunias P, Burrows P, Planet C. Developmental venous anomalies (DVA): the so-called venous angioma. Neurosurg Rev. 1986; 9(3):233–242

[10] McCormick WF. The pathology of vascular ("arteriovenous") malformations. J Neurosurg. 1966; 24(4):807–816

[11] Valavanis A, Wellauer J, Yaşargil MG. The radiological diagnosis of cerebral venous angioma: cerebral angiography and computed tomography. Neuroradiology. 1983; 24(4):193–199

[12] Saito Y, Kobayashi N. Cerebral venous angiomas: clinical evaluation and possible etiology. Radiology. 1981; 139(1):87–94

[13] Rammos SK, Maina R, Lanzino G. Developmental venous anomalies: current concepts and implications for management. Neurosurgery. 2009; 65(1):20–29, discussion 29–30

[14] Truwit CL. Venous angioma of the brain: history, significance, and imaging findings. AJR Am J Roentgenol. 1992; 159(6):1299–1307

[15] Olson E, Gilmor RL, Richmond B. Cerebral venous angiomas. Radiology. 1984; 151(1):97–104

[16] Fierstien SB, Pribram HW, Hieshima G. Angiography and computed tomography in the evaluation of cerebral venous malformations. Neuroradiology. 1979; 17(3):137–148

[17] Chong W, Patel II, Holt M. Developmental venous anomalies (DVA): what are they really? Neuroradiol J. 2011; 24(1):59–70

[18] Pereira VM, Geibprasert S, Krings T, et al. Pathomechanisms of symptomatic developmental venous anomalies. Stroke. 2008; 39(12):3201–3215

[19] Sarwar M, McCormick WF. Intracerebral venous angioma. Case report and review. Arch Neurol. 1978; 35(5):323–325

[20] Gökçe E, Acu B, Beyhan M, Celikyay F, Celikyay R. Magnetic resonance imaging findings of developmental venous anomalies. Clin Neuroradiol. 2014; 24(2):135–143

[21] Pardatscher K, Fiore DL, Galligioni F, Iraci G. Diagnosis of cerebral venous angioma by rapidly enhanced CT scan. Surg Neurol. 1980; 14(2):111–113

[22] Pak H, Patel SC, Malik GM, Ausman JI. Successful evacuation of a pontine hematoma secondary to rupture of a venous angioma. Surg Neurol. 1981; 15(3):164–167

[23] Töpper R, Jürgens E, Reul J, Thron A. Clinical significance of intracranial developmental venous anomalies. J Neurol Neurosurg Psychiatry. 1999; 67(2):234–238

[24] Del Curling O, Jr, Kelly DL, Jr, Elster AD, Craven TE. An analysis of the natural history of cavernous angiomas. J Neurosurg. 1991; 75(5):702–708

[25] Blackmore CC, Mamourian AC. Aqueduct compression from venous angioma: MR findings. AJNR Am J Neuroradiol. 1996; 17(3):458–460

[26] Samadian M, Bakhtevari MH, Nosari MA, Babadi AJ, Razaei O. Trigeminal neuralgia caused by venous angioma: a case report and review of the literature. World Neurosurg. 2015; 84(3):860–864

[27] Peterson AM, Williams RL, Fukui MB, Meltzer CC. Venous angioma adjacent to the root entry zone of the trigeminal nerve: implications for management of trigeminal neuralgia. Neuroradiology. 2002; 44(4):342–346

[28] Yamamoto T, Suzuki M, Esaki T, Nakao Y, Mori K. Trigeminal neuralgia caused by venous angioma: case report. Neurol Med Chir (Tokyo). 2013; 53(1):40–43

[29] Chiaramonte R, Bonfiglio M, D'Amore A, Chiaramonte I. Developmental venous anomaly responsible for hemifacial spasm. Neuroradiol J. 2013; 26(2):201–207

[30] Malinvaud D, Lecanu JB, Halimi P, Avan P, Bonfils P. Tinnitus and cerebellar developmental venous anomaly. Arch Otolaryngol Head Neck Surg. 2006; 132(5):550–553

[31] Bakaç G, Wardlaw JM. Problems in the diagnosis of intracranial venous infarction. Neuroradiology. 1997; 39(8):566–570

[32] Hammoud D, Beauchamp N, Wityk R, Yousem D. Ischemic complication of a cerebral developmental venous anomaly: case report and review of the literature. J Comput Assist Tomogr. 2002; 26(4):633–636

[33] Vishwas MS, Whitlow CT, Haq Iu. An unusual aetiology for internuclear ophthalmoplegia. BMJ Case Rep. 2013; 2013:bcr2013009290

[34] Field LR, Russell EJ. Spontaneous hemorrhage from a cerebral venous malformation related to thrombosis of the central draining vein: demonstration with angiography and serial MR. AJNR Am J Neuroradiol. 1995; 16(9):1885–1888

[35] Koc K, Anik I, Akansel Q, Anik Y, Ceylan S. Massive intracerebral haemorrage due to developmental venous anomaly. Br J Neurosurg. 2007; 21(4):403–405

[36] Agarwal N, Zuccoli G, Murdoch G, Jankowitz BT, Greene S. Developmental venous anomaly presenting as a spontaneous intraparenchymal hematoma without thrombosis. Neuroradiol J. 2016; 29(6):465–469

[37] Meng G, Bai C, Yu T, et al. The association between cerebral developmental venous anomaly and concomitant cavernous malformation: an observational study using magnetic resonance imaging. BMC Neurol. 2014; 14:50

[38] Gross BA, Lin N, Du R, Day AL. The natural history of intracranial cavernous malformations. Neurosurg Focus. 2011; 30(6):E24

[39] Abe T, Singer RJ, Marks MP, Norbash AM, Crowley RS, Steinberg GK. Coexistence of occult vascular malformations and developmental venous anomalies in the central nervous system: MR evaluation. AJNR Am J Neuroradiol. 1998; 19(1):51–57

[40] Dillon WP. Cryptic vascular malformations: controversies in terminology, diagnosis, pathophysiology, and treatment. AJNR Am J Neuroradiol. 1997; 18(10):1839–1846

[41] Rigamonti D, Spetzler RF, Medina M, Rigamonti K, Geckle DS, Pappas C. Cerebral venous malformations. J Neurosurg. 1990; 73(4):560–564

[42] Rigamonti D, Spetzler RF. The association of venous and cavernous malformations. Report of four cases and discussion of the pathophysiological, diagnostic, and therapeutic implications. Acta Neurochir (Wien). 1988; 92(1–4):100–105

[43] Van Roost D, Kristof R, Wolf HK, Keller E. Intracerebral capillary telangiectasia and venous malformation: a rare association. Surg Neurol. 1997; 48(2):175–183

[44] Aksoy FG, Gomori JM, Tuchner Z. Association of intracerebral venous angioma and true arteriovenous malformation: a rare, distinct entity. Neuroradiology. 2000; 42(6):455–457

[45] Uchino A, Hasuo K, Matsumoto S, Ikezaki K, Masuda K. Varix occurring with cerebral venous angioma: a case report and review of the literature. Neuroradiology. 1995; 37(1):29–31

[46] Gabikian P, Clatterbuck RE, Gailloud P, Rigamonti D. Developmental venous anomalies and sinus pericranii in the blue rubber-bleb nevus syndrome. Case report. J Neurosurg. 2003; 99(2):409–411

[47] Cakirer S. De novo formation of a cavernous malformation of the brain in the presence of a developmental venous anomaly. Clin Radiol. 2003; 58(3):251–256

[48] Campeau NG, Lane JI. De novo development of a lesion with the appearance of a cavernous malformation adjacent to an existing developmental venous anomaly. AJNR Am J Neuroradiol. 2005; 26(1):156–159

[49] Chakravarthy H, Lin TK, Chen YL, Wu YM, Yeh CH, Wong HF. De novo formation of cerebral cavernous malformation adjacent to existing developmental venous anomaly: an effect of change in venous pressure associated with management of a complex dural arterio-venous fistula. Neuroradiol J. 2016; 29(6):458–464

[50] Little JR, Awad IA, Jones SC, Ebrahim ZY. Vascular pressures and cortical blood flow in cavernous angioma of the brain. J Neurosurg. 1990; 73(4):555–559

[51] Ciricillo SF, Dillon WP, Fink ME, Edwards MS. Progression of multiple cryptic vascular malformations associated with anomalous venous drainage. Case report. J Neurosurg. 1994; 81(3):477–481

[52] Rothbart D, Awad IA, Lee J, Kim J, Harbaugh R, Criscuolo GR. Expression of angiogenic factors and structural proteins in central nervous system vascular malformations. Neurosurgery. 1996; 38(5):915–924, discussion 924–925

[53] Wilson CB. Cryptic vascular malformations. Clin Neurosurg. 1992; 38:49–84

[54] San Millán Ruíz D, Gailloud P. Cerebral developmental venous anomalies. Childs Nerv Syst. 2010; 26(10):1395–1406

[55] Boon LM, Mulliken JB, Vikkula M, et al. Assignment of a locus for dominantly inherited venous malformations to chromosome 9p. Hum Mol Genet. 1994; 3(9):1583–1587

[56] Gallione CJ, Pasyk KA, Boon LM, et al. A gene for familial venous malformations maps to chromosome 9p in a second large kindred. J Med Genet. 1995; 32(3):197–199

15 Cerebral Cavernous Malformations

Emilio P. Supsupin Jr. and Mark Dannenbaum

15.1 Introduction

Cerebral cavernous malformations (CCMs) are vascular anomalies known as the "popcorn" lesions in the brain. Symptomatic hemorrhage resulting from these lesions is the main reason for imaging and treating them. The epidemiology, natural history, imaging workup, and approach to management of CCMS are addressed.

15.2 Case Presentation

A 30-year-old Hispanic woman sought consult to a primary care provider for headaches. On examination, the patient was neurologically intact without focal deficits. She was referred to our outpatient facility for imaging evaluation.

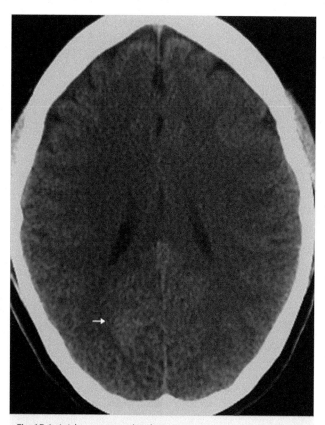

Fig. 15.1 Axial noncontrast head CT.

15.3 Imaging Analysis

15.3.1 Imaging Findings

Noncontrast head CT shows a focal area of increased attenuation in the right occipital lobe without surrounding edema (*arrow* in ▶ Fig. 15.1).

An area of increased attenuation within the brain on CT scan may be due to calcification, an acute hemorrhage, or dense, hypercellular tumor. The lack of surrounding edema makes the possibility of acute hemorrhage unlikely. Therefore, an MRI was recommended for further evaluation.

15.3.2 Additional Imaging

A brain MRI was performed for further evaluation (see ▶ Fig. 15.2).

15.3.3 Imaging Findings

The brain MRI axial T1-weighted image (▶ Fig. 15.2a) demonstrates a mixed signal intensity (SI) lesion with areas of hyperintensity and hypointensity/isointensity relative to the brain parenchyma. The T2-weighted image (▶ Fig. 15.2b) reveals a predominantly hyperintense lesion resembling a "popcorn" ball or mulberry. There is a halo of hypointensity reflecting hemosiderin staining. However, there is no surrounding edema. The GRE sequence (▶ Fig. 15.2c) depicts signal dropout of the lesion. These findings correspond to the localized area of increased attenuation on the reference CT.

15.3.4 Impression

Typical appearing cavernous hemangioma in the right occipital lobe. There is no surrounding edema, to suggest recent or acute hemorrhage.

15.4 Differential Diagnosis

- **Cavernous malformation (CM)**—Classic "popcorn" appearing, round lesion with dark hemosiderin rim on T2-weighted images that "blooms" on GRE sequences. Often a vague surrounding area of T1 shortening (bright signal) in the brain parenchyma may suggest bleeding that originated from an acutely hemorrhagic CM.

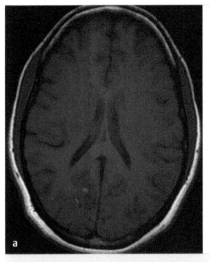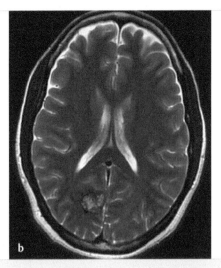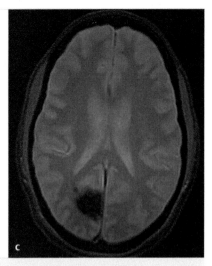

Fig. 15.2 Axial T1-weighted **(a)**, fast-spin echo (FSE) T2-weighted **(b)**, and gradient recalled echo (GRE) images **(c)** of the brain MRI.

- Microhemorrhage associated with shear injury as seen in diffuse axonal injury (DAI)—Clinical history of trauma with severely compromised neurological examination out of proportion to imaging findings. Typical locations include the gray–white matter junction, dorsal brainstem, and corpus callosum. Associated edema is frequent (see Companion Cases 1 and 2: Diffuse Axonal Injury; ▶ Fig. 15.3 and ▶ Fig. 15.4).
- Amyloid angiopathy associated microhemorrhages (see Companion Case 3: Amyloid Angiopathy; ▶ Fig. 15.5).
- Hemorrhagic metastatic disease—surrounding edema and multifocal lesions without hemosiderin rim (see Companion Case 4: Hemorrhagic Metastatic Disease; ▶ Fig. 15.6).
- Arteriovenous malformation (AVM)—Hemorrhage in association with prominent vascular flow voids should prompt consideration of this entity and CTA, MRI/MRA, or DSA performed. This typically lacks hemosiderin rim.

15.5 Diagnostic Imaging Pearls

- "Popcorn" ball (or mulberry) describes the classic appearance of a CM (▶ Fig. 15.2b and ▶ Fig. 15.7, and ▶ Table 15.1)—a well-circumscribed mixed density/SI mass surrounded by hemosiderin rim.[1]
- On T2-weighted MRI, the combination of a reticulated core of mixed SI with a surrounding rim of decreased SI strongly suggests the diagnosis of a CM (▶ Fig. 15.2b and ▶ Fig. 15.7, and ▶ Table 15.1). Smaller lesions appear as areas of decreased SI (*black dots*; ▶ Table 15.1).[2]
- CMs are frequently associated with developmental venous anomalies (DVAs).[3,4,5,6,7]

15.6 Clinical Evaluation and Management

15.6.1 Neurosurgical Evaluation

The patient was neurologically intact. The causal relationship of the lesion to the patient's symptoms (i.e., headaches) was not established given its size, location, and lack of evidence for recent bleeding. Conservative management was elected in this case. Repeat imaging may be performed should the patient develop new neurological symptoms suggesting that CCM has bled. Follow-up imaging may be also considered to reassure the patient about the stability of the lesion.

15.6.2 Essential Diagnostic Imaging Information Regarding Cavernous Malformations

- MRI is particularly sensitive in detecting CMs and is highly specific.[8,9] It is recommended that every symptomatic venous malformation be worked up with a high field strength MR unit.[2,10]
- T2-weighted gradient-echo sequences have been shown to be more sensitive than conventional sequences.[10] More advanced imaging techniques such as high-field and susceptibility-weighted MR imaging have been employed for evaluation of CCMs.[10]
- GRE MRI is a key method for diagnosis of CCMs due to its ability to display hemosiderin-filled brain tissue with a very

distinct hypointensity. GRE MRI not only is more capable of identifying all lesions present, but also delineates them more precisely[11] (see ▶ Table 15.1).

- GRE MRI may show multifocal lesions in elderly patients with hypertension and a history of stroke; however, they must not be mistaken for familial CCMs. They result from hypertensive angiopathy and are located in periventricular areas.[10]
- Susceptibility-weighted imaging (SWI) is very advantageous for detecting CM lesions because it accurately recognizes deoxyhemoglobin and hemosiderin. It is also considered the only method capable of detecting unbled CM lesions.[10] Studies indicate that SWI is more sensitive than GRE in the evaluation of CCMs.[10,12,13,14] This is particularly true in the familial form of the disease where many lesions shown on SWI were not detected on GRE.[10,13,15] It was proposed that the CCMs identified only on SWI and undetectable on GRE be added as a new type (type V) in the Zabramski classification.[16]
- Diffusion tensor imaging (DTI) and functional MR imaging have been applied to the preoperative and intraoperative management of these lesions.[10]

The Zabramski classification system characterizes the varied appearances of CCMs on MRI (▶ Table 15.1),[17] and can help predict the hemorrhage rates of CCMs[18]:

- CCMs *with* acute or subacute blood degradation products have the highest hemorrhage risk (Zabramski types I and II)—23.4%.[18]
- CCMs *without* acute or subacute blood degradation products have an intermediate risk of hemorrhage (Zabramski type III)—3.4%.[18]
- Dot-sized lesions have the lowest hemorrhage rate (Zabramski type IV)—1.3%.[18]
- A simple tripartite classification might be more useful in clinical practice.[18]

15.7 Companion Cases

15.7.1 Companion Cases 1 and 2: Diffuse Axonal Injury

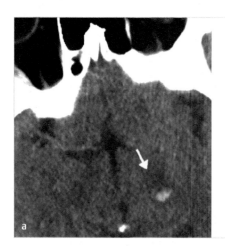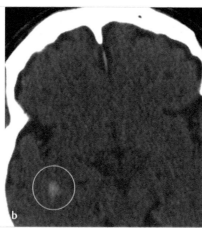

Fig. 15.3 Companion case 1. **(a)** Diffuse axonal injury with a hyperattenuating lesion showing adjacent edema (*arrow*) sustained after motor vehicle collision. **(b)** Another patient with CCM incidentally found on imaging is shown to highlight the differences between CCM and DAI. Note the lack of associated edema (*circle*)

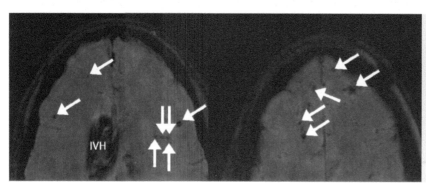

Fig. 15.4 Companion case 2. Diffuse axonal injury (DAI) with multiple susceptibility foci (*arrows*) at and near the gray–white matter interfaces. The black dots (*arrows*) may mimic the findings in multiple CMs (i.e., black dots in Zabramski type IV CCMs). Intraventricular (IVH) hemorrhage is present.

15.7.2 Companion Case 3 : Amyloid Angiopathy

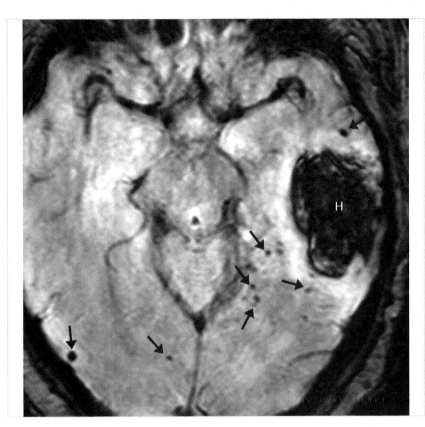

Fig. 15.5 Companion case 3. Lobar hemorrhage (H) associated with multiple black dots (*arrows*) reflecting multiple microhemorrhages in amyloid angiopathy.

15.7.3 Companion Case 4 : Hemorrhagic Metastatic Disease

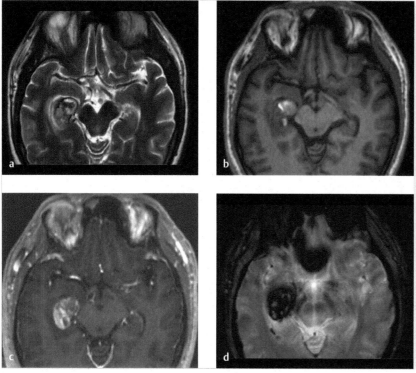

Fig. 15.6 Companion case 4. Hemorrhagic metastasis from renal cell carcinoma. (a) A kidney-shaped mass in the right mesial temporal lobe with mixed SI on T2-weighted sequence. (b) T1-hyperintense components of the lesion representing subacute blood products (methemoglobin). (c) The mass is showing enhancement on the T1 postcontrast study. (d) Signal dropout on GRE sequence reflecting hemorrhage.

15.7.4 Companion Case : Classic "Popcorn" Appearance of CCM

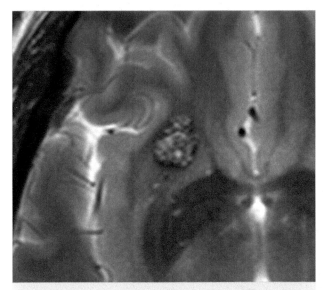

Fig. 15.7 Companion case 5. Classic "popcorn" ball (or mulberry) appearance of CCM with a reticulated core of mixed SI with a surrounding rim of decreased SI. The reticulated appearance of these lesions on MRI, combined with the relatively common finding of calcium, indicates that thrombosis and hemorrhage are an ongoing, repetitive process.[17]

15.8 Neurosurgery Questions and Answers

1. **What is the etiology and histopathology of these lesions?**
   CCMs are vascular abnormalities of the brain that are made up of a cluster of sinusoidal channels with a single endothelial lining.[6,19,20,21,22]
   The lesions are surrounded by hemosiderin deposits and a gliotic margin.[23,24,25,26]
   The vasculature is filled with blood with varying degrees of thrombosis.[26] The tendency of CCMs to leak or bleed results from a dysfunction at the endothelial tight junctions.[27]
   CMs were initially thought to be congenital. There is now compelling evidence that they can arise de novo.[6,28,29] They are also associated with radiation treatment.[30]
   Symptomatic intracerebral hemorrhage is the most feared complication of CCM, and the primary reason for treating them.[9]
   Describe the epidemiology of cavernous malformations.
   CMs occur in two forms: sporadic and familial.[31,32] CCMs are the second most common vascular lesion behind DVAs and account for 10 to 15% of all vascular malformations.[33] Prevalence from multiple reports ranged from 0.4 to 0.6% of the general population.[6,20,34,35,36,37] The lesion tends to be isolated in sporadic or nonhereditary CCM.[9,17] On the contrary, multiple lesions and an autosomal-dominant pattern of inheritance characterize the familial form of the disease.[9,17] The prevalence of CCMs is higher in Hispanic-Americans from the southwest region of the United States and Northern Mexico.[5,9,17]

CMs generally present in the younger population without a gender predilection.[6] Supratentorial lesions most commonly present with seizures, while other modes of presentation include hemorrhage, headache, and focal neurological deficits (FNDs).[6] Lesion distribution generally reflects the distribution of CNS tissue, with the majority in the supratentorial compartment.[6] One-fifth of patients overall will harbor multiple intracranial CMs, increasing to at least four-fifths in familial cases.[6]
An overall annual hemorrhage rate of 2.4% per patient year was seen, with prior hemorrhage and female sex increasing the risk of subsequent hemorrhage.[6] CM size, multiplicity, and location did not affect hemorrhage rates, although deep lesions were more clinically aggressive.[6]

2. **What other vascular anomaly is associated with cavernous malformation?**
   DVAs are present radiographically in approximately 1/10th of cases overall, although they are likely to be more prevalent in aggressive lesions and may play a role in CM development.[6]
   One study demonstrated age-related increase in prevalence of DVA-associated CMs among patients with DVAs.[38] These findings suggest that DVA-associated CMs are acquired lesions.[38]
   It was also reported that familial CCMs are unlikely to be associated with DVAs, while sporadic CCMs are highly associated with DVAs.[7]

3. **How may these lesions present clinically?**
   The most common clinical manifestations of CCMs include seizures, intracranial hemorrhage, and FNDs without radiographic evidence of recent hemorrhage.[39] Up to 20 to 50% of cases are without symptoms, discovered incidentally because of widespread utilization of brain MRI.[40,41]
   CCMs may be an incidental finding when a brain MRI is done for neurologic symptoms not felt to be anatomically related to the discovered lesion.[8]
   Seizures are one of the most common manifestations because CCMs are typically in the supratentorial region.[6,8] The International League Against Epilepsy has published criteria for CM-related epilepsy (▶ Table 15.2).[42] Seizures are more common in patients with supratentorial, cortical lesions.[6,8]
   How is hemorrhage defined in the context of this lesion?
   The definition of hemorrhage varies greatly from study to study, thus creating difficulty in quantifying bleeding rates. Some consider a lesion as having hemorrhaged only when there is a new neurological event in association with positive imaging findings. Others consider only the imaging. Given this, there is a wide range in percentage of patients presenting with hemorrhage.[28]
   A definition of hemorrhage has been proposed by the Angioma Alliance Scientific Advisory Board (▶ Table 15.3).[43]

4. **Does pregnancy increase the risk of symptomatic intracerebral hemorrhage in patients harboring cavernous malformations? Is pregnancy contraindicated?**
   The risk of symptomatic hemorrhage from CCM is *not* increased, and is no different from a nonpregnant state.[44,45]

Table 15.1 The Zabramski classification system of CCMs

Zabramski classification	Features	Imaging	Risk of bleeding
Type I	Subacute hemorrhage: hyperintense on T1- and T2-weighted images (**a,b**) with signal dropout ("blooming") on GRE **(c)**. Surrounding edema may be present **(b)**.		23%[18]
Type II	Typical appearance of CCMs: the classic "popcorn" lesion with reticulated appearance on T1- and T2-weighted sequences (**a,b**) with signal dropout ("blooming") on GRE **(c)**. Surrounding rim of hemosiderin is part of the classic appearance of CCMs.		
Type III	Chronic hemorrhage: hypointense on T1- and T2-weighted images (**a,b**) with signal dropout ("blooming") on GRE **(c)**		3.4%[18]
Type IV	Dot-sized lesions visible on GRE. These are barely or not visible on T1- and T2-weighted sequences.		1.3%[18]

Table 15.2 Criteria for CM-related epilepsy

Definite CM-related epilepsy	Probably CM-related epilepsy	Epilepsy unrelated to CM
• At least one seizure with seizure onset in the immediate vicinity of the CM	• Evidence of focal epilepsy that arises in the same hemisphere as the CM but not necessarily in the same vicinity; no other source of epilepsy found	• Epilepsy is not causally related to the CM

Source: Rosenow et al.[42]

Table 15.3 Definition of CM hemorrhage

A clinical event involving both:
- Acute or subacute onset symptoms (any of headache, epileptic seizure, impaired consciousness, or new/worsened focal neurological deficit referable to the anatomic location of the CM).
- Radiological, pathological, surgical, or rarely only cerebrospinal fluid evidence of recent extra- or intralesional hemorrhage.

The mere existence of a hemosiderin halo, or solely an increase in CM diameter without other evidence of recent hemorrhage, is not considered to constitute hemorrhage.

Source: Al-Shahi Salman et al.[43]

A history of CCM is *not* a contraindication to pregnancy or vaginal delivery.[44,45]

5. **What is the approach in the management of CCMs?**

The management of patients with CCMs includes medical management and treatment aimed at the CM itself.[8] A multidisciplinary team of neurologists, neurosurgeons, and geneticists may be necessary. There are no current clinical trials in medical or surgical management of patients with CM.[8] Thus, guidelines are largely based on uncontrolled case series and expert opinion.[8]

In treating CCMs, the surgical risk must be weighed against the natural history.[8,26] Surgical risk depends on lesion location, proximity to the brain surface, and the expertise of the surgeon.[8]

Surgical removal of the CM is often considered in a symptomatic, surgically accessible lesion.[8] If a CM is in an eloquent region, deep area (e.g., thalamus, basal ganglia), or the brainstem, surgery would generally be considered only in the setting of recurrent hemorrhages or significant and/or worsening morbidity.

In patients with CCM-related epilepsy, surgery may be considered to reduce seizure frequency as well as the risk of hemorrhage.[8] Seizure freedom can be expected in approximately 60 to 80% at 1 to 2 years.[42] Success is higher if the duration of seizures is less than 1 year.[42]

In asymptomatic patients, removal of the CM is generally not recommended because of the benign natural history.[9]

6. **What are the treatment options for cavernous malformation?**

Treatment of the CM may include observation, surgery, or stereotactic radiosurgery (SRS).[8,26]

CMs are resected after patients have experienced multiple hemorrhages in eloquent areas, or a single hemorrhage in a noneloquent area that is associated with deteriorating neurological deficits.[26,46]

Surgery for supratentorial CCMs in noneloquent locations is safe and curative.[34] In CCMs located in deep and eloquent areas and with symptoms including progressive neurological deficits, evidence of hemorrhage, and uncontrolled seizures, surgical treatment according to an integrated plan based on frameless stereotactic guidance and functional MRI is recommended and results in acceptably low morbidity.[47]

While microsurgical resection is the standard treatment for cavernomas, the risk of complication is not negligible when treating deeply located, eloquent CMs. When the lesion is inoperable or surgical risk is high, SRS can be used to prevent the natural progression of the lesion.[26,48,49,50] Radiosurgery is effective in reducing the risk of additional hemorrhages from CCMs that repeatedly bleed.[51]

Due to the potential risks associated with interventional treatment, there have been several studies on the effectiveness of medical management of CMs, allowing lesions to progress naturally and only alleviating the clinical symptoms.[26] A study reported no significant decrease in the risk of future seizures after surgical treatment of CM in patients with nonrefractory epilepsy when compared to conservative management.[52]

7. **Does genetics impact the natural history and treatment of CCMs?**

The genetic basis of CCM has been established. Familial CCMs are multifocal and/or with a family history. Loss of function mutations in one of three genes have been described: CCM1 (KRIT1), CCM2 (MGC4607), and CCM3. The functions of these genes continue to be investigated, including their role as potential therapeutic targets.[8] All of these genes are involved in signaling that genetics is responsible for maintenance of junctional integrity between neighboring vascular endothelial cells.[24,53]

15.9 Key Point Summary

- Clinical and imaging evaluation for hemorrhage of CCMs is undertaken as this is the most feared complication and the primary reason for treating them.[9]
- Brain MRI is recommended for the diagnosis and clinical follow-up of suspected or known CCM. This should include gradient echo or SWI sequences to establish whether there is one, or many, CCMs.[9]
- SWI is preferred over standard GRE-type sequences as it has much greater sensitivity in detecting CCMs, and the ability to distinguish calcification from hemorrhage.
- MRI should ideally be performed within 2 weeks of the onset of a clinical event to demonstrate extracellular methemoglobin, which is high signal on T1- and T2-weighted sequences. SWI or, if not available, GRE sequences tend to demonstrate increasing signal dropout as hemosiderin emerges and may be particularly helpful for identifying small hemorrhages.[9,43]
- Brain imaging should be performed as soon as possible after the onset of clinical symptoms suspicious of hemorrhage.[9] Evidence of acute blood can be easily and accurately identified on CT, which should be performed ideally within 1 week of the onset of a clinical event to reliably demonstrate high density consistent with recent hemorrhage,[9,54] although it may still be apparent for several weeks. To be considered a recent hemorrhage, the high density on CT should be new, when compared to any previous CT imaging of the CM and should have a Hounsfield value consistent with acute blood or should resolve on CT imaging performed at least 2 weeks later.[43]
- Catheter angiography is *not* recommended in the evaluation of CCM, unless a differential diagnosis of arteriovenous malformation is being considered.[9]
- Repeat imaging is recommended if the diagnosis is in question and when there is a negative change in neurologic status, for example, a flurry of seizures or new focal neurologic deficit.[42]

References

[1] Osborn AG, Hedlund GL, Salzman KL. Osborn's Brain: Imaging, Pathology, and Anatomy. 2nd ed. Philadelphia, PA: Elsevier; 2018

[2] Rigamonti D, Drayer BP, Johnson PC, Hadley MN, Zabramski J, Spetzler RF. The MRI appearance of cavernous malformations (angiomas). J Neurosurg. 1987; 67(4):518–524

[3] Perrini P, Lanzino G. The association of venous developmental anomalies and cavernous malformations: pathophysiological, diagnostic, and surgical considerations. Neurosurg Focus. 2006; 21(1):e5

[4] Cakirer S. De novo formation of a cavernous malformation of the brain in the presence of a developmental venous anomaly. Clin Radiol. 2003; 58(3):251–256

[5] Rigamonti D, Spetzler RF. The association of venous and cavernous malformations. Report of four cases and discussion of the pathophysiological, diagnostic, and therapeutic implications. Acta Neurochir (Wien). 1988; 92(1–4):100–105

[6] Gross BA, Lin N, Du R, Day AL. The natural history of intracranial cavernous malformations. Neurosurg Focus. 2011; 30(6):E24

[7] Petersen TA, Morrison LA, Schrader RM, Hart BL. Familial versus sporadic cavernous malformations: differences in developmental venous anomaly association and lesion phenotype. AJNR Am J Neuroradiol. 2010; 31(2):377–382

[8] Flemming KD. Clinical management of cavernous malformations. Curr Cardiol Rep. 2017; 19(12):122

[9] Akers A, Al-Shahi Salman R, A Awad I, et al. Synopsis of guidelines for the clinical management of cerebral cavernous malformations: consensus recommendations based on systematic literature review by the angioma alliance scientific advisory board clinical experts panel. Neurosurgery. 2017; 80(5):665–680

[10] Campbell PG, Jabbour P, Yadla S, Awad IA. Emerging clinical imaging techniques for cerebral cavernous malformations: a systematic review. Neurosurg Focus. 2010; 29(3):E6

[11] Lehnhardt FG, von Smekal U, Rückriem B, et al. Value of gradient-echo magnetic resonance imaging in the diagnosis of familial cerebral cavernous malformation. Arch Neurol. 2005; 62(4):653–658

[12] Lee BC, Vo KD, Kido DK, et al. MR high-resolution blood oxygenation level-dependent venography of occult (low-flow) vascular lesions. AJNR Am J Neuroradiol. 1999; 20(7):1239–1242

[13] de Souza JM, Domingues RC, Cruz LC, Jr, Domingues FS, Iasbeck T, Gasparetto EL. Susceptibility-weighted imaging for the evaluation of patients with familial cerebral cavernous malformations: a comparison with T2-weighted fast spin-echo and gradient-echo sequences. AJNR Am J Neuroradiol. 2008; 29(1):154–158

[14] de Champfleur NM, Langlois C, Ankenbrandt WJ, et al. Magnetic resonance imaging evaluation of cerebral cavernous malformations with susceptibility-weighted imaging. Neurosurgery. 2011; 68(3):641–647, discussion 647–648

[15] Bulut HT, Sarica MA, Baykan AH. The value of susceptibility weighted magnetic resonance imaging in evaluation of patients with familial cerebral cavernous angioma. Int J Clin Exp Med. 2014; 7(12):5296–5302

[16] Kiroglu Y, Oran I, Dalbasti T, Karabulut N, Calli C. Thrombosis of a drainage vein in developmental venous anomaly (DVA) leading venous infarction: a case report and review of the literature. J Neuroimaging. 2011; 21(2):197–201

[17] Zabramski JM, Wascher TM, Spetzler RF, et al. The natural history of familial cavernous malformations: results of an ongoing study. J Neurosurg. 1994; 80(3):422–432

[18] Nikoubashman O, Di Rocco F, Davagnanam I, Mankad K, Zerah M, Wiesmann M. Prospective hemorrhage rates of cerebral cavernous malformations in children and adolescents based on MRI appearance. AJNR Am J Neuroradiol. 2015; 36(11):2177–2183

[19] Awad IA, Robinson JR, Jr, Mohanty S, Estes ML. Mixed vascular malformations of the brain: clinical and pathogenetic considerations. Neurosurgery. 1993; 33(2):179–188, discussion 188

[20] Del Curling O, Jr, Kelly DL, Jr, Elster AD, Craven TE. An analysis of the natural history of cavernous angiomas. J Neurosurg. 1991; 75(5):702–708

[21] McCormick WF, Hardman JM, Boulter TR. Vascular malformations ("angiomas") of the brain, with special reference to those occurring in the posterior fossa. J Neurosurg. 1968; 28(3):241–251

[22] Moriarity JL, Wetzel M, Clatterbuck RE, et al. The natural history of cavernous malformations: a prospective study of 68 patients. Neurosurgery. 1999; 44(6):1166–1171, discussion 1172–1173

[23] Raychaudhuri R, Batjer HH, Awad IA. Intracranial cavernous angioma: a practical review of clinical and biological aspects. Surg Neurol. 2005; 63(4):319–328, discussion 328

[24] Yadla S, Jabbour PM, Shenkar R, Shi C, Campbell PG, Awad IA. Cerebral cavernous malformations as a disease of vascular permeability: from bench to bedside with caution. Neurosurg Focus. 2010; 29(3):E4

[25] Dalyai RT, Ghobrial G, Awad I, et al. Management of incidental cavernous malformations: a review. Neurosurg Focus. 2011; 31(6):E5

[26] Mouchtouris N, Chalouhi N, Chitale A, et al. Management of cerebral cavernous malformations: from diagnosis to treatment. ScientificWorldJournal. 2015; 2015:808314

[27] Clatterbuck RE, Eberhart CG, Crain BJ, Rigamonti D. Ultrastructural and immunocytochemical evidence that an incompetent blood-brain barrier is related to the pathophysiology of cavernous malformations. J Neurol Neurosurg Psychiatry. 2001; 71(2):188–192

[28] Washington CW, McCoy KE, Zipfel GJ. Update on the natural history of cavernous malformations and factors predicting aggressive clinical presentation. Neurosurg Focus. 2010; 29(3):E7

[29] Flemming KD, Bovis GK, Meyer FB. Aggressive course of multiple de novo cavernous malformations. J Neurosurg. 2011; 115(6):1175–1178

[30] Gastelum E, Sear K, Hills N, et al. Rates and characteristics of radiographically detected intracerebral cavernous malformations after cranial radiation therapy in pediatric cancer patients. J Child Neurol. 2015; 30(7):842–849

[31] Hayman LA, Evans RA, Ferrell RE, Fahr LM, Ostrow P, Riccardi VM. Familial cavernous angiomas: natural history and genetic study over a 5-year period. Am J Med Genet. 1982; 11(2):147–160

[32] Rigamonti D, Hadley MN, Drayer BP, et al. Cerebral cavernous malformations. Incidence and familial occurrence. N Engl J Med. 1988; 319(6):343–347

[33] Batra S, Lin D, Recinos PF, Zhang J, Rigamonti D. Cavernous malformations: natural history, diagnosis and treatment. Nat Rev Neurol. 2009; 5(12):659–670

[34] Kim DS, Park YG, Choi JU, Chung SS, Lee KC. An analysis of the natural history of cavernous malformations. Surg Neurol. 1997; 48(1):9–17, discussion 17–18

[35] Otten P, Pizzolato GP, Rilliet B, Berney J. 131 cases of cavernous angioma (cavernomas) of the CNS, discovered by retrospective analysis of 24,535 autopsies. Neurochirurgie. 1989; 35(2):82–83, 128–131

[36] Robinson JR, Awad IA, Little JR. Natural history of the cavernous angioma. J Neurosurg. 1991; 75(5):709–714

[37] Sarwar M, McCormick WF. Intracerebral venous angioma. Case report and review. Arch Neurol. 1978; 35(5):323–325

[38] Brinjikji W, El-Masri AE, Wald JT, Flemming KD, Lanzino G. Prevalence of cerebral cavernous malformations associated with developmental venous anomalies increases with age. Childs Nerv Syst. 2017; 33(9):1539–1543

[39] Al-Shahi Salman R, Hall JM, Horne MA, et al. Scottish Audit of Intracranial Vascular Malformations (SAIVMs) collaborators. Untreated clinical course of cerebral cavernous malformations: a prospective, population-based cohort study. Lancet Neurol. 2012; 11(3):217–224

[40] Morris Z, Whiteley WN, Longstreth WT, Jr, et al. Incidental findings on brain magnetic resonance imaging: systematic review and meta-analysis. BMJ. 2009; 339:b3016

[41] Moore SA, Brown RD, Jr, Christianson TJ, Flemming KD. Long-term natural history of incidentally discovered cavernous malformations in a single-center cohort. J Neurosurg. 2014; 120(5):1188–1192

[42] Rosenow F, Alonso-Vanegas MA, Baumgartner C, et al. Surgical Task Force, Commission on Therapeutic Strategies of the ILAE. Cavernoma-related epilepsy: review and recommendations for management: report of the Surgical Task Force of the ILAE Commission on Therapeutic Strategies. Epilepsia. 2013; 54(12):2025–2035

[43] Al-Shahi Salman R, Berg MJ, Morrison L, Awad IA, Angioma Alliance Scientific Advisory Board. Hemorrhage from cavernous malformations of the brain: definition and reporting standards. Stroke. 2008; 39(12):3222–3230

[44] Kalani MY, Zabramski JM. Risk for symptomatic hemorrhage of cerebral cavernous malformations during pregnancy. J Neurosurg. 2013; 118(1):50–55

[45] Witiw CD, Abou-Hamden A, Kulkarni AV, Silvaggio JA, Schneider C, Wallace MC. Cerebral cavernous malformations and pregnancy: hemorrhage risk and influence on obstetrical management. Neurosurgery. 2012; 71(3):626–630, discussion 631

[46] Steinberg GK, Chang SD, Gewirtz RJ, Lopez JR. Microsurgical resection of brainstem, thalamic, and basal ganglia angiographically occult vascular malformations. Neurosurgery. 2000; 46(2):260–270, discussion 270–271

[47] D'Angelo VA, De Bonis C, Amoroso R, et al. Supratentorial cerebral cavernous malformations: clinical, surgical, and genetic involvement. Neurosurg Focus. 2006; 21(1):e9

[48] Chalouhi N, Jabbour P, Andrews DW. Stereotactic radiosurgery for cavernous malformations: is it effective? World Neurosurg. 2013; 80(6):e185–e186

[49] Lu XY, Sun H, Xu JG, Li QY. Stereotactic radiosurgery of brainstem cavernous malformations: a systematic review and meta-analysis. J Neurosurg. 2014; 120(4):982–987

[50] Lunsford LD, Khan AA, Niranjan A, Kano H, Flickinger JC, Kondziolka D. Stereotactic radiosurgery for symptomatic solitary cerebral cavernous malformations considered high risk for resection. J Neurosurg. 2010; 113(1): 23–29

[51] Niranjan A, Lunsford LD. Stereotactic radiosurgery guidelines for the management of patients with intracranial cavernous malformations. Prog Neurol Surg. 2013; 27:166–175

[52] Fernández S, Miró J, Falip M, et al. Surgical versus conservative treatment in patients with cerebral cavernomas and non refractory epilepsy. Seizure. 2012; 21(10):785–788

[53] Fischer A, Zalvide J, Faurobert E, Albiges-Rizo C, Tournier-Lasserve E. Cerebral cavernous malformations: from CCM genes to endothelial cell homeostasis. Trends Mol Med. 2013; 19(5):302–308

[54] Dennis MS, Bamford JM, Molyneux AJ, Warlow CP. Rapid resolution of signs of primary intracerebral haemorrhage in computed tomograms of the brain. Br Med J (Clin Res Ed). 1987; 295(6594):379–381

16 Colloid Cyst

Christopher R. Conner, Hussein A. Zeineddine, Kaye D. Westmark, and Arthur L. Day

16.1 Introduction

Colloid cysts are histologically benign lesions most often located in the roof of the third ventricle near the foramen of Monro. Although they harbor the dangerous potential to create obstructive hydrocephalus, they may also present as asymptomatic, incidental findings. In this chapter, we discuss imaging and demographic risk factors that may help predict the development of symptoms, including obstructive hydrocephalus. In addition, we demonstrate the varying appearance of colloid cysts and show interesting companion cases in which alternative pathologies mimicked a colloid cyst.

16.2 Case presentation

16.2.1 Clinical History

A 21-year-old man presented to the emergency room after a high-speed motorcycle accident with loss of consciousness at the scene. He complained of back pain but denied headache, nausea, or vomiting. A noncontrast head CT was obtained (see ▸ Fig. 16.1).

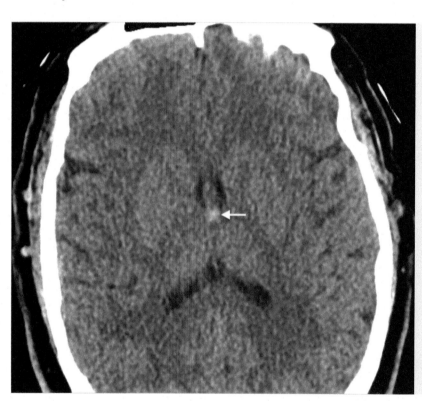

Fig. 16.1 Noncontrast head CT.

16.3 Imaging Analysis

16.3.1 Imaging Findings

The noncontrast head CT (▸ Fig. 16.1) reveals a 3-mm hyperdense lesion in the region of the foramen of Monro. The ventricles are normal in size.

16.3.2 Additional Imaging Performed

An MRI of the brain was performed to evaluate the finding on the head CT. The brain MR imaging findings are shown in ▸ Fig. 16.2.

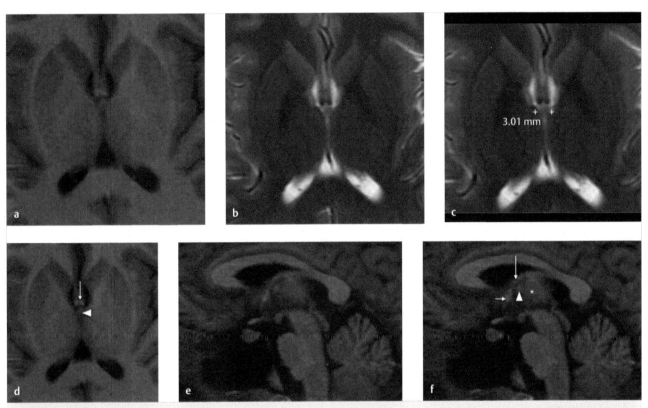

Fig. 16.2 Colloid cyst of the third ventricle. Axial T1-weighted (T1W; **a**) and T2-weighted (T2W; **b, c**) images from a brain MRI reveal a small 3-mm mass in the region of the foramen of Monro. The brain MR axial T1 W image **(d)** reveals that the mass (*arrowhead*) is isointense to the brain, making it very difficult to detect. Columns of the fornix are indicated with the long arrow **(d)**. The mass (*arrowhead*) is best seen on the sagittal T1 W images **(e, f)**, adjacent to the roof of the third ventricle, anterior to the massa intermedia (*asterisk*) and just posterior to the columns of the fornix (*long arrow*), which lie immediately posterior to the anterior commissure (*short arrow*).

16.4 Clinical Evaluation

16.4.1 Neurosurgery Evaluation

The patient denied having a headache (HA) in the ED and had no history of HAs. Neurological examination was normal.

16.4.2 Clinical Management

As this is an incidentally detected, asymptomatic, 3-mm CC with normal-sized ventricles, conservative management with imaging follow-up was elected. The patient was instructed that, although unlikely, the cyst could enlarge. If they experienced a sudden onset of HA or new neurological complaint, they should seek emergency medical attention. If they remained asymptomatic, they were instructed to return to the neurosurgical clinic for a follow-up appointment with a neurosurgeon at which time a follow-up noncontrast head CT would be obtained in 1 year.

16.5 Differential Diagnosis for Masses in the Region of the Foramen of Monro

Cysts

- Colloid cyst (CC):
  - A round or oval shaped, well-defined mass, in the anterosuperior aspect of the third ventricle is virtually pathognomonic of a CC.
  - Majority are hyperdense on CT, which is more sensitive than MRI for small, hyperdense cysts.[1]
- Neurocysticercosis (NCC):
  - Intraventricular, vesicular stage should be considered especially in endemic areas:
    ○ Isointense to cerebrospinal fluid (CSF).
    ○ A hyperintense scolex may be seen, whereas the infrequently reported intracystic nodule of a CC is hypointense on T2 W image.
    ○ NCC vesicular cysts are mobile and most frequently found in the fourth ventricle.
  - Racemose form:
    ○ Numerous cysts, most commonly in the basilar cisterns, that incite inflammatory reaction and cause obstructive hydrocephalus.
- Arachnoid, ependymal, and choroid plexus cysts[2,3,4] have rarely been reported to mimic CC but should follow CSF in signal intensity and density, unlike a CC.

Artifact

- Flow void in the third ventricle on MRI due to CSF pulsation through the foramen of Monro[2] (see "Pearls and Pitfalls" and Companion Case 3").

Vascular

- Dolichoectatic basilar artery or basilar artery aneurysm displacing the floor of the third ventricle superiorly.[2,5]
  - May mimic a CC on a single axial imaging, but its continuity with an ectatic, high-riding basilar artery, or basilar artery aneurysm can be confirmed in the coronal or sagittal plane.
- Cavernous malformation[6] and arteriovenous malformation[7] have been reported to mimic CC but are parenchymal rather than in the third ventricle. Cavernous malformations may have contrast enhancement. The blood products often have a hemosiderin ring appearance on GRE (gradient recalled echo) or susceptibility weighted imaging (SWI) type images with diffuse T1 shortening in the surrounding parenchyma (see Companion Case 7).

Tumor

- Subependymoma:
  - Typically located in the floor of the fourth ventricle or the frontal horn of the lateral ventricle rather than the third ventricle.
- Metastatic disease (see Companion Case 4); intraventricular craniopharyngioma (see Companion Case 8); choroid plexus tumor (primary, secondary); intraventricular meningioma; central neurocytoma; glioma and pituitary adenoma have rarely been reported to mimic CCs.[2,5,8,9]

Inflammatory Reaction

- Xanthogranuloma or xanthogranulomatous change in a CC.[10,11,12]

Miscellaneous

- A punctate (≤ 1 mm) high-attenuation focus that is very well seen despite its small size is likely a tiny calcification within a vessel or choroid plexus (see Companion Case 7).
- Intraventricular hemorrhage:
  - Associated with other areas of intraventricular hemorrhage (IVH).
  - Transient finding associated with other IVH and/or subarachnoid hemorrhage.

Special Considerations in the Pediatric Population

- SEGA (subependymal giant cell astrocytoma; see companion case 6):
  - Most common lesion near the foramen of Monro in children as CCs are rare in the pediatric population.
  - Solid, prominently enhancing mass with calcification.
  - Found in some children with tuberous sclerosis complex (TSC).[5] Images should be inspected for additional associated findings such as cortical tubers and small subependymal hamartomatous nodules although patients presenting with SEGA often will not have other manifestations of the condition even though they carry the genetic mutation in TSC1 and/or TSC2.

- LCH (Langerhans cell histiocytosis) and pilocytic astrocytomas have rarely been reported to mimic CCs.[5,13]

16.6 Pearls and Pitfalls

- CSF flow artifacts represent a major cause of "false-positive" MRI diagnosis of CCs. They are due to rapid or turbulent CSF flow causing signal loss within the ventricles (see Companion Case 3):
  - Flow artifacts occur most commonly on the fluid-attenuated inversion recovery (FLAIR) sequence in the frontal horns of the lateral ventricles and the third ventricle adjacent to the foramen of Monro.[2,5]
  - Inconsistent appearance on multiple sequences, pulsatility artifact, and lack of confirmation on the sagittal T1 W image should raise the possibility of a flow artifact.
  - Confirmation with head CT may be helpful as flow artifacts are not present on CT imaging.
- Initial incidental detection of a CC is often by head CT, which, in almost all cases, is how very small, hyperdense cysts are best seen.[1]
- CCs may be very difficult to see on FLAIR if they are low in signal on T2 W images because they may be isointense to the suppressed CSF.
- CCs do not cause restricted diffusion, create edema in the adjacent brain parenchyma, or have prominent thick, nodular, or homogenous enhancement. Any of these findings should prompt consideration of a broader differential diagnosis.

16.7 Essential Facts about Colloid Cysts

16.7.1 Key Components of the Radiologist's Report

- Size of the cyst is usually measured on the axial imaging sequence on which it is best seen. In oval cysts, with an asymmetrically larger superior to inferior dimension, this may underestimate the cyst's size.
- T2 signal intensity: low signal cysts may be more difficult to aspirate by the surgeon.[14,15]
- FLAIR signal intensity: high signal on FLAIR has been found in some studies to indicate cysts that are more likely to be or become symptomatic.[16]
- Location of the cyst relative to the foramen of Monro[16] (see ▶ Fig. 16.3, third ventricular risk zones).
- Size of ventricles: dilation of temporal horns and rounding of frontal horns are sensitive indicators of early hydrocephalus as is increased signal in the periventricular white matter on FLAIR. Comparison with prior studies, when available, is essential to look for subtle change in the size of the cyst and/or ventricles.
- Presence of a cavum septum pellucidum or cavum vergae should be noted as these anatomic variants may affect the surgical approach.
- Presence of a frontal lobe venous angioma should be noted as this may affect the surgical approach.

16.7.2 Imaging Features of Colloid Cysts

- CCs are well-defined and round or oval in shape, with their signal intensity and density dependent upon their cholesterol content and hydration status.[2]
- Two-thirds are hyperdense on CT. The remainder are iso- to hypodense. Calcification is rare.[17]
- The "black hole" effect on MR is present in 25% (inspissated debris within the cyst forms a center that is black on T2 W images and is surrounded by proteinaceous fluid that is bright).[2]
- Uncommonly, the cyst may be T2 and/or FLAIR "bright" and have a small central or mural nodule that is usually dark. This unusual appearance is reminiscent of a Rathke cleft cyst's mural nodule.[18,19]
- Ninety-nine percent are located in the foramen of Monro. Rarely they have been reported in the lateral and fourth ventricles, frontal lobe, cerebellum, cavum septum pellucidum, and vellum interpositum.[2,20,21,22]

16.7.3 Third Ventricular "Risk" Zones[16]

The precise location of the CC within the third ventricle has been reported by Beaumont et al to be a risk factor for cysts that are or may become symptomatic[16] (see ▶ Fig. 16.3):

- Zone 1: Extending from the lamina terminalis posteriorly to a tangent line between the mammillary bodies and the anterior aspect of the mass intermedia. Cysts in zone 1 are considered at risk of occluding the foramen of Monro.
- Zone 2: Extending from the posterior aspect of zone 1 to the anterior border of the cerebral aqueduct. Cysts in zone 2 are considered at low risk of obstructing CSF flow.
- Zone 3: Extends from the posterior aspect of zone 2 to the posterior border of the third ventricle. Cysts in zone 3 are considered at risk of occluding the cerebral aqueduct.

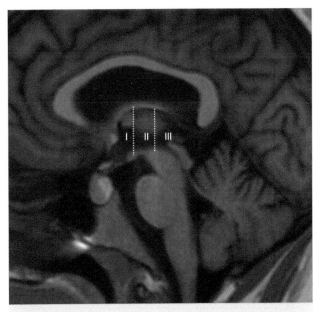

Fig. 16.3 Sagittal T1 W image with dashed lines depicting the third ventricle divided into three anatomic "risk zones." This image is from a 35-year-old pregnant female with an incidental 6 mm, zone I, colloid cyst and physiologic pituitary hypertrophy.

16.8 Companion Cases

16.8.1 Companion Cases Demonstrating Variable Appearances of Third Ventricular Colloid Cysts

Companion Case 1: Variable Signal Intensities of Colloid Cysts on FLAIR Imaging (▶ Fig. 16.4)

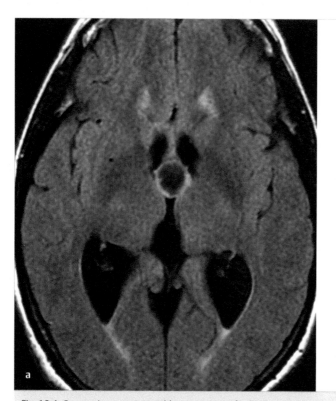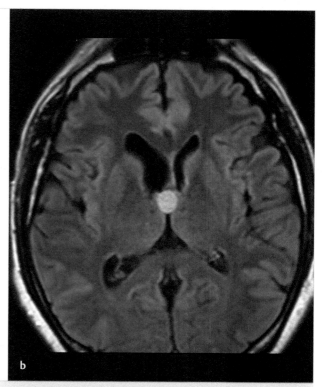

Fig. 16.4 Companion case 1. Variable appearance of colloid cysts. Axial FLAIR images from two different patients, showing colloid cysts with different signal intensity likely due to their hydration state. Note the "black hole" appearance of the cyst in this patient with obstructive hydrocephalus **(a)**. A large, hyperintense, colloid cyst causes asymmetric enlargement of the right lateral ventricle concerning for a trapped ventricle and unilateral hydrocephalus in this patient with worsening headaches **(b)**.

Companion Case 2: The Intracystic Nodule— An Uncommon Appearance, Reminiscent of a Rathke Cleft Cyst

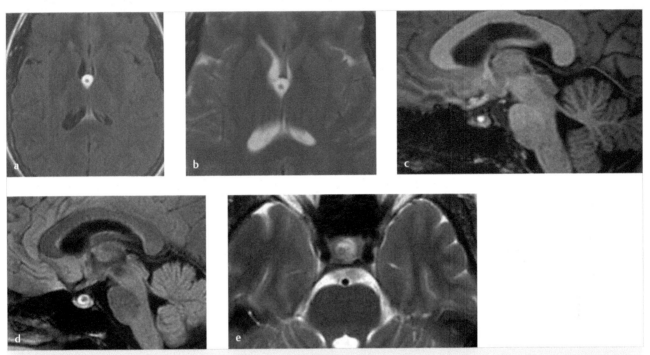

Fig. 16.5 Companion case 2. MRI images of a third ventricular colloid cyst **(a, b)** and a Rathke cleft cyst of the sella **(c–e)**. Axial FLAIR **(a)** and T2 W images **(b)** demonstrate a well-defined intracystic nodule reminiscent of the nodules found with greater frequency in Rathke's cleft cysts of the sella as shown in images c–e. Although this third ventricular colloid cyst was asymptomatic, the surgeon and the patient's family elected to remove the cyst due to the cyst size (7 mm), the patient's young age, and slight asymmetry in the size of the lateral ventricles, which was of uncertain significance.

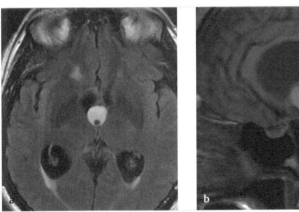

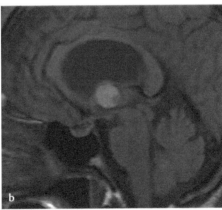

Fig. 16.6 Companion case 2. Third ventricular colloid cyst with intracystic nodule. MR images, axial FLAIR **(a)**, and sagittal T1 W image **(b)** demonstrate a cyst with a small mural nodule appearance. This patient presented with acute obstructive hydrocephalus and underwent surgery to remove the cyst.

16.8.2 Companion Cases of Entities Which May Mimic Third Ventricular Colloid Cysts

Companion Case 3: Cerebrospinal Fluid Flow Artifact

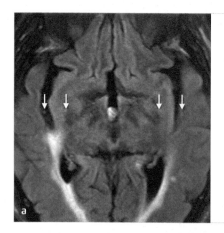 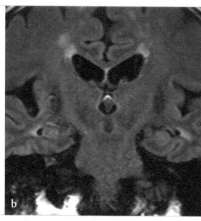

Fig. 16.7 Companion case 3. CSF flow artifact. Axial **(a)** and coronal **(b)** FLAIR images show a possible "lesion" in the third ventricle. Pulsatility artifact in the phase-encoding direction is indicated by *arrows* in **(a)**. Inconsistent signal intensity and lack of confirmation on the sagittal T1 W images (not shown in this case) as well as pulsatility artifact are suggestive of a CSF flow artifact and not a real lesion.

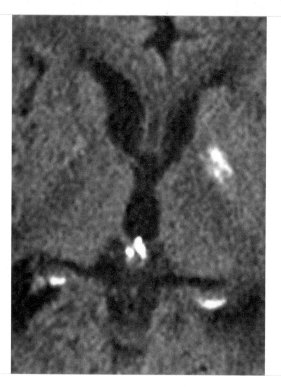

Fig. 16.8 Companion case 3. A follow-up head CT reveals the third ventricle is prominent, but there is no evidence of a mass further confirming the artifactual nature of the "lesion" seen on the MRI. Incidental note is made of dystrophic calcification in the left basal ganglia.

Companion Case 4: Primary CNS Melanoma seeding the cerebrospinal fluid

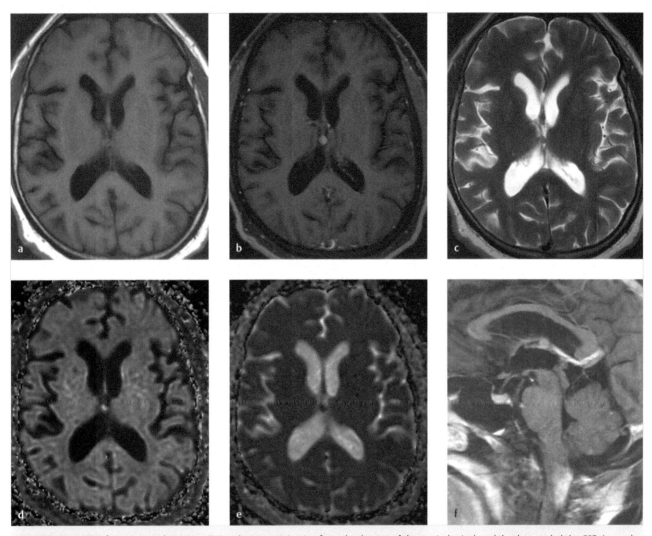

Fig. 16.9 Brain MRI of a patient with primary CNS melanoma originating from the dorsum of the cervical spinal cord that has seeded the CSF. A round, midline, nodular lesion somewhat mimics a colloid cyst on T1 W and T2 W images **(a, c)**. The sagittal T1 W image post contrast **(f)** shows the mass is more posteriorly located than the typical colloid cyst and likely in the vellum interpositum. The lesion enhances homogeneously on the postcontrast T1 W images **(b)**, which is not characteristic of a colloid cyst, which shows, at most, minimal rim enhancement. Marked restriction of diffusion is seen on the diffusion-weighted imaging **(d)** and confirmed on the apparent diffusion coefficient map **(e)** compatible with a highly cellular neoplasm.

Companion Case 5: Low-Grade Glioma

A head CT, performed for headaches in a 13-year-old female, revealed dilation of the lateral and third ventricles. As most colloid cysts are hyperdense on CT and located more anteriorly within the third ventricle, the possibility of a colloid cyst was considered highly unlikely. The MRI appearance is also atypical as the cyst is hypointense on the T1 W images (▶ Fig. 16.10b,c) and appeared adherent to the left thalamus with very slight ependymal thickening in that area (▶ Fig. 16.10d,e). As the lesion did not enhance, and the patient was from central America, the possibility of neurocysticercosis or ependymal cyst was considered most likely. The lesion was biopsied via ventriculoscopy and final pathology revealed a low-grade glioma.

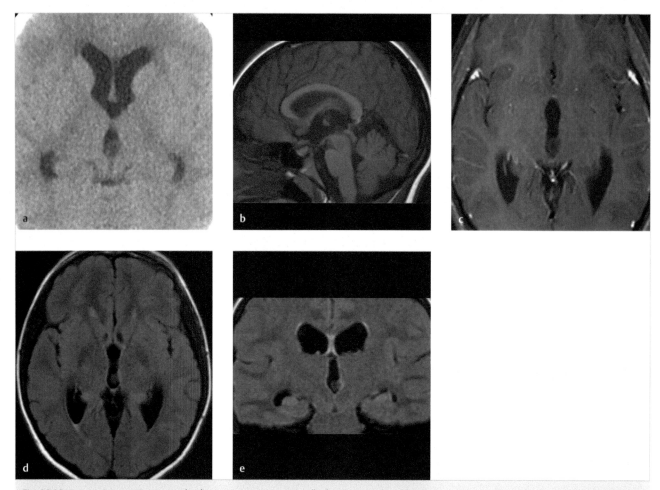

Fig. 16.10 Companion case 5. Low-grade glioma mimics a "zone 3" colloid cyst. A 13-year-old girl with a posterior third ventricular glioma obstructing the cerebral aqueduct. CT scan **(a)** reveals a low-density mass and ventriculomegaly. The sagittal T1 W **(b)** and axial T1 postcontrast **(c)**, and FLAIR images **(d, e)** reveal the nonenhancing mass does not precisely follow CSF signal and is creating obstructive hydrocephalus by occlusion of the cerebral aqueduct.

Companion Case 6: Subependymal Giant Cell Tumor in a Pediatric Patient with TSC

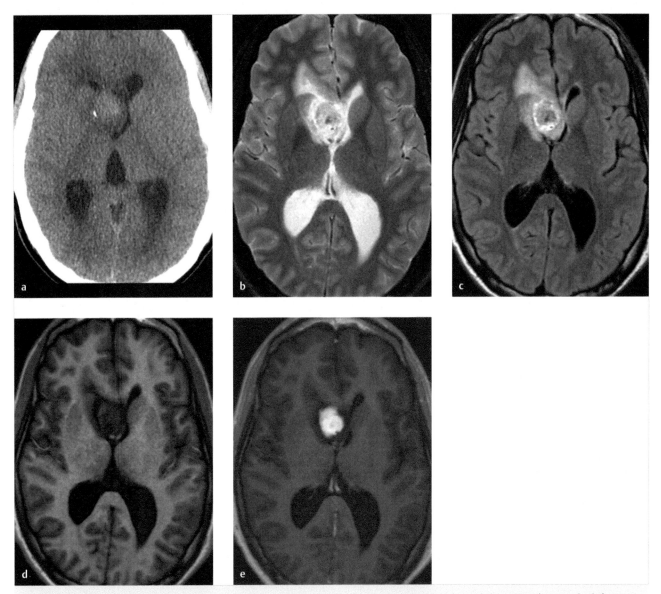

Fig. 16.11 Companion case 6. SEGA in a child with tuberous sclerosis complex. Noncontrast head CT **(a)** revealed a mass with minimal calcification in the region of the foramen of Monro. The MRI **(b–e)** showed the mass to be anterior to the foramen and associated with extensive edema in the surrounding brain with marked, homogenous enhancement, all of which are findings not compatible with a colloid cyst. Although the brain had no additional findings, cutaneous stigmata of tuberous sclerosis complex were present. The patient was found to have a subependymal giant cell tumor (SEGA).

Companion Case 7: Cavernous Malformation

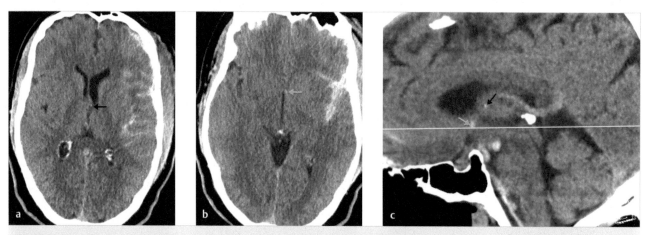

Fig. 16.12 Companion case 7. Axial CT images from a head CT obtained in a patient status post high-speed motor vehicle accident with head injury. Extensive soft-tissue swelling on the left with subarachnoid hemorrhage (SAH) and a small subdural hematoma are present. The left lateral ventricle is asymmetrically larger despite the presence of mass effect in the left hemisphere. A high-density, punctate abnormality in the region of the left foramen of Monro (*black arrow* in **a**) is very well seen despite its small size, indicating that it is likely calcification in a small vein or in the choroid plexus. An axial image 1 cm inferiorly **(b)** shows extensive SAH in the left sylvian fissure and a vague area of increased density (*orange arrow*) inferior to the foramen of Monro. A sagittal midline reformation **(c)** confirms that the punctate calcification in the foramen and parenchymal hyperdense lesion are indeed separate. Subarachnoid blood can be seen in the prepontine and quadrigeminal cisterns.

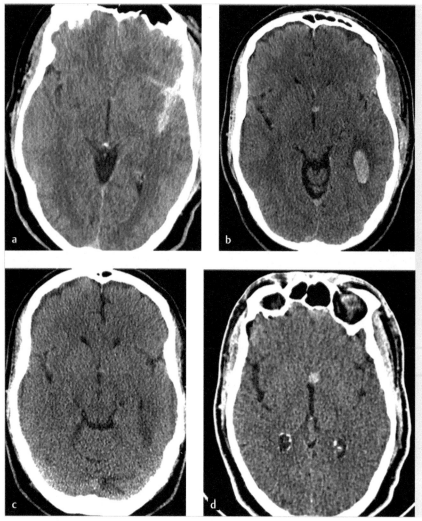

Fig. 16.13 Companion case 7. Initial head CT **(a)** and sequential follow-up head CT 4 days after trauma **(b)** show a left temporal parenchymal hemorrhage with minimal surrounding edema that had been present on the initial examination and was evolving as expected, with decrease in size and better definition. The SAH had significantly resolved. However, the area of increased density, subadjacent to the foramen of Monro, has significantly increased in size. One-month follow-up CT **(c)** shows resorption of the left temporal hematoma and the density in the region of the foramen of Monro. Follow-up examination 1 month later **(d)** for increasing headaches revealed that although the SAH and left temporal lobe hematoma had resolved, the hyperdense lesion in the region of the foramen of Monro had increased significantly in size. An MRI was obtained to evaluate for the possibility of a rapidly enlarging colloid cyst (see ▶ Fig. 16.14).

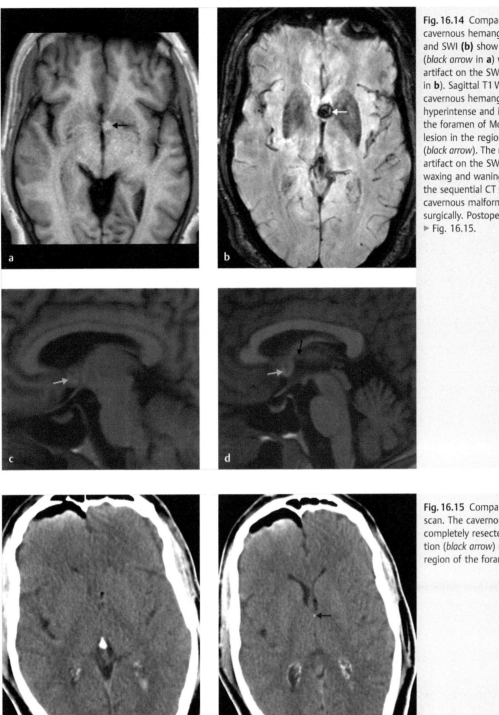

Fig. 16.14 Companion case 7. Brain MRI reveals a cavernous hemangioma. Axial T1 W image **(a)** and SWI **(b)** show a focal area of T1 shortening (*black arrow* in **a**) with marked susceptibility artifact on the SWI that is "ringlike" (*white arrow* in **b**). Sagittal T1 W images **(c, d)** show the cavernous hemangioma (*orange arrow*) is slightly hyperintense and is anterior and inferolateral to the foramen of Monro with a second, smaller lesion in the region of the foramen of Monro (*black arrow*). The marked "ringlike" susceptibility artifact on the SWI sequence as well as the waxing and waning of intra-axial hemorrhage on the sequential CT scans is consistent with a cavernous malformation, which was removed surgically. Postoperative images are shown in ▶ Fig. 16.15.

Fig. 16.15 Companion case 7. Postoperative CT scan. The cavernous malformation **(a)** was completely resected and the punctate calcification (*black arrow*) remained unchanged in the region of the foramen of Monro **(b)**.

Companion Case 8: Third Ventricular Craniopharyngioma

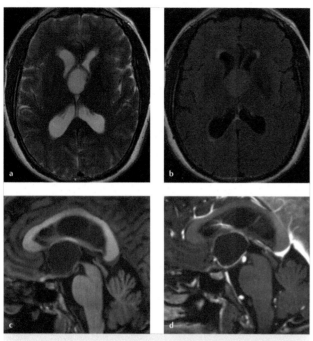

Fig. 16.16 Companion case 8. Anterior third ventricular craniopharyngioma. This 50-year-old male patient presented with memory loss over several weeks with a mass that mimicked a colloid cyst on the axial images **(a, b)** and obstructed the foramen of Monro creating ventriculomegaly. Sagittal T1 W precontrast **(c)** and postcontrast **(d)** images reveal prominent rim enhancement. Very low signal on the T1 W images and prominent wall enhancement are extremely atypical for a colloid cyst, which are usually iso- to hyperintense on T1 W images with minimal, if any, rim enhancement.

16.9 Neurosurgery Questions and Answers

1. **What is the etiology and natural history of a colloid cyst that may assist in clinical decision making?**

   The embryological origin of the colloid cyst is controversial, with competing theories including that it is a remnant of the paraphysis,[23,24] arises from the ependyma of the diencephalon,[25] or is a neuroepithelial cyst of the choroid plexus.[26] More recent ultrastructural analysis and immunohistochemistry support an endodermal derivation similar to that of Rathke's cleft and neurenteric cysts.[24,25,27]

   CCs are unilocular with ciliated and nonciliated cuboidal, columnar, and pseudostratified epithelial cells with interspersed goblet cells. CCs are rarely found in the pediatric population and typically present in the third to fifth decade. It is likely that the endodermal remnants are present congenitally but that the development of an actual cyst occurs over time.[23,28]

   Around half of all colloid cysts are symptomatic at the time of initial evaluation, with the majority of those presenting with HA, nausea, or vomiting.[16] In patients with CCs, estimates vary widely (3–35%) as to the incidence of those presenting with obstructive hydrocephalus.[16] A large cohort

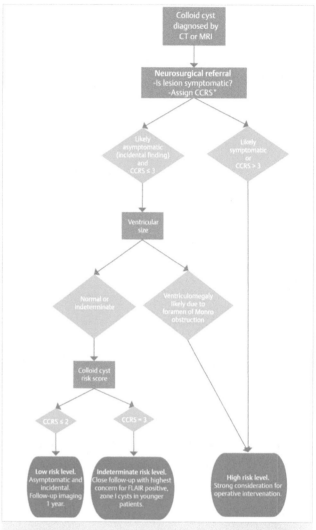

Fig. 16.17 Proposed management decision tree for the incidental colloid cyst. CCRS[16]: one point is awarded for each of the following: age < 65 years; size >= 7 mm; FLAIR hyperintensity; HA possibly due to the cyst; Risk zone location 1 or 3. The CCRS is the sum of the points on a 0 to 5 scale.

study of newly diagnosed CC in the Netherlands estimated a 34% incidence of acute deterioration in those with symptomatic cysts and a 12% mortality despite access to emergency surgery.[29] Fortunately, those found to have an incidental, asymptomatic CCs rarely suffer acute hydrocephalus or sudden death.[16,30,31] Estimates in the literature of the incidence of a CC causing sudden neurological deterioration and death range from 1.2 to 10%.[16,28,32,33]

Several studies have attempted to stratify the risk of a cyst being or becoming symptomatic based on patient demographics and imaging characteristics. Pollock et al found the following factors were associated with cyst-related symptoms: younger age, ventricular dilatation, larger cysts, and high-signal cysts on T2 W MR images.[30,34] More recently, Beaumont et al found that symptomatic cysts were strongly correlated with the following risk factors: younger age (< 65 years old), larger cyst size (≥ 7 mm), complaint of HA at presentation, hyperintense signal on FLAIR imaging, and the cyst being located within a "risk zone" in the third ventricle, practically defined as a location in which it is anatomically capable of obstructing the foramen of Monro or, rarely, the cerebral aqueduct.[16]

2. **In patients in whom a CC has been detected, what specific findings on physical examination and/or elements of the history are important in your determination that this probable incidental finding is truly asymptomatic?**

An incidental finding is an anomaly on imaging that is completely unrelated to the purpose of the examination. In the case of a CC, the determination as to whether the cyst is actually symptomatic is of critical importance. Surgical management is indicated in patients with a symptomatic CC given that the risk of sudden neurological deterioration with high mortality is considered unacceptably high.[16,29] The management of an incidentally detected, truly asymptomatic cyst is often less clear.

HA is one of the most common complaints in patients who have been determined to have symptomatic cysts, occurring in 78 to 89%.[16,30] Although postural HAs are classically described, this presentation is not common.[28,33] Many, if not most authors, have considered any HA at presentation that does not have an alternative explanation, that is, migrainous HAs, to be cyst related.[30] Given the serious nature of a cyst that has become symptomatic, de Witt Hamer et al considered that any unexplained neurological symptom is evidence that the cyst is symptomatic, even if it did not appear related to the cyst.[29] Beaumont et al categorized CCs as incidental if the patient's symptoms could be attributed to an alternative cause and their ventricles were not dilated or were static in size in patients with a diagnosis of NPH (normal-pressure hydrocephalus).[16] Reported symptoms in patients who have had CCs with fatal outcome have included severe episodic HA, nausea and vomiting, gait disturbances, syncopal attacks, blurred vision, dizziness, tinnitus, hypothalamic dysfunction, seizures, mental status change, memory impairment, and incontinence, including an "NPH-like" presentation.[28,33] Although the duration of symptoms before precipitous deterioration and death ranged from several hours to 25 years, the vast majority of patients harboring a benign third ventricular tumor were found to have been symptomatic for at least several days.[32] Rarely, patients with acute worsening may be suffering from "cyst apoplexy" and will have evidence of hemorrhage within the cyst.[35]

Papilledema on fundoscopic examination is an additional sign on physical examination and is seen in up to 70% of patients with symptomatic lesions.[31] The classic postural exacerbation of HAs and positional bradycardia are very uncommon.[16]

3. **What additional testing, if any, is required or recommended in the workup?**

An incidental CC is often detected by CT. MR imaging, both with and without contrast, is the next step in the workup of this finding. For follow-up examinations in the cases undergoing imaging surveillance, no contrast is necessary.

Preoperative imaging for navigation may be used, depending on the surgeon's preference. Lumbar punctures are *contraindicated* given the risk of herniation. Fundoscopic examination can be performed to assess for papilledema.

4. **Are there any American Association of Neurological Surgeons (AANS)/Congress of Neurological Surgeons (CNS) published guidelines for the management of this condition?**

There are no well-defined guidelines.

5. **If electing to follow, what is the suggested time interval and modality?**

Patients without symptoms should have an initial 1-year follow-up visit with the neurosurgeon at which time repeat imaging should be performed and carefully assessed for any possible change in the size of the cyst or of the lateral ventricles. Comparison of the temporal horns of the lateral ventricles is important to detect subtle cases of early ventricular dilatation. Long-term follow-up imaging of the patient will be necessary as there are many case reports of enlargement after many years of interval stability.[28,30,32] Patients should be instructed to return for further evaluation earlier should any symptom develop. A minority of patients (around 10%) will have some progression of cyst size or symptoms requiring surgery.

6. **What are the surgical options and risks?**

Surgical management is recommended in patients with symptomatic CCs and also may be elected should the surgeon assess that the possible benefits outweigh the risks in incidentally detected cysts. Again, factors for consideration would include the patient's age, existing comorbidities, ventricular and cyst size as well as any interval enlargement, and possibly the presence of increased signal on T2 or FLAIR images. In addition, the patient's wishes influence decision-making regarding surgery as concern about having the cyst and undergoing repeat imaging for any new perceived symptom may be a significant personal burden for some. Stereotactic drainage is highly dependent on the viscosity of the fluid within the cyst (lesions hypointense on T2-weighted images are less amenable to aspiration).[14,15,17] Recurrence rates for aspiration can be up to 80%[36] despite a relatively low incidence of morbidity.[37] Endoscopic removal precludes the ability to perform bimanual dissection of the cyst from the wall of the third ventricle, which increases the rate of IVH and lowers the rate of gross total resection.[38,39] Microsurgical transventricular approaches, by either a transcallosal or a transcortical route, when performed by neurosurgeons experienced in these lesions, are associated with low morbidity and the highest likelihood of complete cure.[38] The transcallosal approach often applied to patients without ventriculomegaly. Risks include possible injury of cortical veins, the supplementary motor area, and the anterior cerebral arteries. Memory deficits and disconnection syndrome (greatest for transections > 2.5 cm) may also occur.[31] The transcortical–transventricular approach has a much more direct view into the foramen of Monro for cyst removal, but carries a higher risk of seizures than the other techniques.

7. **What instructions are given regarding return to the neurosurgeon in patients being managed nonoperatively with imaging surveillance?**

Historically, there has been an association with sudden death, which was attributed to acute hydrocephalus following obstruction of the foramen of Monro or hypothalamic dysfunction leading to cardiac arrhythmias.[32] In asymptomatic patients, this risk is considered low. The patient should be informed of the risk for enlargement of the cyst and the possibility of acute hydrocephalus, and that they should return to the ER for assessment if they have any new symptoms.

References

[1] Mamourian AC, Cromwell LD, Harbaugh RE. Colloid cyst of the third ventricle: sometimes more conspicuous on CT than MR. AJNR Am J Neuroradiol. 1998; 19(5):875–878

[2] Osborn AG. "Osborn's Brain." Salt Lake City, UT: AMIRSYS; 2013:803

[3] Gupta A, Nadimpalli SPR, Cavallino RP. Intraventricular neurocysticercosis mimicking colloid cyst. Case report. J Neurosurg. 2002; 97(1):208–210

[4] Wray SD, Ellis TL, Bianco S. Migratory neurocysticercosis mimicking a third ventricular colloid cyst. Case report. J Neurosurg. 2001; 95(1):122–123

[5] Glastonbury CM, Osborn AG, Salzman KL. Masses and malformations of the third ventricle: normal anatomic relationships and differential diagnoses. Radiographics. 2011; 31(7):1889–1905

[6] Longatti P, Fiorindi A, Perin A, Baratto V, Martinuzzi A. Cavernoma of the foramen of Monro. Case report and review of the literature. Neurosurg Focus. 2006; 21(1):e13

[7] Britt RH, Silverberg GD, Enzmann DR, Hanbery JW. Third ventricular choroid plexus arteriovenous malformation simulating a colloid cyst. Case report. J Neurosurg. 1980; 52(2):246–250

[8] Lee YY, Lin SR, Horner FA. Third ventricle meningioma mimicking a colloid cyst in a child. AJR Am J Roentgenol. 1979; 132(4):669–671

[9] Nishio S, Morioka T, Suzuki S, Fukui M. Tumours around the foramen of Monro: clinical and neuroimaging features and their differential diagnosis. J Clin Neurosci. 2002; 9(2):137–141

[10] Swaminathan G, Jonathan GE, Patel B, Prabhu K. Xanthogranulomatous colloid cyst of the third ventricle: Alter your surgical strategy. Neuroradiol J. 2018; 31(1):47–49

[11] Tatter SB, Ogilvy CS, Golden JA, Ojemann RG, Louis DN. Third ventricular xanthogranulomas clinically and radiologically mimicking colloid cysts. Report of two cases. J Neurosurg. 1994; 81(4):605–609

[12] Alugolu R, Chandrasekhar YBVK, Shukla D, Sahu BP, Srinivas BH. Xanthogranulomatous colloid cyst of the third ventricle. J Neurosci Rural Pract. 2013; 4(2):183–186

[13] Sharifi G, Rahmanzadeh R, Lotfinia M, Rahmanzade R. Pilocytic astrocytoma of fornix mimicking a colloid cyst: report of two cases and review of the literature. World Neurosurg. 2018; 109:31–35

[14] Doron O, Feldman Z, Zauberman J. MRI features have a role in pre-surgical planning of colloid cyst removal. Acta Neurochir (Wien). 2016; 158(4):671–676

[15] El Khoury C, Brugières P, Decq P, et al. Colloid cysts of the third ventricle: are MR imaging patterns predictive of difficulty with percutaneous treatment? AJNR Am J Neuroradiol. 2000; 21(3):489–492

[16] Beaumont TL, Limbrick DD, Jr, Rich KM, Wippold FJ, II, Dacey RG, Jr. Natural history of colloid cysts of the third ventricle. J Neurosurg. 2016; 125(6):1420–1430

[17] Kondziolka D, Lunsford LD. Stereotactic management of colloid cysts: factors predicting success. J Neurosurg. 1991; 75(1):45–51

[18] Binning MJ, Gottfried ON, Osborn AG, Couldwell WT. Rathke cleft cyst intracystic nodule: a characteristic magnetic resonance imaging finding. J Neurosurg. 2005; 103(5):837–840

[19] Byun WM, Kim OL, Kim D. MR imaging findings of Rathke's cleft cysts: significance of intracystic nodules. AJNR Am J Neuroradiol. 2000; 21(3):485–488

[20] Müller A, Büttner A, Weis S. Rare occurrence of intracerebellar colloid cyst. Case report. J Neurosurg. 1999; 91(1):128–131

[21] Tanei T, Fukui K, Kato T, Wakabayashi K, Inoue N, Watanabe M. Colloid (enterogenous) cyst in the frontal lobe. Neurol Med Chir (Tokyo). 2006; 46(8):401–404

[22] Morris TC, Santoreneos S. Colloid cyst of velum interpositum: a rare finding. J Neurosurg Pediatr. 2012; 9(2):206–208

[23] Armao D, Castillo M, Chen H, Kwock L. Colloid cyst of the third ventricle: imaging-pathologic correlation. AJNR Am J Neuroradiol. 2000; 21(8):1470–1477

[24] Lach B, Scheithauer BW, Gregor A, Wick MR. Colloid cyst of the third ventricle. A comparative immunohistochemical study of neuraxis cysts and choroid plexus epithelium. J Neurosurg. 1993; 78(1):101–111

[25] Ho KL, Garcia JH. Colloid cysts of the third ventricle: ultrastructural features are compatible with endodermal derivation. Acta Neuropathol. 1992; 83(6):605–612

[26] Gupta JK, Cave M, Lilford RJ, et al. Clinical significance of fetal choroid plexus cysts. Lancet. 1995; 346(8977):724–729

[27] Macaulay RJ, Felix I, Jay V, Becker LE. Histological and ultrastructural analysis of six colloid cysts in children. Acta Neuropathol. 1997; 93(3):271–276

[28] Büttner A, Winkler PA, Eisenmenger W, Weis S. Colloid cysts of the third ventricle with fatal outcome: a report of two cases and review of the literature. Int J Legal Med. 1997; 110(5):260–266

[29] de Witt Hamer PC, Verstegen MJ, De Haan RJ, et al. High risk of acute deterioration in patients harboring symptomatic colloid cysts of the third ventricle. J Neurosurg. 2002; 96(6):1041–1045

[30] Pollock BE, Huston J, III. Natural history of asymptomatic colloid cysts of the third ventricle. J Neurosurg. 1999; 91(3):364–369

[31] Desai KI, Nadkarni TD, Muzumdar DP, Goel AH. Surgical management of colloid cyst of the third ventricle: a study of 105 cases. Surg Neurol. 2002; 57(5):295–302, discussion 302–304

[32] Ryder JW, Kleinschmidt-DeMasters BK, Keller TS. Sudden deterioration and death in patients with benign tumors of the third ventricle area. J Neurosurg. 1986; 64(2):216–223

[33] Little JR, MacCarty CS. Colloid cysts of the third ventricle. J Neurosurg. 1974; 40(2):230–235

[34] Pollock BE, Schreiner SA, Huston J, III. A theory on the natural history of colloid cysts of the third ventricle. Neurosurgery. 2000; 46(5):1077–1081, discussion 1081–1083

[35] Godano U, Ferrai R, Meleddu V, Bellinzona M. Hemorrhagic colloid cyst with sudden coma. Minim Invasive Neurosurg. 2010; 53(5–6):273–274

[36] Mathiesen T, Grane P, Lindquist C, von Holst H. High recurrence rate following aspiration of colloid cysts in the third ventricle. J Neurosurg. 1993; 78(5):748–752

[37] Rajshekhar V. Rate of recurrence following stereotactic aspiration of colloid cysts of the third ventricle. Stereotact Funct Neurosurg. 2012; 90(1):37–44

[38] Sheikh AB, Mendelson ZS, Liu JK. Endoscopic versus microsurgical resection of colloid cysts: a systematic review and meta-analysis of 1,278 patients. World Neurosurg. 2014; 82(6):1187–1197

[39] Horn EM, Feiz-Erfan I, Bristol RE, et al. Treatment options for third ventricular colloid cysts: comparison of open microsurgical versus endoscopic resection. Neurosurgery. 2008; 62(6) Suppl 3:1076–1083

17 Arachnoid Cysts

Phillip A. Choi, Susana Calle, Pejman Rabiei, Shekhar D. Khanpara, Roy F. Riascos, and Dong H. Kim

17.1 Case Presentation

17.1.1 History and Physical Examination

A 35-year-old woman presents with a history of recent-onset headaches.

Neurological examination was normal.

17.2 Imaging Analysis

17.2.1 Imaging Findings and Impression

MRI with and without contrast shows an oblong extra-axial lesion in the left anterotemporal fossa (*asterisks*). The lesion follows cerebrospinal fluid (CSF) signal intensity (hyperintense on T2, hypointense on T1 with suppression of the content on fluid-attenuated inversion recovery [FLAIR]) on all spin-echo sequences (▶ Fig. 17.1a–c). On postcontrast images (▶ Fig. 17.1d,e), the lesion does not demonstrate any enhancement. Findings are consistent with middle cranial fossa arachnoid cyst.

17.2.2 Imaging Guidelines

MRI with and without contrast is the diagnostic examination of choice. Contrast should be administered for initial diagnostic evaluation in the cases in which diagnosis is unclear (atypical findings, edema of the underlying brain, patient symptoms are concerning for infection) to exclude nodular peripheral enhancement.

CT is better for evaluating adjacent bony changes like thinning of overlying skull but not necessary.

Not recommended: CT with contrast (unless MRI with contrast contraindicated).

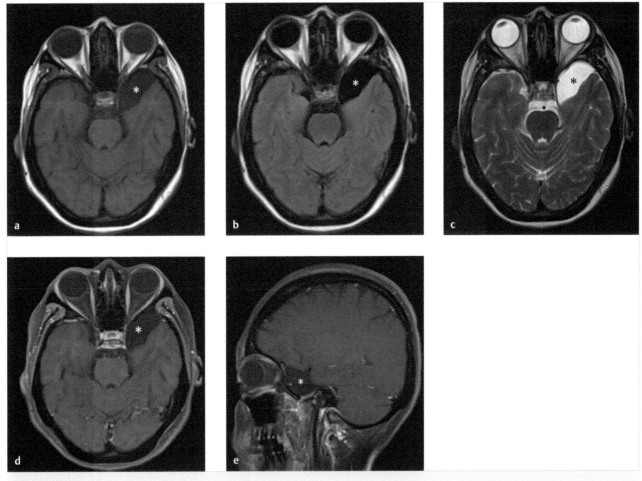

Fig. 17.1 (a–e)

17.3 Clinical Evaluation and Management

This is a young, healthy woman with a small, incidentally found Galassi type I arachnoid cyst. No surgical intervention is needed at this time because the cyst is small without any mass effect and the patient's symptoms cannot be clearly attributed to the cyst. Small arachnoid cysts (< 5 cm) such as this are low risk for rupture or hemorrhage.[1] We would plan to reimage the cyst in 3 months to check for any change in cyst size or morphology. If stable, we would obtain one more MRI in 1 year and then follow the patient clinically and only obtain additional imaging if new symptoms arose.

17.4 Differential Diagnosis

- **Arachnoid cyst:**
  - Well-circumscribed, extra-axial mass that follows CSF signal intensity on MRI and is isodense to CSF on CT with no enhancement identified.[2]
- Epidermoid cyst:
  - It is a congenital lesion occurring due to inclusion of ectodermal elements during neural tube closure.
  - On imaging, it appears as a lobulated extra-axial lesion with a tendency to insinuate between structures rather than cause mass effect in earlier stages.
  - On CT, it may be indistinguishable from an arachnoid cyst as epidermoid cysts exhibit CSF density similar to an arachnoid cyst. Some epidermoid cysts (10–25%) demonstrate internal calcification.
  - On MRI, epidermoid cysts follow CSF signal intensity on T1-weghted image (T1WI) and T2-weghted image (T2WI); however, there is incomplete suppression of the signal on FLAIR, giving a "dirty" CSF appearance.[3]
  - On diffusion-weighted imaging (DWI), it demonstrates bright signal with corresponding dark signal on apparent diffusion coefficient (ADC), due to presence of thick waxy epithelial keratin within the cyst.
  - It may show minimal enhancement around the periphery of the lesion.
- Porencephalic cyst:
  - It occurs after traumatic/ischemic insult to the brain parenchyma.
  - It follows CSF signal intensity on all sequences. However, it is surrounded by gliotic brain.
- Choroid fissure cyst:
  - It has a typical location and is believed to arise from the choroid epithelium.
  - It can be indistinguishable from an arachnoid cyst.
- Racemose neurocysticercosis:
  - It is rare in the western world.
  - There is absence of scolex in racemose neurocysticercosis as opposed to intraparenchymal lesions.
  - They are larger than intraparenchymal lesions since these occur within CSF spaces and their growth is not restricted by relatively noncompliant brain.
  - They may conglomerate to appear as a bunch of grapes.

- Cysts associated with neoplasms:
  - Various tumors like pleomorphic xanthoastrocytoma, ganglioglioma, and dysembryoplastic neuroepithelial tumor (DNET) can present as mixed solid and cystic mass lesions and can mimic an arachnoid cyst when the solid component is negligible.
  - However, these tumors are usually cortical in origin and demonstrate signs of being an intra-axial mass lesion (absence of CSF cleft, absence of buckling of underlying cortex, presence of edema in the surrounding area, etc.).
  - Moreover, these lesions will demonstrate enhancement of the solid component after gadolinium administration.

17.5 Diagnostic Pearls

- CT: Extremely well circumscribed, with an ill-defined wall, and displace adjacent structures. When large, and over time, they can exert a remodeling effect on the bone.
- MRI: Follow CSF signal intensity on all sequences and no enhancement can be identified.[2]
- Magnetic resonance cisternography: high-resolution T2 W sequences help delineate the cyst wall and adjacent anatomic structures.[4]
- Lack of restriction of diffusion on DWI is most important to help distinguish arachnoid cysts of the cerebellar pontine angle from epidermoids.

17.6 Essential information about arachnoid cysts

17.6.1 Etiology

- It is known to arise from within the leaves of arachnoid membrane.
- Arachnoid cysts can occur anywhere within the central nervous system, most frequently (50–60%) located in the middle cranial fossa, where they may invaginate into and widen the sylvian fissure.
- Other locations include the suprasellar cistern, ventricles, posterior fossa, cisterna magna, cerebellopontine angle, and spinal canal.
- They are most frequently solitary.
- Posttrauma, arachnoid cyst can grow in size from increased intracystic fluid accumulation secondary to ball valve mechanism or secretory activity of arachnoid cells.

17.6.2 Galassi Classification

Galassi et al,[5] in 1982, described three types of middle cranial fossa arachnoid cysts based on the size, shape, mass effect on the surrounding brain parenchyma and communication with subarachnoid space on cisternography. It still remains the most widely used classification system in practice.

The three types of arachnoid cysts are as follows:

- **Type I:** These are spindle shaped and smaller in size as compared to the other two types. They are located in anterior most part of temporal fossa and impose minimal to mild mass effect and displacement of the adjacent temporal lobe. On cisternography, they show free communication with the subarachnoid space (▶ Fig. 17.2).
- **Type II:** These are triangular or quadrangular in shape. They occupy the anterior and middle part of the temporal fossa with marked mass effect on the temporal lobe. Slow communication with subarachnoid space can be demonstrated on cisternography (▶ Fig. 17.3).
- **Type III:** These are the most severe form of arachnoid cyst. They are round or oval in shape. They occupy almost the entire temporal fossa with extensive displacement of the temporal lobe and even frontal and parietal lobes to some extent. Little communication with subarachnoid space is seen on cisternography (▶ Fig. 17.4).

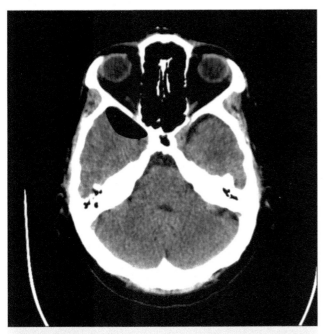

Fig. 17.2 Type I.

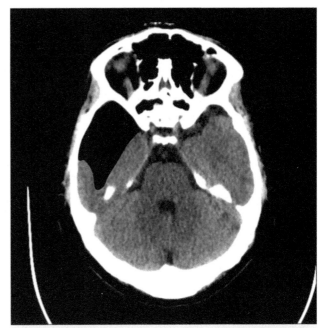

Fig. 17.3 Type II.

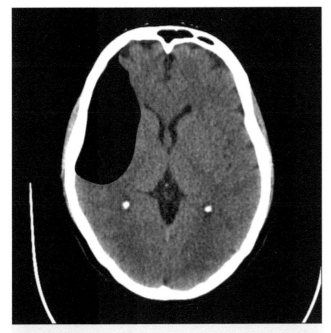

Fig. 17.4 Type III.

17.7 Companion Case

17.7.1 History

A 12-year-old boy presented to the ED after a head trauma while playing football.

17.7.2 Imaging Findings and Impression

Axial and coronal CT scan of the head shows a large hypodense extra-axial lesion of approximate size 6 × 8 cm within the right middle cranial fossa with scalloping of the underlying bone (*asterisks* in ▶ Fig. 17.5).

Diagnosis: arachnoid cyst.

17.7.3 Neurosurgical Consultation

This is a young boy with a normal neurological examination who has an incidentally discovered Galassi type III arachnoid cyst. This cyst exerts significant mass effect on the brain with compression of the lateral ventricle, midline shift, and erosion of the skull. Although the cyst is asymptomatic at this time and unlikely to grow given the patient's age, the cyst is at risk of rupture or hemorrhage. There is also a risk of developing hydrocephalus from compression of normal CSF pathways. We would recommend endoscopic or open craniotomy as initial treatment of the cyst depending on the individual surgeon's comfort level with both procedures. If either of these approaches fails, then a cystoperitoneal shunt can be placed.

17.8 Neurosurgery Questions and Answers

1. **What are the etiology and natural history of arachnoid cyst that may assist in clinical decision-making?**

   Arachnoid cysts can form from a congenital malformation of the arachnoid or due to trauma.[6] Congenital arachnoid cysts form due to splitting of the arachnoid membrane and trapping of fluid between an outer and inner leaflet of the arachnoid.[7,8] Multiple hypotheses have been proposed regarding the formation and growth of arachnoid cysts: (1) ball-valve mechanism with one-way CSF flow between the cyst and the subarachnoid space; (2) formation of an osmotic gradient between the fluids inside and outside the cyst wall; (3) congenital malformation of the arachnoid; and (4) hypersecretion by cells lining the cyst wall. Arachnoid cysts account for 1% or less of all intracranial masses.[6,9] The majority of arachnoid cysts are found in the middle cranial fossa, but they can also be found in other locations arachnoid is present such as the posterior fossa, the suprasellar cistern, the prepontine cistern, or the spine.[6,9] There is a 2:1 male-to-female predominance of arachnoid cysts.[6,10,11,12] Arachnoid cysts are often detected in the first two decades of life.[6,10,12]

   The majority of arachnoid cysts (78%) remain stable over time, while a smaller percentage either increases (10%) or decreases (12%) in size.[10] Younger age of presentation correlates with cyst growth. Patients older than 4 years of age are unlikely to have cyst enlargement, development of new symptoms, or to required surgical intervention.[10] Although rare, arachnoid cysts can rupture or hemorrhage and cause subdural hygromas, subdural hematomas, or intracranial hypertension.[6] Recent cranial trauma and larger cyst size (maximal diameter greater than 5 cm) have been associated with a higher risk of cyst rupture or hemorrhage.[1]

2. **In patients in whom an arachnoid cyst has been detected, what specific findings on physical examination and/or elements of the history are important in your determination that this problematic incidental finding is truly asymptomatic?**

   Signs or symptoms of a symptomatic arachnoid cyst are dependent on the location of the lesion. Headache is a common, but nonspecific, symptom that can be caused by arachnoid cysts in any location. Middle fossa cysts can cause contralateral weakness, seizures, proptosis, developmental delay, and asymmetric development of the skull.[11,12,13,14,15,16] Arachnoid cysts of the sella can cause hydrocephalus, visual dysfunction, and endocrine dysfunction.[12,17,18] Posterior fossa arachnoid cysts can present as hydrocephalus with

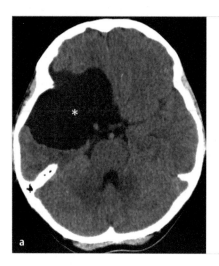
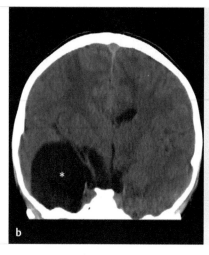

Fig. 17.5 Companion case. **(a)** Axial and **(b)** coronal CT scan of the head.

macrocrania, nystagmus, and upper cervical cord dysfunction with gait instability and myelopathy.[12,19,20]

3. **What additional testing is needed and are there any management guidelines?**

No additional diagnostic testing is needed after brain MRI with and without gadolinium for asymptomatic lesions with the typical appearance of an arachnoid cyst.

There are no published guidelines by the American Association of Neurological Surgeons (AANS)/Congress of Neurological Surgeons (CNS).

4. **If electing to follow, what is the suggested time interval and modality?**

Initial follow-up imaging in 3 months with an MRI of the brain is recommended to assess for rapid growth. If initial follow-up imaging is stable, then one more follow-up MRI can be obtained at 1 year.

5. **What are the surgical options and risks?**

Surgical options for arachnoid cysts include stereotactic endoscopic fenestration, endoscopic fenestration, craniotomy for marsupialization of the cyst, and cystoperitoneal shunt placement. Treatment of a symptomatic arachnoid cyst can relieve focal neurological deficits. However, headaches and seizures often persist despite treatment.[21] Dysfunctional development of adjacent temporal lobe may contribute to continued seizures.

Ali et al analyzed a series of 27 pediatric patients with surgical management of arachnoid cysts and found that there was no difference in symptom resolution, need for additional surgery, change in cyst size, or morbidity/mortality between endoscopic fenestration, cystoperitoneal shunting, and craniotomy.[11] Approximately two-thirds of patients had decrease in cyst size and two-thirds of patients had symptom resolution within 6 months. Complications were rare, but included CSF leak (19%), infection (11%), and hemorrhage (4%). Couvreur et al described endoscopic treatment of arachnoid cysts in 34 patients. They noted that 91% of patients had decreased cyst size and clinical improvement in 76% of cases.[13] Patients with intracranial hypertension and acute neurological deficits had the most benefit, while those with congenital syndromes and developmental delay had the least benefit. The complication rate was 29%, but only 2 patients required subsequent shunting. Craniotomy for marsupialization of the cyst can provide durable results, but introduces greater surgical risk than other options. Cystoperitoneal shunting provides consistent decrease in the cyst size but introduces the risk of hardware infection or failure and the possibility of overdrainage. No clear consensus exists in the literature regarding the optimal surgical management of arachnoid cysts.[16]

6. **What instructions are given to patients regarding return to neurosurgeon in the patient being managed nonoperatively with imaging surveillance?**

Patients are instructed to watch for signs of increased intracranial pressure such as persistent headaches, nausea, and vomiting. Any new neurological symptoms such as weakness, seizures, or visual changes warrant reimaging and evaluation by a neurosurgeon. Development of new symptoms after a traumatic brain injury is particularly concerning and warrants immediate evaluation in an emergency room.

References

[1] Cress M, Kestle JRW, Holubkov R, Riva-Cambrin J. Risk factors for pediatric arachnoid cyst rupture/hemorrhage: a case-control study. Neurosurgery. 2013; 72(5):716–722, discussion 722

[2] Osborn AG, Preece MT. Intracranial cysts: radiologic-pathologic correlation and imaging approach. Radiology. 2006; 239(3):650–664

[3] Horowitz BL, Chari MV, James R. MR of intracranial epidermoid tumors: correlation of in vivo imaging with in vitro 13c spectroscopy. AJNR Am J Neuroradiol. 1990; 11(2):299–302

[4] Yildiz H, Erdogan C, Yalcin R, et al. evaluation of communication between intracranial arachnoid cysts and cisterns with phase-contrast cine MR imaging. AJNR Am J Neuroradiol. 2005; 26(1):145–151

[5] Galassi E, Tognetti F, Gaist G, Fagioli L, Frank F, Frank G. CT scan and metrizamide CT cisternography in arachnoid cysts of the middle cranial fossa: classification and pathophysiological aspects. Surg Neurol. 1982; 17(5):363–369

[6] Pradilla G, Jallo G. Arachnoid cysts: case series and review of the literature. Neurosurg Focus. 2007; 22(2):E7

[7] Miyagami M, Tsubokawa T. Histological and ultrastructural findings of benign intracranial cysts. Noshuyo Byori. 1993; 10(2):151–160

[8] Rengachary SS, Watanabe I. Ultrastructure and pathogenesis of intracranial arachnoid cysts. J Neuropathol Exp Neurol. 1981; 40(1):61–83

[9] Basaldella L, Orvieto E, Dei Tos AP, Della Barbera M, Valente M, Longatti P. Causes of arachnoid cyst development and expansion. Neurosurg Focus. 2007; 22(2):E4

[10] Al-Holou WN, Yew AY, Boomsaad ZE, Garton HJL, Muraszko KM, Maher CO. Prevalence and natural history of arachnoid cysts in children. J Neurosurg Pediatr. 2010; 5(6):578–585

[11] Ali M, Bennardo M, Almenawer SA, et al. Exploring predictors of surgery and comparing operative treatment approaches for pediatric intracranial arachnoid cysts: a case series of 83 patients. J Neurosurg Pediatr. 2015; 16(3): 275–282

[12] Gosalakkal JA. Intracranial arachnoid cysts in children: a review of pathogenesis, clinical features, and management. Pediatr Neurol. 2002; 26(2): 93–98

[13] Couvreur T, Hallaert G, Van Der Heggen T, et al. Endoscopic treatment of temporal arachnoid cysts in 34 patients. World Neurosurg. 2015; 84(3):734–740

[14] Krupp W, Döhnert J, Kellermann S, Seifert V. Intradiploic arachnoid cyst with extensive deformation of craniofacial osseous structures: case report. Neurosurgery. 1999; 44(4):868–870

[15] Koch CA, Moore JL, Voth D. Arachnoid cysts: how do postsurgical cyst size and seizure outcome correlate? Neurosurg Rev. 1998; 21(1):14–22

[16] Tamburrini G, Dal Fabbro M, Di Rocco C. Sylvian fissure arachnoid cysts: a survey on their diagnostic workout and practical management. Childs Nerv Syst. 2008; 24(5):593–604

[17] Adan L, Bussières L, Dinand V, Zerah M, Pierre-Kahn A, Brauner R. Growth, puberty and hypothalamic-pituitary function in children with suprasellar arachnoid cyst. Eur J Pediatr. 2000; 159(5):348–355

[18] Mohn A, Schoof E, Fahlbusch R, Wenzel D, Dörr HG. The endocrine spectrum of arachnoid cysts in childhood. Pediatr Neurosurg. 1999; 31(6):316–321

[19] Erdinçler P, Kaynar MY, Bozkus H, Ciplak N. Posterior fossa arachnoid cysts. Br J Neurosurg. 1999; 13(1):10–17

[20] Shukla R, Sharma A, Vatsal DK. Posterior fossa arachnoid cyst presenting as high cervical cord compression. Br J Neurosurg. 1998; 12(3):271–273

[21] Levy ML, Wang M, Aryan HE, Yoo K, Meltzer H. Microsurgical keyhole approach for middle fossa arachnoid cyst fenestration. Neurosurgery. 2003; 53(5):1138–1144, discussion 1144–1145

18 Mega Cisterna Magna

Cole T. Lewis, Octavio Arevalo, Rajan P. Patel, and David I. Sandberg

18.1 Case Presentation

18.1.1 History

A 15-year-old female patient presents with a history of a one-time seizure episode.

18.2 Imaging Analysis

18.2.1 Imaging Findings and Impression

Brain MR images sagittal T1 (▶ Fig. 18.1a), axial T1 (▶ Fig. 18.1b), axial T2 (▶ Fig. 18.1c), and axial T2 fluid-attenuated inversion recovery (FLAIR; (▶ Fig. 18.1d) images are displayed. There is widening of the subarachnoid spaces posterior and inferior to the vermis (*asterisk*), without any mass effect or displacement of the falx cerebelli (*black arrow*). The cerebellar vermis and fourth ventricle are normal. Findings are consistent with a mega cisterna magna (MCM).

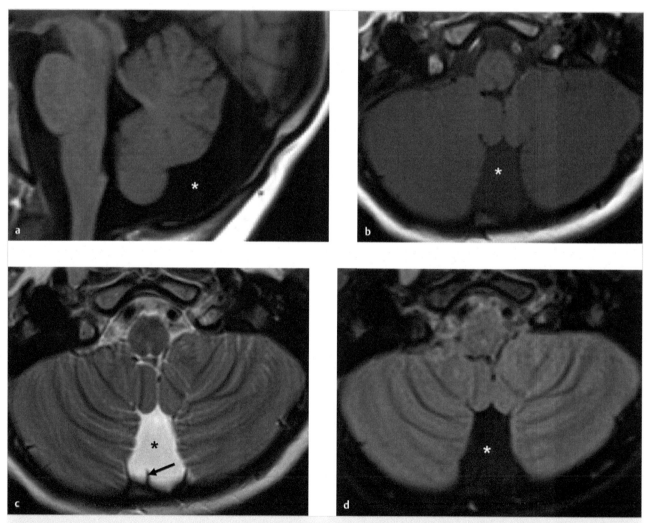

Fig. 18.1 (a–d)

18.3 Differential Diagnosis

- **MCM:**
  - It is a normal variant and corresponds to a focal enlargement of subarachnoid space in the posterior and inferior midline posterior fossa.
- Posterior fossa arachnoid cyst:
  - It is an extra-axial collection of cerebrospinal fluid (CSF) delineated by arachnoid that does not directly communicate with the ventricular system or the subarachnoid space.
  - Retrocerebellar arachnoid cyst pushes the vermis forward, whereas an MCM pushes the vermis up from foramen magnum.[1,2,3]
  - Midline arachnoid cyst demonstrates mass effect and deviation of the falx cerebelli.
- Dandy–Walker malformation and variants:
  - Cystic dilatation of the fourth ventricle, enlarged posterior fossa, small hypoplastic vermis superiorly rotated, and elevated torcula are some symptoms.
  - In MCM, there is no malformation of vermis, cerebellum, or other posterior fossa components.[3,4,5]
- Blake's pouch cyst:
  - Persistent Blake's pouch cysts occur due to a failed perforation of the foramen of Magendie.
  - Findings include an infravermian cyst that communicates with the fourth ventricle without communication with the cisterna magna posteriorly.
  - It is often associated with mild upward displacement and rotation of vermis but normally formed vermis, normally positioned torcula.
  - Choroid plexus can extend from the fourth ventricle into the superior portion of the cyst.

18.4 Diagnostic Pearls

- Inside the MCM, tiny veins and falx cerebelli are seen. There should not be any deviation of falx cerebelli.
- There should be normal-appearing cerebellar vermis and fourth ventricle.[1,4,6]

18.5 Essential Information about Mega Cisterna Magna

- **Etiology:**
  - Delayed Blake's pouch fenestration.
- **Follow-up:**
  - No follow up is needed.

18.6 Companion Case

Dandy–Walker malformation. Sagittal T1-weighted (▶ Fig. 18.2a) and axial T2-weighted (▶ Fig. 18.2b) images of brain MRI of a 12-month-old infant showing a midline cystic lesion in the posterior cranial fossa (*asterisk*), which is in continuity with the fourth ventricle (4). The cystic lesion causes enlargement of the posterior cranial fossa evidenced by elevation of torcula (*arrow* in ▶ Fig. 18.2a). Hypoplastic and cephalad rotated vermis (V) is a cornerstone in the diagnosis of this congenital malformation.

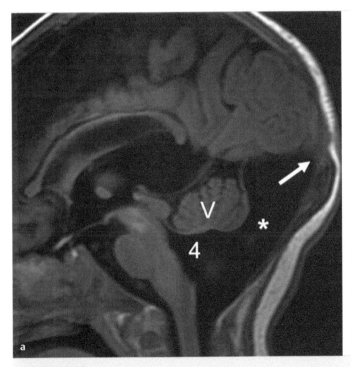
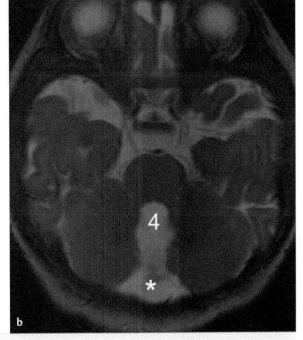

Fig. 18.2 (a, b)

18.7 Neurosurgery Questions and Answers

1. **Given the presentation and imaging findings, what specific findings on physical examination and/or elements of the history are important in your determination of the diagnosis and, more importantly, in the determination as to if this probable incidental finding is truly asymptomatic?**

   MCM is an incidental finding and is typically asymptomatic.[7] The presence of MCM can be found during evaluation of trauma, stroke, or headaches. MCM consists of an enlarged cisterna magna without evidence of hydrocephalus or other posterior fossa abnormalities.[7] Patients are typically asymptomatic and do not exhibit physical examination findings.

2. **What additional testing, if any, is required or recommended in the workup?**

   No additional workup is required.

3. **If electing to follow, what is the suggested time interval and modality?**

   No follow-up is required.

4. **If electing surgical (or medical) management, then why and what are the surgical options and risks?**

   No surgical intervention is indicated.

5. **If following, what restrictions are placed on the patient?**

   There are no restrictions.

References

[1] Jones BV. Arachnoid cyst. In: Barkovich J, ed. Diagnostic Imaging Pediatric Neuroradiology. Salt Lake City, UY: Amirsys; 2007:I-6–2

[2] Bosemani T, Orman G, Boltshauser E, Tekes A, Huisman TAGM, Poretti A. Congenital abnormalities of the posterior fossa. Radiographics. 2015; 35(1): 200–220

[3] Kollias SS, Ball WS, Jr, Prenger EC. Cystic malformations of the posterior fossa: differential diagnosis clarified through embryologic analysis. Radiographics. 1993; 13(6):1211–1231

[4] Blaser SI. Dandy Walker spectrum. In: Barkovich J, ed. Diagnostic Imaging Pediatric Neuroradiology. Salt Lake City, UT: Amirsys; 2007:I-4–22

[5] Estroff JA, Scott MR, Benacerraf BR. Dandy-Walker variant: prenatal sonographic features and clinical outcome. Radiology. 1992; 185(3):755–758

[6] Zimmer EZ, Lowenstein L, Bronshtein M, Goldsher D, Aharon-Peretz J. Clinical significance of isolated mega cisterna magna. Arch Gynecol Obstet. 2007; 276 (5):487–490

[7] Shekdar K. Posterior fossa malformations. Semin Ultrasound CT MR. 2011; 32(3):228–2–41

19 Benign Enlargement of Subarachnoid Spaces

Cole T. Lewis, Octavio Arevalo, Rajan P. Patel, and David I. Sandberg

19.1 Case Presentation

19.1.1 History

A 14-month-old female patient presents with a history of macrocephaly and emesis.

19.2 Imaging Analysis

19.2.1 Imaging Findings and Impression

Brain MRI axial T2-weighted (T2w; ▶ Fig. 19.1a,b), axial T2*GRE (gradient recalled echo; ▶ Fig. 19.1c,d), and coronal T1-weighted (T1w) with gadolinium (▶ Fig. 19.1e) images show prominence of the subarachnoid spaces overlying the anterior cerebral convexities (*asterisks*) consistent with benign enlargement of subarachnoid spaces (BESS) of infancy, which is a normal variant. Note the presence of small bridging veins crossing the subarachnoid spaces (*white arrow* in ▶ Fig. 19.1e). Lack of susceptibility signal from blood degradation products on T2*GRE images (▶ Fig. 19.1c,d) further supports diagnosis of BESS.

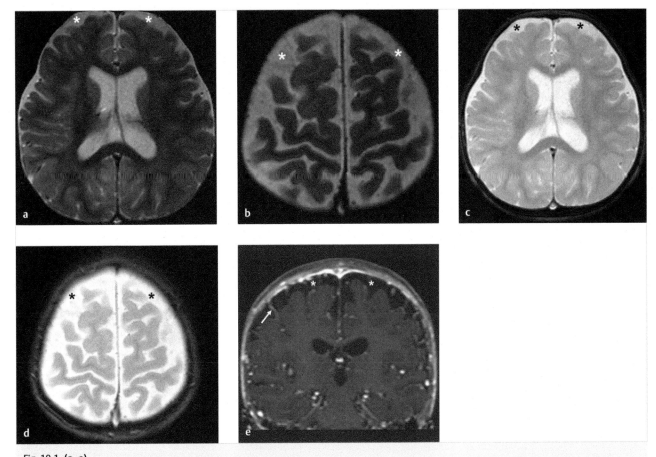

Fig. 19.1 (a–e)

19.3 Differential Diagnosis

- **BESS:**
  - Normal transient enlargement of the subarachnoid spaces associated with macrocephaly.
- Chronic subdural hematoma:
  - It should be suspected if the collection thickness is wider than 6 mm, shows higher T2 fluid-attenuated inversion recovery (FLAIR) signal as compared to cerebrospinal fluid (CSF), and displays hemorrhagic staining on T2*GRE.[1]
  - The collection is usually asymmetric, displaces the bridging veins toward the brain surface, and has mass effect.
- Cerebral volume loss/brain atrophy:
  - When present, it is usually accompanied by small head circumference, and "pointed" forehead due to early metopic suture fusion.
  - Benign enlargement of subarachnoid spaces causes an increase of the head circumference and a flat forehead due to frontal bossing.
- Acquired communicating hydrocephalus:
  - It usually is caused by a hemorrhagic, inflammatory, or neoplastic process.
  - Some congenital causes include achondroplasia due to narrow foramen magnum and jugular foramina.
  - Density or signal intensity of extra-axial collection does not follow the CSF.

19.4 Diagnostic Pearls

- Widening of the vertical distance between calvarium and brain frontal parenchyma ≥ 5 mm.
- It is usually accompanied by enlarged cisterns (suprasellar and suprachiasmatic) and mildly enlarged ventricles (66%).
- Normal veins are traversing subarachnoid space, the fluid in subarachnoid space follow the CSF signal on all sequences, and there is no abnormal meningeal enhancement.[2,3,4,5,6]

19.5 Essential information about Benign Enlargement of Subarachnoid Spaces

- **Etiology:**
  - Immature CSF drainage pathways.
- **Imaging Pitfalls:**
  - Gibbs' truncation artifact: parallel lines that appear when the interface between high and low signal intensities occurs in the same plane, that is, brain cortex–CSF interface.
- **Follow-up:**
  - Head circumference measurement is the best follow-up. No follow-up imaging is needed if head circumference remains in normal range.

19.6 Companion Case

19.6.1 Benign Enlargement of Subarachnoid Spaces versus Chronic Subdural Hematomas

▶ Fig. 19.2 shows axial CT brain images from different patients. On the left image, there is widening of the subarachnoid space of the frontal convexity compatible with BESS; note that the width of the sulci is proportional to the enlargement of the frontal subarachnoid space, and there are little dots in the subarachnoid space corresponding to bridging veins (*arrows*) suggestive of "the cortical vein sign."[7] On the other hand, the right image shows bilateral chronic subdural hematomas. The mass effect of hematomas is depicted by the mismatch between the distance from the brain surface to the diploe and the width of the sulci. No bridging veins are seen within the hematoma. (The *white arrow* in ▶ Fig. 19.2b shows displacement of bridging vein toward the brain surface and the *arrowheads* point out the effacement of sulci.)

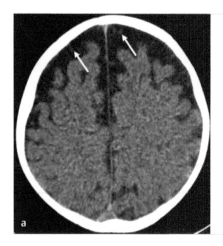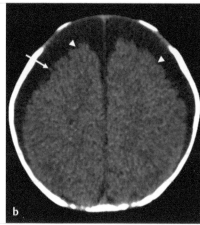

Fig. 19.2 (a, b) Companion case.

19.7 Neurosurgery Questions and Answers

1. **Given the presentation and imaging findings, what specific findings on physical examination and/or elements of the history are important in your determination of the diagnosis and, more importantly, in the determination as to if this probable incidental finding is truly asymptomatic?**

   BESS is a common cause of macrocephaly. Patients will typically have head circumferences that cross percentile lines, often above the 95th percentile. They are otherwise neurologically normal. The fontanelle is typically open and soft.[8,9]

2. **What are the etiology and natural history of the condition that would assist in decision-making?**

   BESS has an unclear etiology, but it is thought to be due to immature arachnoid granulations reducing CSF absorption.[5,10]

3. **If electing to follow, what is the suggested time interval and modality?**

   The patient should be followed by his pediatrician at their regularly scheduled appointments with continued trending of the fronto-occipital circumference (FOC).

4. **Does the patient need to return to neurosurgeon/ENT, neurology, etc., or, if normal variant, benign finding, etc., can follow-up be with the primary care doctor?**

   No. FOC typically stabilizes and the enlargement of the subarachnoid space often resolves.[5] Patients with BESS are at a higher risk of developing spontaneous subdural hemorrhage than other children, even with minor trauma.[11] In these instances, the patient should return for evaluation by a neurosurgeon.

There is no surgical or medical management required for these patients.

5. **If following, what restrictions are placed on the patient?**
   There are no restrictions.

References

[1] McNeely PD, Atkinson JD, Saigal G, O'Gorman AM, Farmer J-P. Subdural hematomas in infants with benign enlargement of the subarachnoid spaces are not pathognomonic for child abuse. AJNR Am J Neuroradiol. 2006; 27(8): 1725–1728

[2] Blaser SI. Enlarged subarachnoid spaces. In: Barkovich J, ed. Diagnostic Imaging Pediatric Neuroradiology. Salt Lake City, UT: Amirsys; 2007:I-5-I-30

[3] Zahl SM, Egge A, Helseth E, Wester K. Benign external hydrocephalus: a review, with emphasis on management. Neurosurg Rev. 2011; 34(4): 417–432

[4] Hamza M, Bodensteiner JB, Noorani PA, Barnes PD. Benign extracerebral fluid collections: a cause of macrocrania in infancy. Pediatr Neurol. 1987; 3(4): 218–221

[5] Suara RO, Trouth AJ, Collins M. Benign subarachnoid space enlargement of infancy. J Natl Med Assoc. 2001; 93(2):70–73

[6] Tucker J, Choudhary AK, Piatt J. Macrocephaly in infancy: benign enlargement of the subarachnoid spaces and subdural collections. J Neurosurg Pediatr. 2016; 18(1):16–20

[7] McCluney KW, Yeakley JW, Fenstermacher MJ, Baird SH, Bonmati CM. Subdural hygroma versus atrophy on MR brain scans: "the cortical vein sign.". AJNR Am J Neuroradiol. 1992; 13(5):1335–1339

[8] Ment LR, Duncan CC, Geehr R. Benign enlargement of the subarachnoid spaces in the infant. J Neurosurg. 1981; 54(4):504–508

[9] Tucker J, Choudhary AK, Piatt J. Macrocephaly in infancy: benign enlargement of the subarachnoid spaces and subdural collections. J Neurosurg Pediatr. 2016; 18(1):16–20

[10] Halevy A, Cohen R, Viner I, Diamond G, Shuper A. Development of infants with idiopathic external hydrocephalus. J Child Neurol. 2015; 30(8): 1044–1047

[11] Ravid S, Maytal J. External hydrocephalus: a probable cause for subdural hematoma in infancy. Pediatr Neurol. 2003; 28(2):139–141

20 Pituitary Incidentaloma and Incidental Silent Macroadenoma

Wesley H. Jones, Katie B. Guttenberg, Kaye D. Westmark, and Spiros L. Blackburn

20.1 Pituitary Incidentaloma

20.1.1 Introduction

A pituitary incidentaloma (PI) refers to a small, potential mass within the gland detected by an imaging study that was performed for reasons, a priori, unrelated to pituitary dysfunction or suspected dysfunction. Constant improvement in the sensitivity of MR has outpaced specificity, which may result in a diagnostic dilemma for the primary care physician.

In this chapter, we will first present a classic case of a PI that illustrates the diagnostic imaging and clinical evaluation. Important guidelines as to which tests are needed and appropriate imaging follow-up intervals will be given as well as imaging protocols for optimal evaluation of the sella.

An interesting companion case is shown to demonstrate a common incidental cystic lesion of the pituitary gland, Rathke's cleft cyst.

A final companion case is shown to demonstrate that endocrine dysfunction is not always readily apparent and some conditions, such as acromegaly, may present insidiously and, in most cases, require surgical management. Therefore, when an incidental pituitary lesion is discovered, a detailed history and physical examination is paramount as is clinical laboratory testing.

20.1.2 Case Presentation

History

A 36-year-old woman presents with a history of left retro-orbital pain, nausea, and vomiting. Routine MRI revealed a prominent pituitary gland with a superiorly convex margin. Therefore, a dedicated pituitary MR was performed. The images are shown in ▶ Fig. 20.1.

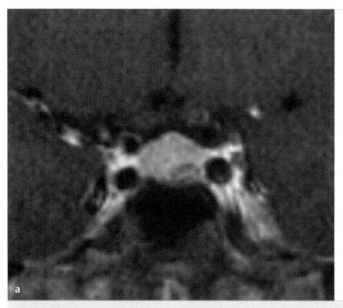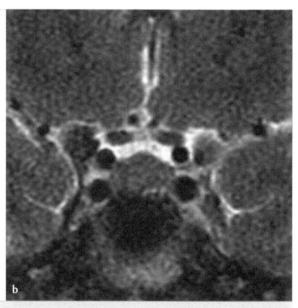

Fig. 20.1 MRI coronal contrast-enhanced **(a)** T1-weighted imaging and **(b)** fast spin echo T2-weighted imaging.

20.1.3 Imaging Analysis

Imaging Findings

There is a small area of heterogeneous signal intensity in the left side of the pituitary gland (see *arrows* ▶ Fig. 20.2a-c) measuring 4.6 × 3.76 × 4.84 mm, which was not well seen on the precontrast T1-weighted (T1W) images (not shown) but is well defined postcontrast as it enhances to a lesser degree than the remainder of the gland (▶ Fig. 20.2a). The gland is slightly prominent with a superiorly convex margin, measuring 9 mm in maximum height. The cavernous sinuses are symmetric, the gland does not contact the optic chiasm, and the pituitary stalk is midline.

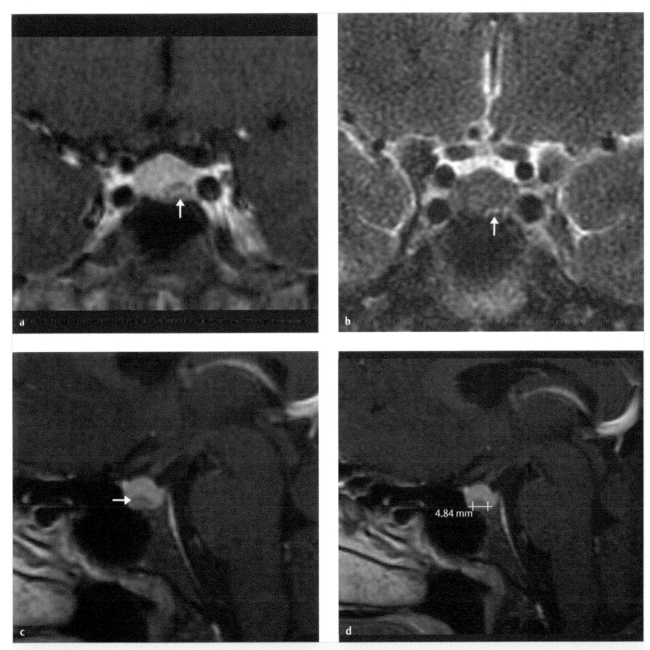

Fig. 20.2 (a–d)

Imaging Impression

Probable pituitary microadenoma.

Recommendation

Clinical evaluation is recommended to determine if this is a functioning or nonfunctioning microadenoma. No additional imaging is needed. When evaluating a possible PI found on a routine brain MRI in a patient with no evidence of endocrinological dysfunction, dynamic contrast-enhanced (DCE) pituitary MRI may increase the incidence of false-positive results.

20.1.4 Clinical Evaluation

Endocrinology Evaluation

This is a 36-year-old woman with an incidentally discovered pituitary mass. She denies galactorrhea or breast tenderness. Menses are regular. There has been no change in the size of shoes, rings, or gloves, change in voice, sleep apnea, or carpal tunnel–like symptoms. There is no new sleep disturbance, excessive skin fragility, difficulty climbing stairs or rising out of the chair, lower extremity swelling, weight gain, or history of kidney stones. There is no history of diabetes, hypertension, or cardiovascular disease.

Physical Examination

Physical examination was unremarkable.

Additional Testing Results

- Prolactin: 16.2 ng/mL (3–30 ng/mL).
- Insulin-like growth factor 1 (IGF-1): 178 ng/mL (126–291 ng/mL).

Clinical Impression

No evidence of prolactinoma or growth hormone (GH) secreting tumor in this normal-appearing 36-year-old woman with a small pituitary mass. Most small (< 6 mm) incidentally detected lesions in the pituitary gland are nonfunctioning microadenomas or cysts.[1] At a minimum, a prolactin (PRL) and IGF-1 level are recommended. If normal, no additional workup is necessary.

Neurosurgery and Endocrinology Recommendation

The overwhelming majority of incidental microadenomas are nonfunctioning pituitary adenomas (NFPAs) that will either remain stable or decrease in size. A follow-up MR of the pituitary gland should be obtained in 1 year. Unless there is a clinical change, no follow-up laboratory testing is necessary. The recommendations made above for laboratory testing and follow-up imaging are based on current Endocrine Society and American Association of Neurological Surgeons (AANS)/Congress of Neurological Surgeons (CNS) guidelines.[2,3] Guidelines vary between publishing society (see ▸ Table 20.1).

20.1.5 Imaging Differential Diagnosis of Intrasellar Lesions

Common solid lesions:
- Pituitary micro-/macroadenoma:
  - The most common solid lesion of the pituitary gland in adults, but rare in children.
  - Usually enhances less than the normal gland but may become hyperintense on delayed postcontrast imaging.
- Pituitary hyperplasia:
  - Homogeneous enhancing, enlarged gland most often associated with normal physiologic hypertrophy.

Common cystic lesions:
- Rathke's cleft cyst (RCC):
  - Midline, nonenhancing mass, between the anterior and posterior lobes of the pituitary gland.
  - Often hyperintense on T1 precontrast images.
  - Small nodule within a cyst is considered characteristic but not always seen.
- Pituitary adenoma with cystic/necrotic change:
  - Usually off-midline with septations or fluid–fluid levels.
- Empty sella:
  - Pituitary infundibulum seen traversing the "empty" sella without mass effect.

Less common lesions:
- Craniopharyngioma:
  - Nodular enhancement and calcification in a sellar/suprasellar mass are highly suggestive of this lesion. Presentation as a purely intrasellar mass is rare.
- Aneurysm:
  - A mass that is dark on T1 W and T2 W images and in continuity with the cavernous carotid artery should raise concern and MR or CT angiography performed.
- Meningioma:
  - Isointense to the brain on T1 W and T2 W images with homogeneous enhancement. Usually centered outside the sella. Pure, intrasellar presentation is rare.
- Metastatic disease:
  - Rapidly enlarging mass, frequently associated with destruction of the bony sella.
- Granulomatous disease:
  - Pituitary stalk is enlarged and abnormally enhancing.
  - Posterior lobe bright spot may be absent.

20.1.6 Diagnostic Imaging Pearls

- Attempt to identify the "lesion" in both sagittal and coronal planes on a dedicated high-field MR examination to increase confidence that the lesion is not artifactual.
- Although a small, solid mass in the pituitary gland most likely represents a pituitary adenoma (PA), clinical correlation is extremely important as microcysts, asymptomatic hemorrhage, infarcts, and nonfunctioning microadenomas are common.[7]
- Deviation of the pituitary stalk away from the "lesion" may be helpful but not definitive as "tilting" of the stalk is reported as a normal variant.[8]

Table 20.1 Initial evaluation and follow-up testing of a pituitary incidentaloma

Author/society	Size	Initial	1st follow-up (f/u)	Subsequent follow-up
Paschou et al[4]	≤4 mm	Hypersecretion testing	1 y f/u MRI	None if stable
	>4 mm	Hypersecretion and hypopituitarism testing	1 y f/u MRI	Every 2 y × 4 y MRI
	≥10 mm	Hypersecretion and hypopituitarism testing	6 mo f/u MRI; plus hypopituitarism testing with MRI; ±visual field testing (VF)	Every y × 3 y; then every 2 y × 6 y; then every 5 y MRI; plus hypopituitarism testing with MRI; ±VF
Freda et al[2]/Endocrine Society	<10 mm	Hypersecretion testing and hypopituitarism testing if 6–9 mm	1-y f/u MRI	1–2 y × 3 y; then every 2 y × 6 y; then every 5 y MRI
	≥10 mm	Hypersecretion and hypopituitarism testing	6 mo f/u MRI; plus hypopituitarism testing with MRI; ±VF	Every 1 y × 3 y; then every 2 y × 6 y; then every 5 y MRI; plus hypopituitarism testing with MRI; ±VF
Hoang et al[5]/ACR	"Simple cyst" that is not large without mass effect or surrounding structure invasion	No additional testing	None	None
	<5 mm	No testing unless clinical history suggests otherwise	None	None
	5–10 mm	No testing unless clinical history suggests hypersecretion or hypopituitarism	None	None
	≥10 mm	Endocrine function testing recommended	6 mo or 1 y f/u MRI	Not addressed
CNS/AANS Guidelines[6]	Pituitary lesion ("nonfunctioning pituitary adenoma")	Hypersecretion and hypopituitarism testing	Not addressed	Not addressed

Note: Testing for hypersecretion, as discussed in the Endocrine Society guidelines, is recommended even in the completely asymptomatic patient and involves, at a minimum, PRL and IGF-1 levels.
Recommended screening labs for hypopituitarism vary. Minimal screening as stated by the Endocrine Society involves free T4, morning cortisol, and testosterone levels (in males). Visual field testing is recommended only if the tumor abuts or compresses the optic chiasm or nerves.

- Even small, 4- to 6-mm, microadenomas will usually distort the contour of the gland, creating an upper surface bulge or depression of the sellar floor.[7]
- Contrast may not be necessary. Most adenomas, especially the common prolactinoma, are most frequently hypointense on *non-contrast* T1 W images and hyperintense on T2 W images relative to the normal pituitary gland.

20.1.7 Diagnostic Imaging Pitfalls: Artifacts and "Overcalls"

Computed tomography pitfalls:
- In addition to radiation exposure, a major drawback to CT is the creation of artifactual areas of low density within the gland due to beam hardening creating streak artifact, which has been reported in 65% of CT scans of the sella, especially on the reformatted images.[9,10,11]

Magnetic resonance pitfalls:
- Susceptibility artifact: Prominently aerated sinus adjacent to the sella or metal within the patient's mouth may create local magnetic field inhomogeneity that causes areas of falsely decreased signal within the adjacent skull base and sella, generating both false-positive and false-negative examinations.[12] This phenomenon is worse at higher field strength and on gradient recall echo (GRE) type images but less noticeable on fast spin echo (FSE) T2 W images.
- Motion artifact: Pulsatility from cavernous carotid and patient motion artifact may create ghosting throughout the gland.
- Volume averaging: Routine brain MRIs, which often employ 5-mm-thick sagittal T1W images, may create the false impression of a lesion within the pituitary gland by volume averaging pituitary tissue with the adjacent cavernous carotid artery or bony sella. Volume averaging occurs when different anatomic structures are present within the same voxel. The dedicated pituitary MR protocol uses thinner imaging cuts and allows confirmation of a lesion in two planes.
- False-positive examinations for very small lesions: Diagnosing small lesions as adenomas within the gland that may be areas of normal heterogeneity is well reported.[13] Chong et al found small microlesions in the pituitaries of 40% of normal volunteers on 3-mm noncontrast T1 W images (well above the average 10–14% incidence reported in autopsy series[14]), leading them to state that a "hypodensity in the pituitary gland

was recognized as consistent with the diagnosis of a pituitary microadenoma but not in itself diagnostic of such."[15] Microlesions may also be caused by cysts, infarcts, metastases, voxel-to-voxel heterogeneity in normal tissue, and MR system noise.[15] Teramoto et al calculated that there was a 6.1% false-positive rate when the "diagnosis of pituitary microadenoma" was made on imaging alone.[16]

- Is the lesion possibly vascular? Small cavernous carotid aneurysm projecting medially into the region of the sella could appear as a "lesion" that is very dark on the T1 W and T2 W images. Close inspection of the continuity of the flow void with the cavernous carotid on the coronal high-resolution T2 W images is helpful. Circle of Willis MRA or CTA is important to obtain if there is suspicion the lesion could be vascular in nature.

20.1.8 Additional Information Regarding Pituitary Lesion Imaging

Having dedicated imaging protocols for the evaluation of the pituitary gland and parasellar region is very important when a possible lesion of the gland is suspected.

Recommended imaging: dedicated pituitary magnetic resonance:

- Pre- and postcontrast sagittal and coronal T1 W images, ≤ 3 mm image slice thickness with a minimal interslice gap and a small, < 23 cm, field of view. Coronal high-resolution, FSE T2 W images are important to obtain through the sella.

Optional sequence: dynamic contrast-enhanced imaging:

- DCE images are acquired during the infusion of contrast at four to six locations repetitively.
- Immediately after contrast administration, at 15 to 30 seconds, adenomas enhance less than the normal gland and become progressively isointense at approximately 60 seconds. On delayed imaging, 30 to 40 minutes after contrast injection, some adenomas may be hyperintense.
- DCE-MR is a highly sensitive sequence that may detect an additional 5 to 14% of very small lesions not visualized on routine pituitary MRI.[17,18,19,20,21] As 8 to 9% of lesions are seen only on routine postcontrast imaging and not seen on

the dynamic study, routine postcontrast T1 W images are still recommended in two planes following the dynamic sequence.[19]

- DCE is not recommended routinely due to an increased rate of false-positive results and is best reserved for cases in which the endocrinologist or neurosurgeon strongly suspect a secreting microadenoma (commonly a corticotroph), which is not apparent on the routine pituitary MRI.[13,22,23]

Optional advanced MR sequences: The following techniques are described in the literature but are not currently part of most imaging centers' dedicated pituitary protocol.

- VIBE (volume interpolated breath hold): T1 W volumetric examination may yield superior resolution and improved contrast between the gland and the cavernous sinus in comparison to routine postcontrast T1 W images. It has also been reported to have greater sensitivity for detection of small adrenocorticotropic hormone (ACTH) secreting tumors.[24,25]
- VIBE with GRASP (golden angle radial sparse parallel imaging): This 3D GRE imaging technique acquires all dynamic information in a single continuous scan giving greater temporal resolution for DCE.[26]
- Two-plane DCE: Acquiring DCE images in two planes may provide greater confidence in diagnosing a very small microadenoma.[18]
- FIESTA (fast imaging employing steady-state acquisition) postcontrast for determining if pituitary mass is more likely to be soft or firm.[27]

Computed tomography imaging:

- Useful in patients in whom MR is contraindicated.
- Superior sensitivity for calcification and therefore useful to help differentiate a craniopharyngioma from an RCC and adenoma, which rarely calcify.[28]
- Preferred modality for surgical navigation.
- Preoperative planning sinus CT should note the following: asymmetric septation of the sphenoid sinus, attachment of septation to the optic canal, and abnormally medial position of the carotid arteries.

20.1.9 Companion Cases

Companion Case 1

Case Presentation

History

A 20-year-old man presented with a history of long-standing headaches from 6 years of age. The pituitary gland appeared prominent on routine brain MR; therefore, a dedicated pituitary MR was performed.

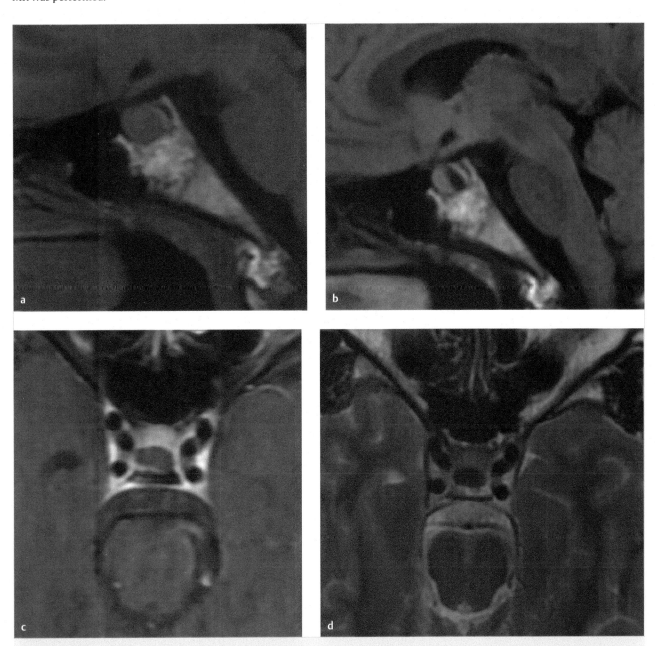

Fig. 20.3 Companion case 1. Precontrast sagittal T1 W image **(a)**, postcontrast sagittal **(b)** and axial **(c)** T1 W images, and axial T2 W **(d)** image from a dedicated pituitary MRI.

Imaging Analysis of Companion Case 1

Imaging Findings

There is a kidney bean–shaped lesion in the region of the pars intermedia, which is isointense on T1 W (► Fig. 20.4a) and dark on T2 W (*arrowhead* in ► Fig. 20.4c) images. It appears dark on the postcontrast T1 W image (*arrow* in ► Fig. 20.4b) because it does not enhance unlike the remainder of the gland. There is no nodular enhancing component and no septation. The gland is not significantly enlarged given the size of the lesion, 3 mm × 8 mm × 6 mm. Incidental note is made of heterogeneous marrow signal in the floor of the sella, which is bright on the T1 W images (*asterisk* in ► Fig. 20.4a).

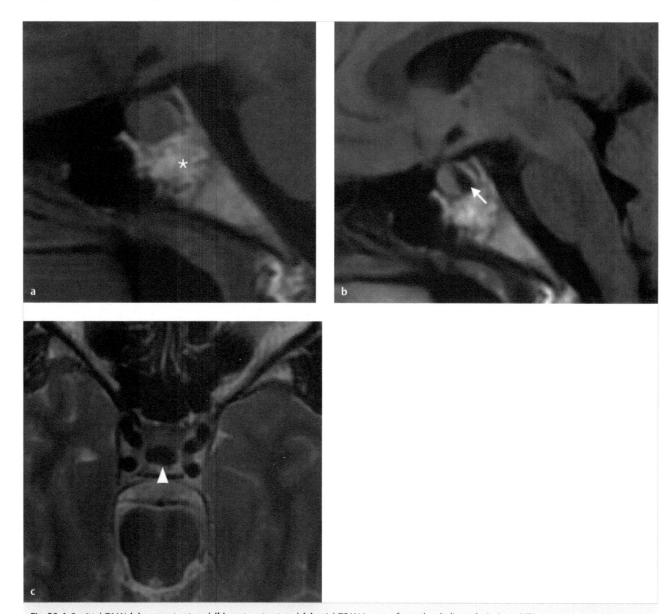

Fig. 20.4 Sagittal T1 W **(a)** precontrast and **(b)** postcontrast and **(c)** axial T2 W images from the dedicated pituitary MRI.

Impression

Probable Rathke's cleft cyst and skull base hemangioma.

Differential diagnosis: See Differential Diagnosis of Intrasellar Lesions (Section 20.1.5).

Clinical Evaluation of Companion Case 1

Endocrinology Evaluation

An RCC is often an incidental finding with no additional imaging or laboratory testing needed. However, an RCC may cause pituitary hypofunction or, more rarely, coexist with a PA.[29,30] Therefore, testing for hypopituitarism is recommended in patients with larger cystic lesions (≥ 6 mm).[2] In this case, early morning serum cortisol, free T4, and testosterone were normal. No additional endocrine function testing is required in the absence of the development of signs or symptoms of pituitary dysfunction. As these cysts may enlarge, follow-up MRI is recommended in 1 year, with subsequently less frequent imaging in smaller lesions that are stable and more closely spaced imaging in those with larger cysts that have suprasellar extension and approach the optic chiasm. These guidelines are based on current Endocrine Society and AANS/CNS guidelines.[2,3] Laboratory testing and follow-up imaging guidelines vary by publishing society (see ▶ Table 20.1). The recently published American College of Radiology (ACR) guidelines do not recommend either laboratory testing for endocrine dysfunction or follow-up imaging if the lesion is a "simple cyst" that is small, without mass effect or invasion of surrounding structures.[5]

Neurosurgery Evaluation

Surgical decision-making for the incidental, small RCC is similar to that of an incidental pituitary microadenoma. Observation is the treatment of choice for small, clinically asymptomatic lesions without evidence of pituitary dysfunction and in elderly patients. It is reasonable to offer surgical resection for larger RCCs in young, otherwise healthy patients. RCCs have a high rate of recurrence and aggressive surgical resection is associated with a higher rate of complication in comparison to PAs.

Imaging Pearls and Pitfalls of Rathke's Cleft Cysts (RCC)

- A thickened, enhancing cyst wall or calcification is atypical and should suggest the possibility of a craniopharyngioma. In the appropriate clinical setting, infection of an RCC has also been reported to cause increased pituitary dysfunction, a thickened, enhancing cyst wall, and restricted diffusion, all of which are not seen in an uncomplicated RCC.
- Septation, fluid/fluid levels, or off-midline location suggest that the lesion is more likely a hemorrhagic PA than an RCC.[31]
- The differentiation between a small RCC and nonfunctioning cystic pituitary microadenoma is not always possible but is not of immediate clinical importance as neither would mandate surgical treatment.
- An RCC may coexist with a PA. A lesion exerting mass effect upon a midline T1 "bright" cyst may suggest this unusual diagnosis.[7]

Essential Facts about Rathke's Cleft Cysts

- RCC is derived from embryologic remnants of Rathke's pouch, an outpouching of the stomatodeum, in the region of the pars intermedia, which lies between the pars distalis of the adenohypophysis and the pars nervosa (see ▶ Fig. 20.5).[32]
- Most commonly intrasellar but may extend into the suprasellar region or, rarely, be completely suprasellar.[28]
- Majority have increased signal relative to cerebrospinal fluid (CSF) on both T1 W and T2 W images.[28,33]
- The presence of an intracystic nodule, high in signal on T1 W images and dark on T2 W images, has been reported in up to 77% of RCCs and is pathognomonic.[34]
- Homogeneous hypointense signal intensity on the T2 W images within a nonenhancing, midline pituitary cyst is highly suggestive of an RCC.[35]
- The "egg-in-a-cup" appearance of a well-defined oval, T1WI hyperintense mass located in a depression in the superior aspect of the pituitary gland is highly suggestive of an RCC.

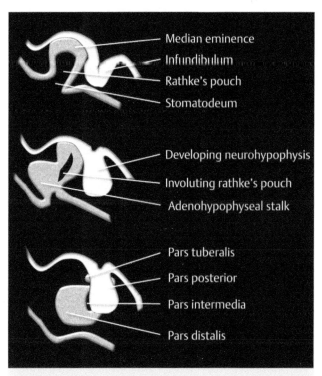

Fig. 20.5 Embryologic development of the pituitary gland. (Illustration courtesy of Dr. Roy F. Riascos.)

Companion Case 2

Case Presentation

History

A 53-year-old woman underwent a brain MR during the evaluation of a syncopal episode. Although the normal gland was displaced to the right, there was asymmetric fullness in the left side of the gland. Therefore, a dedicated pituitary MR was performed; the images are shown in ▶ Fig. 20.6 and ▶ Fig. 20.7.

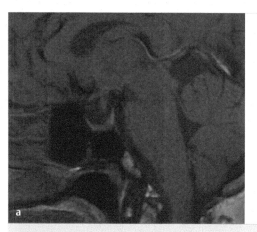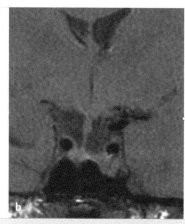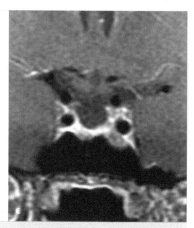

Fig. 20.6 Companion case 2. Pituitary MRI. **(a)** Precontrast sagittal T1 W midline image, **(b)** precontrast and **(c)** postcontrast coronal T1 W images of the sella.

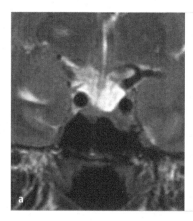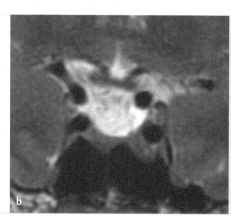

Fig. 20.7 Companion case 2. MRI. Coronal T2 W images posteriorly through the gland **(a)** at the insertion of the pituitary stalk and, more anteriorly, **(b)** at the optic chiasm.

Imaging Analysis of Companion Case 2

Imaging Findings

Images reveal a partially empty sella (*asterisk* in ▶ Fig. 20.8a), which distorts the normal anatomy and may be contributing to subtle deviation of the pituitary stalk (*arrow* in ▶ Fig. 20.8b) and normal gland to the right. There is a small mass contiguous with the left side of the gland (*arrowheads* in ▶ Fig. 20.8a–c),

filling the inferior aspect of the cavernous sinus. The dura of the medial cavernous sinus wall is normal and well seen on the right (*short arrows* in ▶ Fig. 20.8c) but not seen between the tumor and the normal gland within the left side of the sella. Important note is made of asymmetric expansion of the floor of the sella on the left, inferior to the left intracavernous carotid artery (*asterisk* in ▶ Fig. 20.8b).

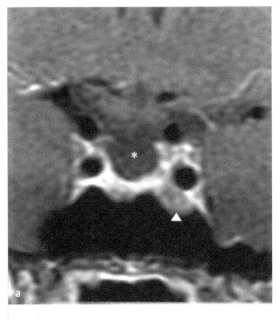
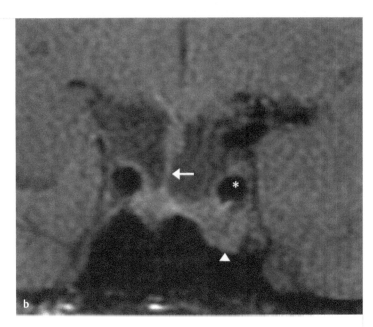
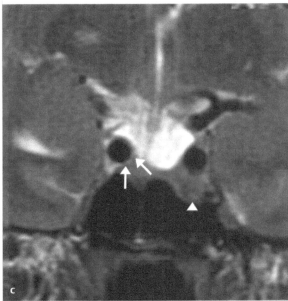

Fig. 20.8 (a–c)

Imaging Diagnosis

Probable microadenoma involving the left cavernous sinus. Clinical correlation is needed to determine if this is a functioning or nonfunctioning adenoma.

Recommendation

Referral to an endocrinologist.

Clinical Evaluation of Companion Case 2

Endocrinology Evaluation

This is a 53-year-old woman who presents with an incidental finding of a sellar mass during evaluation of syncope. She was diagnosed with atrioventricular block and subsequently received a permanent pacemaker. Left heart catheterization showed nonobstructive coronary artery disease. She reports no change in the size of shoes, rings, or gloves, sleep apnea, carpal tunnel–like symptoms, difficultly sleeping, or lower extremity swelling. Menopause occurred at age 50 years. Her medical history includes hypertension and nephrolithiasis. Medications include hydrochlorothiazide, amlodipine, and propranolol.

Physical Examination

Her blood pressure is 152/88 mm Hg and her pulse rate is 72 bpm. She has prominent facial features, including a slightly wide nasal bridge.

Additional Testing Results (Sample Obtained at 8 a.m.)

- IGF-1: 948 ng/mL (50–317 ng/mL).
- Prolactin: 42.0 ng/mL (4.8–23.3 ng/mL).
- Cortisol: 19.0 μg/dL (5–25 μg/dL).
- Free T4: 1.0 ng/dL (0.8–1.8 ng/dL).

Clinical Impression and Further Management

The IGF-1 is abnormally elevated; therefore, a GH suppression test was performed. Her nadir GH was 2.2 ng/mL, which is abnormal as a normal individual will suppress less than 1 ng/mL after a 75-g oral glucose load.[36]

Even though overt physical features of acromegaly were absent, and the tumor considered, a priori, an incidental finding, endocrinology evaluation revealed the presence of a GH–secreting microadenoma. Acromegalic features typically develop insidiously; therefore, a delay in diagnosis is common, averaging 6 years.[37] Common manifestations of acromegaly present in this case include hypertension and kidney stones. In addition, long-term GH excess likely resulted in atrioventricular block. Cardiovascular disease is highly prevalent in patients with acromegaly and is the primary cause of increased mortality in this population. The most common cardiovascular abnormalities include hypertension and myocardial hypertrophy. Valvular heart disease and arrhythmias may also be observed.[38]

Neurosurgical consultation is recommended for a GH-secreting tumor.

Neurosurgery Evaluation

Surgical resection is the standard of care and most definitive treatment for GH-secreting tumors and provides better long-term outcomes compared with medical therapy.[39] Endoscopic transsphenoidal resection has superseded microscopic transsphenoidal or transcranial surgery as the primary surgical approach. Endoscopic surgery improves direct tumor visualization, allowing for greater extent of tumor removal, with up to 90% remission rates in microadenomas. In comparison to the microscopic approach, there is a lower incidence of septal perforation and a complication rate of less than 5% if performed by an expert, experienced endoscopic pituitary surgeon.[40] The most common complication is panhypopituitarism and/or diabetes insipidus (DI), which can occur in 7.2 and 7.6% of patients, respectively.[41] Delayed syndrome of inappropriate antidiuretic hormone (SIADH) beginning approximately 7 days postoperatively occurs in 4 to 12% of patients.[42] Rare complications include CNS injury, vision loss, carotid injury, meningitis, and death.

Transsphenoidal surgery was performed in this case, which confirmed a PA with immunoreactivity for GH and PRL. Her serum IGF-1 was normal 12 weeks after surgery.

20.2 Incidental Silent Macroadenoma

20.2.1 Introduction

In this section, we present two cases of incidentally discovered nonfunctioning pituitary macroadenomas. We review the differential diagnosis of a large sellar mass and highlight imaging features that help distinguish a pituitary macroadenoma from a nonpituitary sellar mass, most commonly a meningioma. Next, we review the clinical evaluation and recommendations for laboratory testing, including assessment of hormonal hypersecretion and hypopituitarism. Finally, we discuss indications for surgical management and provide recommendations for patients in whom imaging and clinical surveillance is favored.

20.2.2 Case Presentation

History and Physical Examination

The patient is a 71-year-old man with MR brain performed for right-sided hearing loss. The regions of the temporal bones and brainstem were unremarkable. Sagittal T1 W images were noted to be abnormal (▶ Fig. 20.9).

Physical examination was unremarkable.

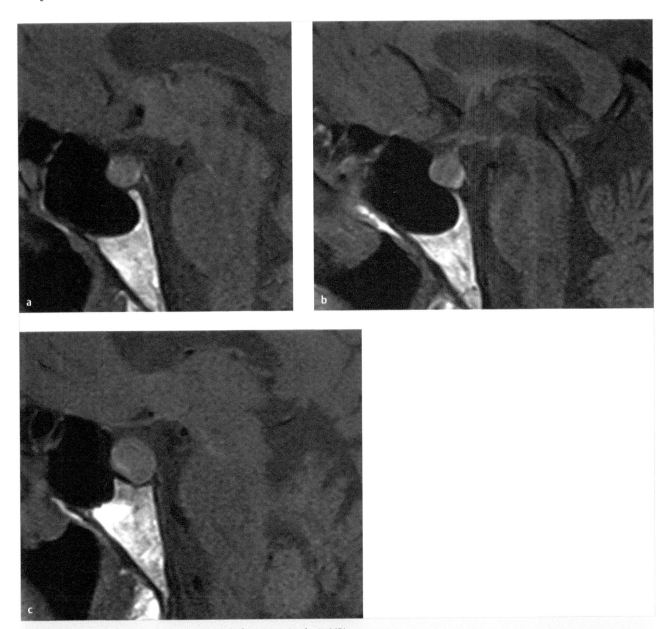

Fig. 20.9 (a–c) Right to left sagittal T1 W images from a routine brain MRI.

20.2.3 Imaging Analysis

Imaging Findings

Sagittal midline and left parasagittal T1 W images reveal a prominent pituitary gland with asymmetric enlargement of the left side of the gland. The superior aspect of the gland is convex, which is abnormal in a 71-year-old man.

Recommended Additional Imaging

Dedicated pituitary MR with and without contrast, which is shown in ▶ Fig. 20.10. DCE images were obtained during administration of contrast.

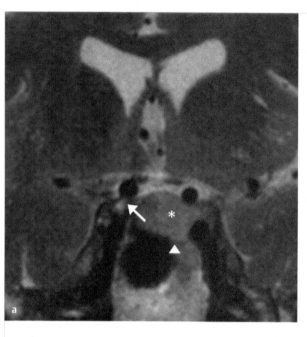
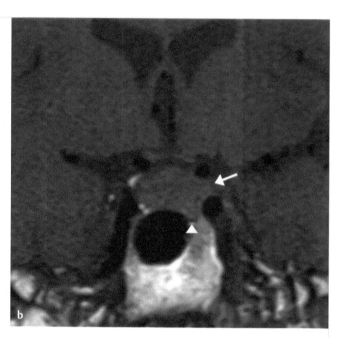
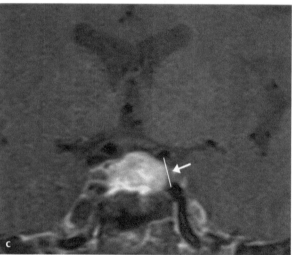

Fig. 20.10 Coronal T2 W image **(a)** and precontrast **(b)** and postcontrast **(c)** T1 W images. The coronal T2 W image **(a)** shows that the enlargement of the gland is due to a 1.4 × 1.2 × 1.2 cm mass in the left side of the sella (*asterisk*). Note the convex appearance of the superior aspect of the gland and the subtle asymmetric expansion of the floor of the sella on the left (*arrowhead* in **a** and **b**). The mass is isointense to the normal gland on the pre- and postcontrast T1 W images and is therefore best seen on the T2 W image (*asterisk* in **a**) where it is slightly hyperintense relative to the normal gland, which is displaced to the patient's right. Note extension of the mass lateral to the intercarotid line (see ▶ Fig. 20.16 and *white line* in **c**)[43,44] into the region of the left cavernous sinus (*arrow* in **b** and **c**). The normally identified black line of the dura between the sella and cavernous sinus on the left is not seen on the coronal high-resolution T2 W images **(a)**. Note normal appearance of the black dural line between the right side of the gland and the cavernous sinus (*arrow* in **a**). The mass does not contact the optic chiasm.

Dynamic Contrast-Enhanced Magnetic Resonance of the Pituitary

Impression

Pitutary macroadenoma in the left side of the gland with possible cavernous sinus invasion and displacement of the residual normal gland to the right. Displacement of the residual normal gland to the right.

Recommendation

Referral to neurosurgeon and endocrinologist.

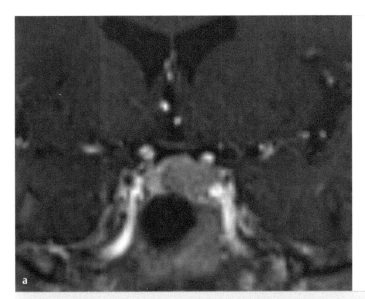 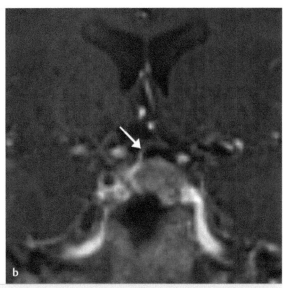

Fig. 20.11 Coronal T1 W images during the early phase of dynamic contrast enhancement through the mid **(a)** and posterior aspect of the sella **(b)**, respectively. Note the displacement of the normal enhancing pituitary stalk to the patient's right (*arrow* in **b**). The mass enhances to a lesser degree than the normal pituitary gland and cavernous sinus during this early phase of contrast enhancement.

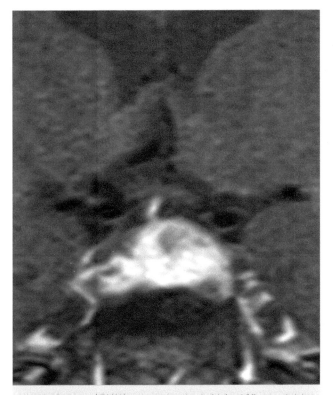

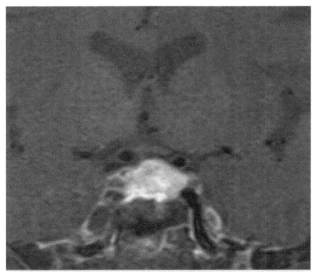

Fig. 20.13 Routine postcontrast T1 W coronal image reveals an asymmetrically enlarged, but more homogeneous gland.

Fig. 20.12 Coronal T1 W image postcontrast obtained 10 seconds later during the dynamic postcontrast acquisition reveals a heterogenous enhancing mass within the left side of the sella. The normal pituitary gland is not as well seen separate from the mass in comparison to images obtained in an earlier phase of contrast enhancement.

20.2.4 Clinical Evaluation

Endocrinology Evaluation

This is a 71-year-old man with an incidentally detected sellar mass during an evaluation for right-sided hearing loss. He has normal energy, muscle strength, and libido. He denies dizziness, nausea, loss of appetite, cold intolerance, or dry skin. There is no polyuria, nocturia, or dry mouth. He reports no change in the size of shoes or gloves, lower extremity swelling, or weight gain. He denies headaches or changes in vision. There is no history of diabetes, hypertension, or kidney stones.

Physical Examination

Physical examination is unremarkable.

Additional Testing Results (Sample Obtained at 8 a.m.)

- Cortisol: 16.2 µg/dL (5–25 µg/dL).
- Free T4: 1.1 ng/dL (0.8–1.8 ng/dL).
- Prolactin: 4.8 ng/mL (2.0–18.0 ng/mL).
- IGF-1: 78 ng/mL (62–184 ng/mL).

As the tumor does not abut the optic chiasm or optic nerves, formal visual field testing was not recommended.

Clinical Impression

Incidentally detected silent macroadenoma.

Neurosurgery Consultation

This is an elderly male patient with a clinically asymptomatic macroadenoma. In a younger, otherwise healthy individual, it would be reasonable to offer surgical intervention. Cavernous sinus invasion with lack of neurological deficits does not warrant surgical resection. In this case, nonoperative management was elected with follow-up pituitary MRI and laboratory testing for hypopituitarism (serum cortisol, free T4, and testosterone) in 6 months. Subsequent monitoring can be performed at increasing time intervals if the radiographic appearance, endocrine evaluation, and neurological status remain unchanged. These recommendations follow the current Endocrine Society and AANS/CNS guidelines (see ▶ Table 20.1).[2,3]

20.2.5 Differential Diagnosis of Sellar/Parasellar Masses

Common:
- Pituitary macroadenoma.
- Meningioma.

Less common/rare:
- RCC.
- Schwannoma.
- Aneurysm.
- Craniopharyngioma.
- Sarcoid.
- Germinoma.
- Tuberculosis.
- Langerhans cell histiocytosis (LCH)/eosinophilic granuloma (EG).
- Pilocytic astrocytoma.
- Metastatic disease.
- Arachnoid cyst.
- Lymphocytic/granulomatous hypophysitis.

20.2.6 Diagnostic Imaging and Clinical Pearls and Pitfalls

Pituitary macroadenoma:
- Should always be high in the differential diagnosis for a sellar region mass in an adult.
- Rarely found in the pediatric population; consider alternative diagnoses.
- Rarely presents with DI; consider alternative diagnoses.
- Sellar enlargement strongly favors PA.
- The gland appears heterogeneous.
- Normal gland and stalk may be displaced by the mass, often posteriorly and superiorly out of the sella, with very large pituitary macroadenomas.
- "Snowman" appearance with a "waist" due to compression from the diaphragm sella.
- Mucosal thickening of the paranasal sinuses is associated with PAs.

Meningioma[45,46]:
- Tuberculum sella meningiomas may mimic PAs.
- The center of the lesion is located outside the confines of the sella but may involve it secondarily.
- A prominent enhancing dural tail has been described but is not diagnostic as it is also seen in lymphocytic hypophysitis (LH), PAs, lymphoma, and metastatic disease.
- CT scan showing hyperostosis, dilatation of the adjacent paranasal sinus, and/or calcification.
- Narrowing or occlusion of an encased cavernous carotid artery is often seen with meningiomas and is not a feature of PAs.

Lymphocytic hypophysitis[47,48]:
- Although rare and never found incidentally, this entity is important to consider as it may mimic a pituitary macroadenoma.
- Symmetrically enlarged gland.
- Pituitary stalk enlargement.
- Loss of the posterior pituitary bright spot.
- Prominent homogeneous enhancement of an enlarged gland with less enhancement of the cavernous sinus.
- Rim of marked decrease signal on T2 W images about the periphery of the gland.
- Importantly, LH is not an incidental finding! Typical clinical scenario is in the peripartum female with headaches, visual changes, and possibly DI.

20.2.7 Companion Case

Companion Case 1

Case Presentation

History

The patient is a 55-year-old woman who was found to have sellar mass during evaluation for headaches.

Physical Examination

Physical examination was unremarkable.

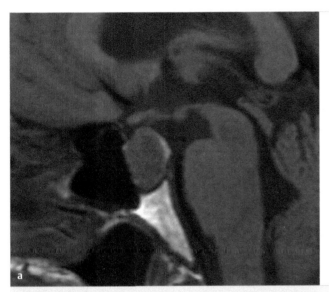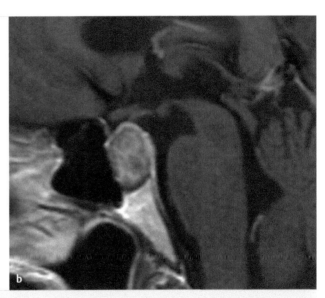

Fig. 20.14 (a, b)

Imaging Analysis for Companion Case 1

Imaging Findings

There is a large 1.7 × 1.2 × 1.1 cm heterogeneous mass that is centered within the sella, displacing the pituitary stalk to the left (*arrow* in ▶ Fig. 20.15a). As is often noted in macroadeno-mas, the posterior pituitary bright spot is displaced superiorly up out of the sella (*arrow* in ▶ Fig. 20.15b). Although the mass bulges into the superior aspect of the cavernous sinus on the right (see *arrow* in ▶ Fig. 20.15c), it does not extend lateral to the intercarotid line (see ▶ Fig. 20.16).[43,44] The mass does not contact the optic chiasm (*asterisk* in ▶ Fig. 20.15d).

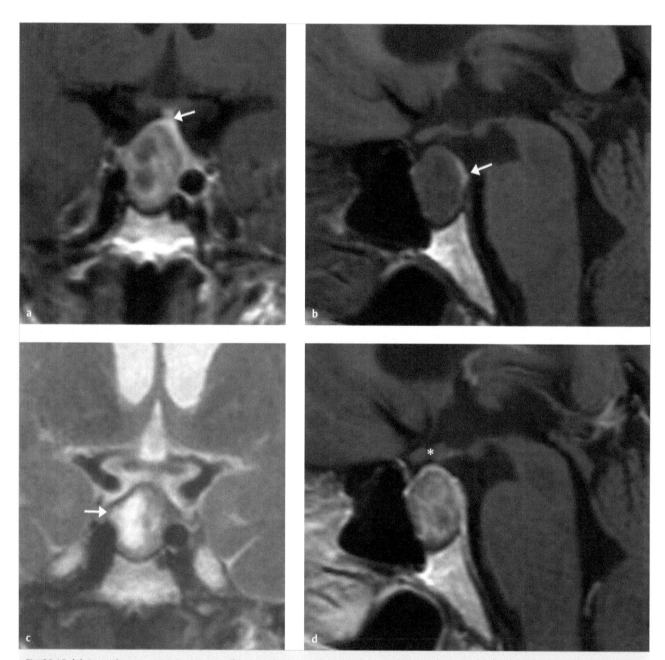

Fig. 20.15 (a) Coronal postcontrast T1 W image, **(b)** sagittal precontrast T1 W image and **(c)** coronal T2 W image and **(d)** postcontrast sagittal T1 W image.

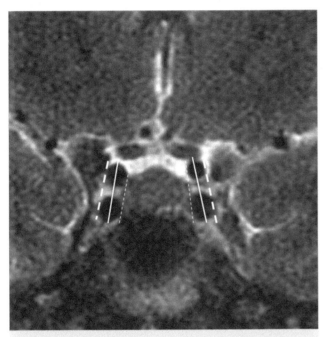

Fig. 20.16 Divisions of the cavernous sinus by medial and lateral tangent lines and intercarotid line.[43,44] (Tangent lines are constructed with respect to the supra- and intracavernous internal carotid artery. *Thin dotted line* = medial tangent line; *thick dotted line* = lateral tangent line; *solid line* = intercarotid line.)

Imaging Diagnosis

Probable pituitary macroadenoma in the right side of the sella. Referral to neurosurgeon and endocrinologist is recommended.

Clinical Evaluation and Management

Endocrinology Evaluation

As typically the case in an incidentally detected macroadenoma, this is most likely a nonfunctioning lesion. Routine laboratory testing for hormone hypersecretion should still include measurement of serum PRL and IGF-1 levels.

In addition, testing for hypopituitarism should be performed in all macroadenomas. In this case, the lesion does not abut the optic chiasm; therefore, formal visual field testing is not required.

Physical examination and review of systems were normal. However, she did note that she has had fatigue and dry skin. Menopause occurred at age 51 years.

Additional Testing Results (Sample Obtained at 8 a.m.)

- Cortisol: 13.2 µg/dL (5–25 µg/dL).
- Thyroid-stimulating hormone (TSH): 1.3 mIU/L (0.5–5.0 mIU/L).
- Free T4: 0.6 ng/dL (0.8–1.8 ng/dL).
- Prolactin: 26.4 ng/mL (2–20 ng/mL).
- IGF-1: 122 ng/mL (62–184 ng/mL).

Clinical Impression

This is most likely a nonfunctioning macroadenoma. Her low free T4 level in association with an inappropriately normal TSH

confirms a diagnosis of central hypothyroidism. She was subsequently started on thyroid replacement therapy.

Neurosurgical Consultation

A 55-year-old woman with an incidentally discovered macroadenoma with no mass effect upon the optic chiasm or evidence of cavernous sinus invasion. Endocrine workup reveals central hypothyroidism for which the patient has begun replacement therapy. The presence of hypopituitarism is a relative indication for surgical resection via endoscopic transsphenoidal approach. There is a paucity of evidence regarding the utility of surgical resection of macroadenomas for the treatment of headaches. This large macroadenoma does not currently contact the optic chiasm; however, minimal growth could result in mass effect. Therefore, surgical resection was offered with the option of close observation with repeat imaging at 6 months. If the patient should develop any new neurological symptoms or should repeat imaging reveal interval growth, surgical intervention would be recommended.

20.2.8 Neurosurgery and Endocrinology Questions and Answers

1. **What is the etiology and natural history of the condition that would assist in decision-making?**

   Although most PIs do not receive a pathological diagnosis, in autopsy series, the majority are clinically NFPAs.[49] Pituitary adenomas have been found to be quite common with a prevalence of 14.4% at autopsy and 22.5% in radiologic studies.[14] Macroadenomas, defined as tumors greater than or equal to 1 cm in size, are far less common with a reported prevalence of 0 to 1.3% in autopsy studies. The most common nonpituitary sellar masses are RCCs, craniopharyngiomas, and meningiomas.[50,51,52]

   Although limited evidence exists regarding the natural history of PIs, the majority of tumors remain stable or demonstrate very slow growth and are therefore unlikely to become clinically relevant.[53] However, a systematic review and meta-analysis showed that the incidence of growth is higher in macroadenomas (12.5 per 100 person-years) compared to microadenomas and cystic lesions (3.3 and 0.05 per 100 person-years, respectively).[54]

   A major complication of PAs is the development of pituitary apoplexy, a clinical syndrome of headaches and acute visual change due to rapid growth and/or hemorrhage into the tumor. Fortunately, this complication is uncommon and is estimated to occur in 1.8 to 12.6% of patients with pituitary macroadenomas. The occurrence of apoplexy in microadenomas is considered to be exceedingly rare.[55,56]

2. **Given the presentation and imaging findings, what specific findings on the history and physical examination are important in your determination of the diagnosis and if it is truly asymptomatic?**

   The vast majority of PAs that present incidentally do so because they are clinically nonfunctioning adenomas and therefore do not cause a hypersecretion syndrome. Interestingly, however, the majority of these "silent" tumors, or NFPA, will stain positively by immunohistochemistry: 44% null cell; 44% gonadotroph (follicle-stimulating hormone

[FSH], LH-secreting); 5% corticotroph (ACTH-secreting); 2 to 4% somatotroph (GH-secreting); 2% lactotroph (PRL-secreting); 1% thyrotroph (TSH-secreting), and 2% plurihormonal.[57,58] This positive staining has important implications in management, as silent corticotroph and somatotroph adenomas are associated with higher rates of recurrence compared to other nonfunctioning adenomas.[59,60,61] In addition, some of these adenomas may transform into functioning tumors that cause Cushing's disease or acromegaly.[62,63]

As the majority of PIs are microadenomas, it is not surprising that most lack overt signs and symptoms of mass effect that usually lead to detection of an nonfunctioning pituitary macroadenoma.

It is important to recognize, however, that a patient with an incidentally discovered PA may, on further evaluation, exhibit evidence of hormone hypersecretion that is not recognized a priori because the clinical signs and symptoms are subtle. Prolactinomas, the most common type of functioning PA, typically cause symptoms in most patients, such as menstrual cycle dysfunction or galactorrhea in premenopausal women.[64] However, in postmenopausal women, they may present incidentally. In men, a prolactinoma may present with vague complaints of decreased libido and energy as other symptoms, such as gynecomastia and galactorrhea, are rarely present.

Corticotroph and somatotroph adenomas appear to present with a spectrum of clinical manifestations. For example, in subclinical Cushing's disease the patient does not appear overtly Cushingoid even though conditions associated with cortisol excess (e.g., diabetes mellitus, hypertension) are present.[65,66] Somatotroph adenomas may present a priori as an incidental finding as features of acromegaly may be insidious with changes in facial features and ring or shoe size occurring over many years. In a recent study, 18% of patients with acromegaly were diagnosed as the result of unrelated physical or radiographic evaluations.[67]

In the case of an incidentally discovered macroadenoma, it is important to consider the possibility of subtle hypopituitarism. Signs of pituitary hyposecretion include fatigue, intolerance to cold, constipation, weight gain, hair loss, and slowed thinking. Formal visual field testing should be performed proactively when there is compression of the optic chiasm, since some patients may not be aware of their vision loss.[2] The classic visual field deficit due to chiasmatic compression from a macroadenoma is bitemporal hemianopia, typically beginning in the superotemporal visual field quadrant.

3. **What additional testing, if any, is required or recommended in the workup of a micro- or macroadenoma?**

   Hormone hypersecretion: The Endocrine Society and the CNS recommend assessment of PRL and IGF-1 levels for all PIs.[2,3] The ACR recommends routine testing for hormone hypersecretion in patients with macroadenomas.[5] A prolactinoma must be distinguished from hyperprolactinemia caused by pituitary stalk effect. The PRL level should be interpreted in the context of tumor size. Macroprolactinomas are typically associated with PRL levels over 200 ng/mL. A PRL level below 100 ng/mL may be due to pituitary stalk effect or caused by a microprolactinoma.[68,69]

   As mentioned previously, acromegalic features typically develop insidiously. The best initial test is serum IGF-1 because levels remain constant during the day and reflect integrated GH secretion. A normal age-adjusted IGF-1 excludes a diagnosis of acromegaly. In patients with elevated or equivocal IGF-1, the diagnosis is confirmed by lack of GH suppression to less 1 µg/L during an oral glucose tolerance test.[36]

   If the patient, on further evaluation, exhibits subtle manifestations of cortisol excess, additional testing should be obtained, including urine-free cortisol, late-night salivary cortisol, or the low-dose dexamethasone suppression test.[70] A significant proportion of corticotroph macroadenomas are clinically nonfunctioning, whereas the majority of corticotroph microadenomas cause Cushing's disease, which is not unexpected as silent tumors typically reach larger size and come to attention due to mass effect. Some silent corticotroph macroadenomas may be identified by elevated levels of plasma ACTH,[59,60,71] suggesting that the ACTH produced by these adenomas is biologically inactive.[72,73]

   Hypopituitarism: Hypopituitarism has been identified in 37 to 85% of patients with NFPAs, which may be artificially inflated due to the fact that these estimates are primarily derived from surgical series, which therefore include a high proportion of macroadenomas.[74,75,76,77,78,79] The true prevalence of hypopituitarism in patients with microadenomas is unknown considering the very small number of cases reported.[76,80,81]

   Given the fact that larger tumors are more likely to result in hypopituitarism,[74,75,76,77,78,79] evaluation for hypopituitarism should be considered based on size along a continuum of both micro- and macroadenomas. The Endocrine Society and the ACR recommend routine testing for hypopituitarism in patients with macroadenomas.[2,5] The Endocrine Society also recommends testing for hypopituitarism in patients with larger microadenomas (6–9 mm).[2] The CNS recommends routine testing of all anterior pituitary hormones, given the overall prevalence of hypopituitarism.[3]

   Testing for hypopituitarism includes measurement of serum cortisol, free T4, and testosterone levels in men. An early morning (8–9 a.m.) serum cortisol level of less than 3 µg/dL is consistent with adrenal insufficiency, whereas a cortisol level greater than 15 µg/dL excludes the diagnosis. A corticotropin stimulation test is recommended for patients with an indeterminate cortisol level. If hormonal deficiencies are detected, additional testing is needed to confirm a central etiology. For example, central hypothyroidism is confirmed with a low free T4 in association with an inappropriately low or normal TSH. Testing in premenopausal women with oligomenorrhea or amenorrhea includes serum FSH, LH, and estradiol. Low gonadotropin levels in postmenopausal women provide evidence of hypopituitarism. Considering variability in clinical practice, testing for GH deficiency, including serum IGF-1 and stimulation testing, should be guided by anticipated management.[2,82]

4. **If electing to follow, what is the suggested time interval and modality?**

   The Endocrine Society, AANS/CNS, and ACR have all released recommendations for laboratory testing and imaging, which are not uniform (see ► Table 20.1).[2,3,4,5] The Endocrine

Society acknowledges that some studies distinguish between cystic and solid lesions but has issued uniform guidelines for all incidentalomas regardless of imaging characteristics. The Endocrine Society recommends testing for hormone hypersecretion even if patients are clinically asymptomatic, consisting of PRL and IGF-1 levels. Screening for hyperprolactinemia is considered essential because prolactinomas may be treated medically. Serum IGF-1 is recommended because early detection of a GH-secreting adenoma is likely to improve surgical outcomes and reduce long-term morbidity. They also note that some endocrinologists measure ACTH because some silent corticotroph adenomas may be identified by elevated ACTH levels,[59,70,71] even though there are no clinical manifestations of cortisol excess. The Endocrine Society recommends routine testing for hypopituitarism in patients with macroadenomas and larger microadenomas (6–9 mm).[2] The AANS/CNS recommends routine testing for hormonal hypersecretion and hypopituitarism in all patients, regardless of adenoma size. The AANS/CNS provides treatment guidelines for symptomatic lesions but does not provide recommendations for lesions selected for observation.[3]

In patients with microadenomas, long-term radiographic surveillance is unlikely to affect clinical outcomes given the low incidence of tumor growth in this population.[54,81] In a meta-analysis, new endocrine dysfunction developed in 2.4% of patients per year.[54] In patients with microadenomas, the Endocrine Society recommends repeat testing for hypopituitarism in the setting of significant tumor growth or changes in the clinical picture. Formal visual field testing is recommended if the PI abuts the optic nerves or chiasm at the initial evaluation or during follow-up.[2]

5. **If electing surgical (or medical) management, then why … and what are the surgical options and risks?**

Indications for surgical intervention include (1) visual field deficits, (2) neurological abnormalities due to tumor expansion (pituitary apoplexy), and (3) hypersecreting adenomas, except prolactinomas.[2]

Dopamine agonists are recommended as initial therapy for prolactinomas given their effect on both hormonal secretion and tumor size. Cabergoline is more effective with fewer adverse effects than bromocriptine. Treatment aims to restore gonadal function and reduce tumor size in macroprolactinomas. Medication may be tapered and possibly discontinued after 2 years of therapy, if the PRL level remains normal and the adenoma is no longer visible on MRI.[83] Long-term remission following withdrawal of therapy may be achieved in 30 to 40% of patients.[84,85] Surgical treatment is offered if patients cannot tolerate the medication side effects, although chemical cure rates decrease with increasing serum PRL level.

In patients with acromegaly, surgery yields a higher remission rate compared to medical therapy (67 vs. 45%).[39] In patients with Cushing's disease, the reported remission rate after resection is 73% for microadenomas and 43% for macroadenomas.[86] Patients with residual tumor or persistent hormone hypersecretion after surgical or medical therapy may be treated with radiation. Stereotactic radiosurgery results in faster reduction of hormone secretion with fewer adverse effects compared to conventional radiotherapy; however, radiosurgery cannot be used if the tumor is close to or abutting the optic nerves due to the risk of radiation-induced vision loss. The risk of hypopituitarism after radiation therapy is approximately 20% by 5 years and increases to 80% by 10 to 15 years.[87]

In a meta-analysis, transsphenoidal surgery was associated with low perioperative mortality (< 1%) and complications (< 5%), including CSF leakage, meningitis, new visual field defects, and persistent DI.[40] The rate of new anterior pituitary insufficiency ranged from 7 to 20% in a large survey.[41] Delayed SIADH beginning approximately 5 to 8 days postoperatively occurs in 4 to 12% of patients.[42]

6. **Are there any special circumstances that would lead the surgeon to consider being more proactive?**

The age of the patient, comorbidities, proximity of the tumor to the optic chiasm, planned pregnancy, and patient preference may all influence the decision to perform surgery. Surgery is recommended for patients with tumors abutting the optic chiasm, given the risk of future visual field loss. Women planning pregnancy may elect to have surgery if the tumor is close to the optic chiasm, as physiologic hyperplasia may lead to neurologic decline.[2] Surgery may be considered in the setting of hypopituitarism. Pituitary function may improve postoperatively in up to 30% of patients.[40]

7. **What instructions are given to the patient regarding follow-up? That is, the risks associated with following the lesion.**

Given the risk of tumor growth and pituitary apoplexy, patients should seek immediate neurosurgical evaluation if they experience severe headaches, vision loss, or symptoms of hypopituitarism, particularly nausea, vomiting, loss of appetite, and dizziness, which may be due to acute adrenal insufficiency.

20.3 Key Point Summary

- The majority of PIs are clinically NFPAs.
- An RCC is a common incidental cystic lesion of the pituitary gland. A kidney bean–shaped lesion which is midline, between the anterior and posterior lobes of the pituitary gland, homogeneously bright on T1W images, with a small intracystic nodule is virtually pathognomonic.
- According to the Endocrine Society and AANS/CNS guidelines, PRL and IGF-1 levels should be obtained for all PIs.
- According to the Endocrine Society guidelines, laboratory testing for hypopituitarism should be obtained for macroadenomas and larger microadenomas (6–9 mm).
- Indications for surgical intervention include (1) visual field deficits, (2) neurological abnormalities due to tumor expansion (pituitary apoplexy), and (3) hypersecreting adenomas, except prolactinomas.
- For those who favor active surveillance, recommendations should be guided by tumor size. Note that recommendations for the time interval and future laboratory testing vary by publishing society (see ► Table 20.1).

References

[1] Sanno N, Oyama K, Tahara S, Teramoto A, Kato Y. A survey of pituitary incidentaloma in Japan. Eur J Endocrinol. 2003; 149(2):123–127

[2] Freda PU, Beckers AM, Katznelson L, et al. Endocrine Society. Pituitary incidentaloma: an endocrine society clinical practice guideline. J Clin Endocrinol Metab. 2011; 96(4):894–904

[3] Fleseriu M, Bodach ME, Tumialan LM, et al. Congress of Neurological Surgeons Systematic Review and Evidence-Based Guideline for Pretreatment Endocrine Evaluation of Patients with Nonfunctioning Pituitary Adenomas. Neurosurgery. 2016; 79(4):E527–E529

[4] Paschou SA, Vryonidou A, Goulis DG. Pituitary incidentalomas: a guide to assessment, treatment and follow-up. Maturitas. 2016; 92:143–149

[5] Hoang JK, Hoffman AR, González RG, et al. Management of incidental pituitary findings on CT, MRI, and 18F-fluorodeoxyglucose PET: a white paper of the ACR Incidental Findings Committee. J Am Coll Radiol. 2018; 15(7):966–972

[6] Aghi MK, Chen CC, Fleseriu M, et al. Congress of Neurological Surgeons systematic review and evidence-based guidelines on the management of patients with nonfunctioning pituitary adenomas: executive summary. Neurosurgery 2016;79(4):521–523

[7] Bonneville JF, Bonnevile F, Cattin F, et al, eds. MRI of the Pituitary Gland. New York, NY: Springer; 2016

[8] Ahmadi H, Larsson EM, Jinkins JR. Normal pituitary gland: coronal MR imaging of infundibular tilt. Radiology. 1990; 177(2):389–392

[9] Kulkarni MV, Lee KF, McArdle CB, Yeakley JW, Haar FL. 1.5-T MR imaging of pituitary microadenomas: technical considerations and CT correlation. AJNR Am J Neuroradiol. 1988; 9(1):5–11

[10] Guy RL, Benn JJ, Ayers AB, et al. A comparison of CT and MRI in the assessment of the pituitary and parasellar region. Clin Radiol. 1991; 43(3):156–161

[11] Earnest F, IV, McCullough EC, Frank DA. Fact or artifact: an analysis of artifact in high-resolution computed tomographic scanning of the sella. Radiology. 1981; 140(1):109–113

[12] Sakurai K, Fujita N, Harada K, Kim SW, Nakanishi K, Kozuka T. Magnetic susceptibility artifact in spin-echo MR imaging of the pituitary gland. AJNR Am J Neuroradiol. 1992; 13(5):1301–1308

[13] Hall WA, Luciano MG, Doppman JL, Patronas NJ, Oldfield EH. Pituitary magnetic resonance imaging in normal human volunteers: occult adenomas in the general population. Ann Intern Med. 1994; 120(10):817–820

[14] Ezzat S, Asa SL, Couldwell WT, et al. The prevalence of pituitary adenomas: a systematic review. Cancer. 2004; 101(3):613–619

[15] Chong BW, Kucharczyk W, Singer W, George S. Pituitary gland MR: a comparative study of healthy volunteers and patients with microadenomas. AJNR Am J Neuroradiol. 1994; 15(4):675–679

[16] Teramoto A, Hirakawa K, Sanno N, Osamura Y. Incidental pituitary lesions in 1,000 unselected autopsy specimens. Radiology. 1994; 193(1):161–164

[17] Lee HB, Kim ST, Kim HJ, et al. Usefulness of the dynamic gadolinium-enhanced magnetic resonance imaging with simultaneous acquisition of coronal and sagittal planes for detection of pituitary microadenomas. Eur Radiol. 2012; 22(3):514–518

[18] Gao R, Isoda H, Tanaka T, et al. Dynamic gadolinium-enhanced MR imaging of pituitary adenomas: usefulness of sequential sagittal and coronal plane images. Eur J Radiol. 2001; 39(3):139–146

[19] Bartynski WS, Lin L. Dynamic and conventional spin-echo MR of pituitary microlesions. AJNR Am J Neuroradiol. 1997; 18(5):965–972

[20] Vasilev V, Rostomyan L, Daly AF, et al. Management of endocrine disease: pituitary "incidentaloma"—neuroradiological assessment and differential diagnosis. Eur J Endocrinol. 2016; 175(4):R171–R184

[21] Rumboldt Z. Pituitary adenomas. Top Magn Reson Imaging. 2005; 16(4):277–288

[22] Potts MB, Shah JK, Molinaro AM, et al. Cavernous and inferior petrosal sinus sampling and dynamic magnetic resonance imaging in the preoperative evaluation of Cushing's disease. J Neurooncol. 2014; 116(3):593–600

[23] Tabarin A, Laurent F, Catargi B, et al. Comparative evaluation of conventional and dynamic magnetic resonance imaging of the pituitary gland for the diagnosis of Cushing's disease. Clin Endocrinol (Oxf). 1998; 49(3):293–300

[24] Davis MA, Castillo M. Evaluation of the pituitary gland using magnetic resonance imaging: T1-weighted vs. VIBE imaging. Neuroradiol J. 2013; 26(3):297–300

[25] Grober Y, Grober H, Wintermark M, Jane JA, Jr, Oldfield EH. Comparison of MRI techniques for detecting microadenomas in Cushing's disease. J Neurosurg. 2018; 128(4):1051–1057

[26] Rossi Espagnet MC, Bangiyev L, Haber M, et al. High-resolution DCE-MRI of the pituitary gland using radial k-space acquisition with compressed sensing reconstruction. AJNR Am J Neuroradiol. 2015; 36(8):1444–1449

[27] Yamamoto J, Kakeda S, Shimajiri S, et al. Tumor consistency of pituitary macroadenomas: predictive analysis on the basis of imaging features with contrast-enhanced 3D FIESTA at 3 T. AJNR Am J Neuroradiol. 2014; 35(2):297–303

[28] Osborn AG. Osborn's Brain: Imaging, Pathology, and Anatomy. 1st ed. Salt Lake City, UT: Amirsys Pub.; 2013

[29] Babu R, Back AG, Komisarow JM, Owens TR, Cummings TJ, Britz GW. Symptomatic Rathke's cleft cyst with a co-existing pituitary tumor; Brief review of the literature. Asian J Neurosurg. 2013; 8(4):183–187

[30] Eguchi K, Uozumi T, Arita K, et al. Pituitary function in patients with Rathke's cleft cyst: significance of surgical management. Endocr J. 1994; 41(5):535–540

[31] Park M, Lee SK, Choi J, et al. Differentiation between cystic pituitary adenomas and Rathke cleft cysts: a diagnostic model using MRI. AJNR Am J Neuroradiol. 2015; 36(10):1866–1873

[32] Ramji S, Touska P, Rich P, MacKinnon AD. Normal neuroanatomical variants that may be misinterpreted as disease entities. Clin Radiol. 2017; 72(10):810–825

[33] Bonneville F, Cattin F, Bonneville JF, et al. Rathke's cleft cyst. J Neuroradiol. 2003; 30(4):238–248

[34] Byun WM, Kim OL, Kim D. MR imaging findings of Rathke's cleft cysts: significance of intracystic nodules. AJNR Am J Neuroradiol. 2000; 21(3):485–488

[35] Bonneville F, Chiras J, Cattin F, Bonneville JF. T2 hypointense signal of rathke cleft cyst. AJNR Am J Neuroradiol. 2007; 28(3):397

[36] Katznelson L, Laws ER, Jr, Melmed S, et al. Endocrine Society. Acromegaly: an endocrine society clinical practice guideline. J Clin Endocrinol Metab. 2014; 99(11):3933–3951

[37] Reid TJ, Post KD, Bruce JN, Nabi Kanibir M, Reyes-Vidal CM, Freda PU. Features at diagnosis of 324 patients with acromegaly did not change from 1981 to 2006: acromegaly remains under-recognized and under-diagnosed. Clin Endocrinol (Oxf). 2010; 72(2):203–208

[38] Ramos-Leví AM, Marazuela M. Cardiovascular comorbidities in acromegaly: an update on their diagnosis and management. Endocrine. 2017; 55(2):346–359

[39] Abu Dabrh AM, Mohammed K, Asi N, et al. Surgical interventions and medical treatments in treatment-naïve patients with acromegaly: systematic review and meta-analysis. J Clin Endocrinol Metab. 2014; 99(11):4003–4014

[40] Murad MH, Fernández-Balsells MM, Barwise A, et al. Outcomes of surgical treatment for nonfunctioning pituitary adenomas: a systematic review and meta-analysis. Clin Endocrinol (Oxf). 2010; 73(6):777–791

[41] Ciric I, Ragin A, Baumgartner C, Pierce D. Complications of transsphenoidal surgery: results of a national survey, review of the literature, and personal experience. Neurosurgery. 1997; 40(2):225–236, discussion 236–237

[42] Cote DJ, Alzarea A, Acosta MA, et al. Predictors and rates of delayed symptomatic hyponatremia after transsphenoidal surgery: a systematic review [corrected]. World Neurosurg. 2016; 88:1–6

[43] Knosp E, Steiner E, Kitz K, Matula C. Pituitary adenomas with invasion of the cavernous sinus space: a magnetic resonance imaging classification compared with surgical findings. Neurosurgery. 1993; 33(4):610–617, discussion 617–618

[44] Micko AS, Wöhrer A, Wolfsberger S, Knosp E. Invasion of the cavernous sinus space in pituitary adenomas: endoscopic verification and its correlation with an MRI-based classification. J Neurosurg. 2015; 122(4):803–811

[45] Cattin F, Bonneville F, Andréa I, Barrali E, Bonneville JF. Dural enhancement in pituitary macroadenomas. Neuroradiology. 2000; 42(7):505–508

[46] Young SC, Grossman RI, Goldberg HI, et al. MR of vascular encasement in parasellar masses: comparison with angiography and CT. AJNR Am J Neuroradiol. 1988; 9(1):35–38

[47] Gutenberg A, Larsen J, Lupi I, Rohde V, Caturegli P. A radiologic score to distinguish autoimmune hypophysitis from nonsecreting pituitary adenoma preoperatively. AJNR Am J Neuroradiol. 2009; 30(9):1766–1772

[48] Nakata Y, Sato N, Masumoto T, et al. Parasellar T2 dark sign on MR imaging in patients with lymphocytic hypophysitis. AJNR Am J Neuroradiol. 2010; 31(10):1944–1950

[49] Buurman H, Saeger W. Subclinical adenomas in postmortem pituitaries: classification and correlations to clinical data. Eur J Endocrinol. 2006; 154(5):753–758

[50] Kovacs K, Ryan N, Horvath E, Singer W, Ezrin C. Pituitary adenomas in old age. J Gerontol. 1980; 35(1):16–22

[51] Parent AD, Bebin J, Smith RR. Incidental pituitary adenomas. J Neurosurg. 1981; 54(2):228–231

[52] Molitch ME, Russell EJ. The pituitary "incidentaloma.". Ann Intern Med. 1990; 112(12):925–931

[53] Honegger J, Zimmermann S, Psaras T, et al. Growth modelling of non-functioning pituitary adenomas in patients referred for surgery. Eur J Endocrinol. 2008; 158(3):287–294

[54] Fernández-Balsells MM, Murad MH, Barwise A, et al. Natural history of non-functioning pituitary adenomas and incidentalomas: a systematic review and metaanalysis. J Clin Endocrinol Metab. 2011; 96(4):905–912

[55] Semple PL, Jane JA, Lopes MB, Laws ER. Pituitary apoplexy: correlation between magnetic resonance imaging and histopathological results. J Neurosurg. 2008; 108(5):909–915

[56] Möller-Goede DL, Brändle M, Landau K, Bernays RL, Schmid C. Pituitary apoplexy: re-evaluation of risk factors for bleeding into pituitary adenomas and impact on outcome. Eur J Endocrinol. 2011; 164(1):37–43

[57] Saeger W, Lüdecke DK, Buchfelder M, Fahlbusch R, Quabbe HJ, Petersenn S. Pathohistological classification of pituitary tumors: 10 years of experience with the German Pituitary Tumor Registry. Eur J Endocrinol. 2007; 156(2):203–216

[58] Yamada S, Ohyama K, Taguchi M, et al. A study of the correlation between morphological findings and biological activities in clinically nonfunctioning pituitary adenomas. Neurosurgery. 2007; 61(3):580–584, discussion 584–585

[59] Ioachimescu AG, Eiland L, Chhabra VS, et al. Silent corticotroph adenomas: Emory University cohort and comparison with ACTH-negative nonfunctioning pituitary adenomas. Neurosurgery. 2012; 71(2):296–303, discussion 304

[60] Jahangiri A, Wagner JR, Pekmezci M, et al. A comprehensive long-term retrospective analysis of silent corticotrophic adenomas vs hormone-negative adenomas. Neurosurgery. 2013; 73(1):8–17, discussion 17–18

[61] Langlois F, Lim DST, Varlamov E, et al. Clinical profile of silent growth hormone pituitary adenomas; higher recurrence rate compared to silent gonadotroph pituitary tumors, a large single center experience. Endocrine. 2017; 58(3):528–534

[62] Righi A, Faustini-Fustini M, Morandi L, et al. The changing faces of corticotroph cell adenomas: the role of prohormone convertase 1/3. Endocrine. 2017; 56(2):286–297

[63] Daems T, Verhelst J, Michotte A, Abrams P, De Ridder D, Abs R. Modification of hormonal secretion in clinically silent pituitary adenomas. Pituitary. 2009; 12(1):80–86

[64] Ciccarelli A, Daly AF, Beckers A. The epidemiology of prolactinomas. Pituitary. 2005; 8(1):3–6

[65] Toini A, Dolci A, Ferrante E, et al. Screening for ACTH-dependent hypercortisolism in patients affected with pituitary incidentaloma. Eur J Endocrinol. 2015; 172(4):363–369

[66] Tamada D, Kitamura T, Otsuki M, Oshino S, Saitoh Y, Shimomura I. Clinical significance of screening for subclinical Cushing's disease in patients with pituitary tumors. Endocr J. 2016; 63(1):47–52

[67] Nachtigall L, Delgado A, Swearingen B, Lee H, Zerikly R, Klibanski A. Changing patterns in diagnosis and therapy of acromegaly over two decades. J Clin Endocrinol Metab. 2008; 93(6):2035–2041

[68] Hong JW, Lee MK, Kim SH, Lee EJ. Discrimination of prolactinoma from hyperprolactinemic non-functioning adenoma. Endocrine. 2010; 37(1):140–147

[69] Pinzone JJ, Katznelson L, Danila DC, Pauler DK, Miller CS, Klibanski A. Primary medical therapy of micro- and macroprolactinomas in men. J Clin Endocrinol Metab. 2000; 85(9):3053–3057

[70] Nieman LK, Biller BM, Findling JW, et al. The diagnosis of Cushing's syndrome: an Endocrine Society Clinical Practice Guideline. J Clin Endocrinol Metab. 2008; 93(5):1526–1540

[71] Guttenberg KB, Mayson SE, Sawan C, et al. Prevalence of clinically silent corticotroph macroadenomas. Clin Endocrinol (Oxf). 2016; 85(6):874–880

[72] Tateno T, Izumiyama H, Doi M, Akashi T, Ohno K, Hirata Y. Defective expression of prohormone convertase 1/3 in silent corticotroph adenoma. Endocr J. 2007; 54(5):777–782

[73] Matsuno A, Okazaki R, Oki Y, Nagashima T. Secretion of high-molecular-weight adrenocorticotropic hormone from a pituitary adenoma in a patient without Cushing stigmata. Case report. J Neurosurg. 2004; 101(5):874–877

[74] Webb SM, Rigla M, Wägner A, Oliver B, Bartumeus F. Recovery of hypopituitarism after neurosurgical treatment of pituitary adenomas. J Clin Endocrinol Metab. 1999; 84(10):3696–3700

[75] Drange MR, Fram NR, Herman-Bonert V, Melmed S. Pituitary tumor registry: a novel clinical resource. J Clin Endocrinol Metab. 2000; 85(1):168–174

[76] Nomikos P, Ladar C, Fahlbusch R, Buchfelder M. Impact of primary surgery on pituitary function in patients with non-functioning pituitary adenomas: a study on 721 patients. Acta Neurochir (Wien). 2004; 146(1):27–35

[77] Del Monte P, Foppiani L, Ruelle A, et al. Clinically non-functioning pituitary macroadenomas in the elderly. Aging Clin Exp Res. 2007; 19(1):34–40

[78] Fatemi N, Dusick JR, Mattozo C, et al. Pituitary hormonal loss and recovery after transsphenoidal adenoma removal. Neurosurgery. 2008; 63(4):709–718, discussion 718–719

[79] Berkmann S, Fandino J, Müller B, Kothbauer KF, Henzen C, Landolt H. Pituitary surgery: experience from a large network in Central Switzerland. Swiss Med Wkly. 2012; 142:w13680

[80] Yuen KC, Cook DM, Sahasranam P, et al. Prevalence of GH and other anterior pituitary hormone deficiencies in adults with nonsecreting pituitary microadenomas and normal serum IGF-1 levels. Clin Endocrinol (Oxf). 2008; 69(2):292–298

[81] Imran SA, Yip CE, Papneja N, et al. Analysis and natural history of pituitary incidentalomas. Eur J Endocrinol. 2016; 175(1):1–9

[82] Fleseriu M, Hashim IA, Karavitaki N, et al. Hormonal replacement in hypopituitarism in adults: an Endocrine Society clinical practice guideline. J Clin Endocrinol Metab. 2016; 101(11):3888–3921

[83] Melmed S, Casanueva FF, Hoffman AR, et al. Endocrine Society. Diagnosis and treatment of hyperprolactinemia: an Endocrine Society clinical practice guideline. J Clin Endocrinol Metab. 2011; 96(2):273–288

[84] Biswas M, Smith J, Jadon D, et al. Long-term remission following withdrawal of dopamine agonist therapy in subjects with microprolactinomas. Clin Endocrinol (Oxf). 2005; 63(1):26–31

[85] Kharlip J, Salvatori R, Yenokyan G, Wand GS. Recurrence of hyperprolactinemia after withdrawal of long-term cabergoline therapy. J Clin Endocrinol Metab. 2009; 94(7):2428–2436

[86] Alexandraki KI, Kaltsas GA, Isidori AM, et al. Long-term remission and recurrence rates in Cushing's disease: predictive factors in a single-centre study. Eur J Endocrinol. 2013; 168(4):639–648

[87] Loeffler JS, Shih HA. Radiation therapy in the management of pituitary adenomas. J Clin Endocrinol Metab. 2011; 96(7):1992–2003

21 Pituitary Gland: Diffuse Enlargement

Saint-Aaron L. Morris, Kaye D. Westmark, Spiros L. Blackburn, and Katie B. Guttenberg

21.1 Introduction

Unlike pituitary micro- and macroadenomas, there are no well-established guidelines for the evaluation of an incidentally detected, diffusely enlarged pituitary gland. Consideration of the age and sex of the patient is a key factor in determining the differential diagnosis and deciding whether any further investigation is warranted. In this chapter, we will discuss the normal appearance of the pituitary gland and the most common underlying conditions that are associated with diffuse enlargement.

21.2 Case Presentation

21.2.1 History

A 29-year-old woman presented with headaches. Dedicated pituitary images were performed for "prominence of the pituitary gland" detected on a routine brain MRI (▶ Fig. 21.1).

21.3 Imaging Analysis

21.3.1 Imaging Findings and Impression

The pituitary gland appears mildly enlarged and homogeneously enhancing, measuring 11 mm in height × 10 mm in transverse dimension. No focal area of heterogeneity is seen on the T1- or T2 W images. It is convex superiorly where it contacts but does not compress the optic chiasm. The gland is symmetric and the stalk midline. The cavernous sinuses are normal (▶ Fig. 21.2).

Incidentally detected, mild pituitary enlargement that is homogenous and symmetric most often represents physiologic hyperplasia or secondary pituitary hypertrophy. Convexity of the superior aspect of the gland is normal in peripubescent females but atypical for a 29-year-old woman. Considerations include pregnancy as well as other causes of physiologic hyperplasia and secondary hypertrophy.

21.3.2 Additional Imaging Recommended

None. Clinical correlation is needed.

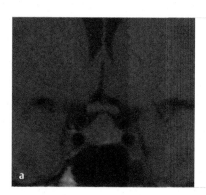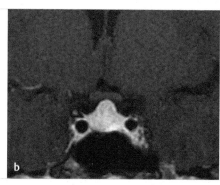

Fig. 21.1 MRI of the sella: coronal T1-weighted (T1W) (a) pre- and (b) postcontrast images.

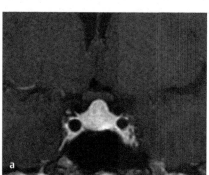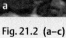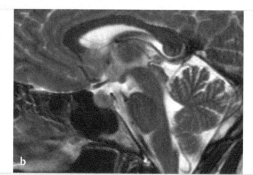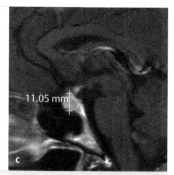

Fig. 21.2 (a–c)

21.4 Clinical Evaluation

21.4.1 Endocrinologist Evaluation

This is a 29-year-old woman who presents with an incidentally detected, enlarged pituitary gland. She denies galactorrhea or breast tenderness. Menses are regular. There is no fatigue, constipation, dry skin, nausea, or loss of appetite. She denies polydipsia or nocturia.

The physical examination is unremarkable.

21.4.2 Recommended Laboratory Testing and Results

- Pregnancy test: negative.
- PRL: 28.2 ng/mL (3–30 ng/mL).
- Thyroid-stimulating hormone (TSH): 0.6 mIU/L (0.5–5.0 mIU/L).
- Free T4: 1.4 ng/dL (0.8–1.8 ng/dL).

21.4.3 Clinical Impression

This is a well-appearing woman without signs or symptoms of hormonal dysfunction. It was important to exclude pregnancy, which would be the most common cause of this finding. In this asymptomatic patient, this mildly enlarged gland is most likely a normal variant of physiologic hyperplasia. A follow-up MR was performed 5 months later and showed a completely stable appearance of the pituitary gland.

21.4.4 Recommendations

No further testing was recommended.

21.5 Differential Diagnosis of Diffuse Enlargement of the Pituitary Gland

Common

- True physiologic hyperplasia:
  - In the female, normal physiologic change during puberty may cause the superior aspect of the gland to become convex. Pregnancy should also be considered during which pituitary volume increases due to lactotroph and gonadotroph hyperplasia. Milder enlargement due to gonadotroph hyperplasia may occur during the perimenopausal period due to estrogen deficiency.
- Pathological hyperplasia:
  - This is most commonly secondary to end organ failure, specifically hypothyroidism or hypogonadism.
- Macroadenoma/microadenoma:
  - Rarely, the lesion may be of similar signal intensity to the normal gland with homogeneous enhancement, making the tumor difficult to detect as a separate entity.

Uncommon

- Congenitally small sella:
  - If the sella is congenitally small, the gland may bulge superiorly but not actually be increased in volume.

- Tortuous cavernous carotid arteries:
  - If the cavernous carotids are tortuous and converge medially, they may cause the gland to project superiorly but not be increased in overall volume.

Uncommon Causes in Which the Pituitary Enlargement Is a Nonincidental, Important Finding

- Cerebrospinal fluid (CSF) hypotension.
- Lymphocytic hypophysitis.
- Langerhans cell histiocytosis (LCH).
- Neurosarcoidosis.
- Pituicytoma.
- Lymphoma/leukemia.
- Metastatic disease.

21.6 Clinical and Diagnostic Imaging Pearls

Know What Is Normal

- Prepuberty: ≤ 6 mm.
- Postmenopausal females and males: ≤ 8 mm.
- Premenopausal females: ≤ 9 mm.
- In females during puberty, the superior margin of the gland may become convex.
- The gland enlarges throughout pregnancy and may rarely reach 12 to 15 mm in height but usually does not exceed 10 to 11 mm.

Correlate Clinically

- A peripartum female who is asymptomatic with a diffusely enlarged gland most likely has normal physiologic hypertrophy.
- Pregnancy should always be considered in a female with a diffusely enlarged gland.
- A diffusely enlarged gland in a male child is most likely due to pituitary hyperplasia resulting from end organ failure (i.e., hypothyroidism) as pituitary adenomas are rare in this population.
- A peripartum female, or patient on immune therapy for malignancy and/or with a history of autoimmune disorders (i.e., thyroiditis) who is not asymptomatic but has headaches and visual complaints and confusion secondary to low serum sodium, may have lymphocytic hypophysitis. MR in these patients often reveals diffuse enlargement of the pituitary gland, loss of the normal posterior pituitary bright spot, and thickening of the stalk. Associated clinical abnormalities include adrenal insufficiency, diabetes insipidus, prolactin (PRL) elevation, and hypopituitarism.
- If a patient is symptomatic with postural headaches, consider CSF hypotension. Important additional findings on MR may include tonsillar ectopia, distended dural sinuses, enhancing subdural "collections," decreased CSF cisterns about the brainstem, and anteroposterior elongation of the midbrain.

21.7 Companion Cases

21.7.1 Companion Case 1

Case Presentation

History

The patient is a 42-year-old woman with a possible pituitary lesion seen on routine brain MR for headaches.

Imaging Analysis

MRI Findings

On the dedicated pituitary protocol MR performed for further evaluation, an ill-defined "lesion" was called on the postcontrast sagittal T1 W images, which could not be confirmed on the coronal pre- or postcontrast T1 W nor the T2 W images. Note is made of the normal midline position of the pituitary stalk and overall normal shape and size of the gland without expansion of the sellar floor.

A follow-up MR was recommended.

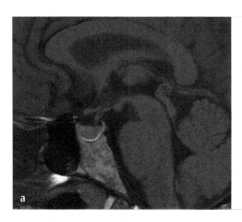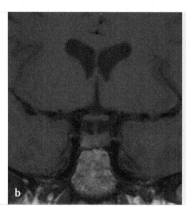

Fig. 21.3 (a, b) Sella MRI: sagittal and coronal noncontrast T1 W images.

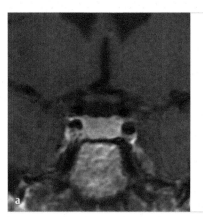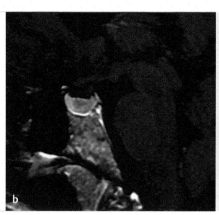

Fig. 21.4 (a, b) Postcontrast coronal and sagittal T1 W images.

Follow-up MRI

The recommended 1-year follow-up MR for the "possible incidental microadenoma" is shown in ▸ Fig. 21.5.

Follow-up MRI Findings and Impression

There has been interval enlargement of the pituitary gland, which remains homogeneous without a discrete lesion. The stalk is midline and the cavernous sinuses are normal. The previously identified "incidental pituitary microadenoma" is no longer seen and was probably not a true abnormality but rather mild heterogeneity in the enhancement of the gland, the appearance of which can be accentuated by technical factors such as narrowing the display window or by dynamic imaging after the administration of contrast.

This interval development of diffuse enlargement of the pituitary gland in a 43-year-old woman is of uncertain significance; clinical correlation will be needed. The patient reported prior to the MR that she was not pregnant, which was verified by subsequent testing.

Clinical Evaluation

Endocrinology Evaluation

This is a 43-year-old woman who initially presented for evaluation of a possible pituitary microadenoma. Her medical history includes hypothyroidism, which was diagnosed 10 years ago.

Initial Testing Performed for Possible "Microadenoma" 1 Year Ago When Patient Was Asymptomatic

- PRL: 23.2 ng/mL (4.8–23.3 ng/mL).
- Insulin-like growth factor 1 (IGF-1): 125 ng/mL (98–261 ng/mL).

- TSH: 2.3 mIU/L (0.5–5.0 mIU/L).
- Free T4: 1.2 ng/dL (0.8–1.8 ng/dL).

One-year Follow-up Evaluation

Since the prior evaluation, she reports new constipation and fatigue. Physical examination is notable for dry skin and slightly delayed relaxation of deep tendon reflexes in her upper and lower extremities.

Additional Testing Results:

- Pregnancy test: negative.
- TSH: 214 mIU/L (0.5–5.0 mIU/L).
- Free T4: 0.5 ng/dL (0.8–1.8 ng/dL).
- Cortisol: 14.5 μg/dL (5–25 μg/dL).

Clinical Diagnosis

Hypothyroidism with secondary hypertrophy of the pituitary gland.

There is no evidence of a microadenoma, which was most likely an "overcall" on the prior study and due to normal heterogeneity in enhancement of the gland.

Impression and Management

The initial presentation demonstrates the limits of MR specificity for small microadenomas and therefore the importance of clinical correlation. The follow-up imaging provided a fortuitous MR image of diffuse hypertrophy of the gland secondary to interval development of hypothyroidism in this patient. The patient began daily oral thyroid hormone supplementation.

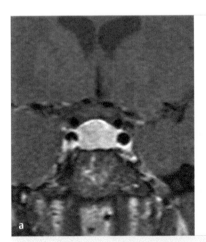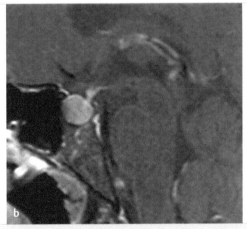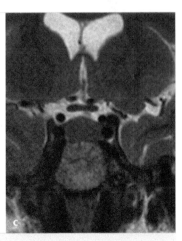

Fig. 21.5 (a) Coronal and (b) sagittal postcontrast T1 W images and (c) coronal T2 W image.

21.7.2 Companion Case 2

Case Presentation

History

This is a 72-year-old woman with a history of melanoma who presents with headache and fatigue.

Imaging Analysis

Imaging Findings

The gland appears slightly enlarged for a 72-year-old woman with a convex superior border. The pituitary stalk is abnormally thickened but remains midline. Diffuse enlargement of the gland in this patient with primary melanoma is of uncertain significance. Considerations include hypertrophy due to "end organ failure" (i.e., hypothyroidism), hypophysitis and, less likely, metastatic disease. Clinical correlation is recommended.

Clinical Evaluation

Endocrinologist Evaluation

This is a 72-year-old woman who was recently diagnosed with metastatic melanoma. Immunotherapy was initiated 3 months ago with the anti-CTLA-4 antibody, ipilimumab. She reports new headache, fatigue, and nausea for the last month. There is no polydipsia or polyuria.

Physical Examination

Her blood pressure is 98/65 mm Hg and pulse rate is 92 bpm. She appears cachectic.

Testing Results

- Sodium: 135 mEq/L (135–145 mEq/L).
- TSH: 0.9 mIU/L (0.5–5.0 mIU/L).
- Free T4: 0.3 ng/dL (0.8–1.8 ng/dL).
- Adrenocorticotropic hormone (ACTH): 8 pg/mL (10–60 pg/mL).
- Cortisol: 2.2 µg/dL (5–25 µg/dL).
- PRL: 3.1 ng/mL (2–20 ng/mL).

Clinical Findings and Diagnosis

Ipilimumab-induced hypophysitis (IH) presenting with headache and hypopituitarism.

Her low free T4 in association with an inappropriately normal TSH confirms a diagnosis of central hypothyroidism. Similarly, her low cortisol level in association with a low ACTH confirms central adrenal insufficiency. She was subsequently started on thyroid hormone replacement and high-dose glucocorticoid therapy.

Diffuse enlargement of the pituitary gland in this case was clearly not an incidental finding but is included to demonstrate a case of hypophysitis. The most common form of hypophysitis is lymphocytic hypophysitis, which often occurs during pregnancy or postpartum. In addition, hypophysitis is a known complication of immunotherapy.

Hypophysitis is an important cause of diffuse enlargement of the pituitary gland, which is often accompanied by a prominently enhancing and thickened stalk. In immunotherapy-induced hypophysitis, pituitary gland enlargement is typically mild, whereas in lymphocytic hypophysitis, patients may develop severe pituitary hyperplasia, frequently resulting in visual abnormalities.

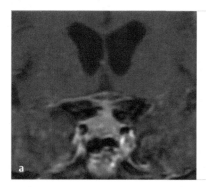 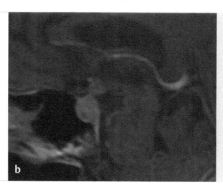

Fig. 21.6 (a) Coronal and **(b)** sagittal T1 W images postcontrast.

21.7.3 Companion Case 3

Case Presentation

History

A 13-year-old adolescent girl with history of a ventriculoperitoneal shunt and headaches.

Imaging Analysis

Imaging Findings

There is evidence of mild tonsillar descent and a prominent appearing pituitary gland. However, the actual size of the gland measures only 8 × 6 mm, which is within normal limits. The CT scan confirms that the bony sella is congenitally shallow.

Imaging Diagnosis

Mild intracranial hypotension in combination with a congenitally small sella leading to prominence of the pituitary gland.

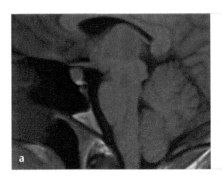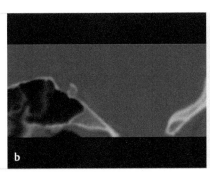

Fig. 21.7 (a) Sagittal T1 W noncontrast image. **(b)** CT scan sagittal midline reformation.

21.8 Neurosurgery and Endocrinology Questions and Answers

1. **What are the most common causes of diffuse enlargement of the pituitary gland?**

   Pituitary gland enlargement may be due to physiologic changes or, less commonly, end organ insufficiency. Physiologic hyperplasia occurs in women during pregnancy, peripubescence, and perimenopause. The gland increases in volume throughout pregnancy but usually does not exceed 10 to 11 mm in height. Maximum height of the gland is reached in the immediate postpartum period when it rarely may enlarge up to 12 to 15 mm. Gland size, shape, and volume return to normal within 6 months postpartum.[1,2,3] The pituitary typically appears enlarged in peripubescent females with a frequently convex superior margin and in perimenopausal women due to declining ovarian function.[4,5] Incidentally detected pituitary hyperplasia in postmenopausal women or men should prompt further evaluation.

   Pathologic hyperplasia most commonly occurs in long-standing primary hypothyroidism due to loss of negative feedback inhibition on thyrotropin-releasing hormone. This response is typically reversible with the initiation of thyroid replacement hormone.[6] Although less common, gonadotroph and corticotroph hyperplasia have been described in patients with long-standing primary hypogonadism and primary adrenal insufficiency, respectively.[7,8]

2. **Will oral contraceptives increase the size of the pituitary gland on MR and is there an increased risk of pituitary adenoma?**

   No, oral contraceptives have not been shown to cause pituitary hyperplasia or an increase in the incidence of pituitary adenomas.[9]

3. **What labs should be performed and in which patient demographic(s) that present with diffuse enlargement?**

   There are no established guidelines for the evaluation of pituitary hyperplasia. Laboratory testing should be guided by the clinical scenario.

   - In the first case, a young well-appearing woman was found to have pituitary gland enlargement during the evaluation of headaches. Clinical evaluation did not reveal any evidence of hormonal dysfunction. Thyroid function tests were obtained to exclude the possibility of pathologic hyperplasia due to primary hypothyroidism.[6] Patients with lymphocytic hypophysitis often present with headache. However, there was no evidence of hypopituitarism, diabetes insipidus, or hyperprolactinemia to support a diagnosis of lymphocytic hypophysitis in this case.[10] Ultimately, her pituitary gland enlargement was considered a normal variant of physiologic hyperplasia.
   - In the second case, a woman with untreated hypothyroidism was found to have pathologic hyperplasia. Patients may develop new anterior pituitary hormone deficiencies as a result of the hyperplasia.[11] A serum cortisol was

   obtained to confirm normal adrenal function before restarting thyroid replacement hormone.
   - In the final case, a woman with metastatic melanoma was diagnosed with IH. Pituitary gland enlargement is often mild, and a thickened pituitary stalk is found in some patients. Most patients present with headache and evidence of hypopituitarism. In contrast to lymphocytic hypophysitis, which also causes diffuse enlargement of the gland, diabetes insipidus and hyperprolactinemia are rare in patients with IH.[12,13]

4. **It is known that many medications can cause PRL increase. What are the most common culprits? Is the gland enlarged on MR when PRL increase is medication related?**

   The medications that most commonly cause hyperprolactinemia include antipsychotic medications, metoclopramide, verapamil, and some antidepressant medications (▶ Table 21.1).[14,15,16,17,18] PRL levels are typically less than 100 ng/mL. In patients taking phenothiazines, risperidone and metoclopramide PRL levels may exceed 200 ng/mL.[14,19,20] Typical antipsychotic medications cause mild pituitary gland enlargement.[21]

5. **If no cause is found for the apparent pituitary enlargement, is imaging follow-up recommended and, if so, at what interval?**

   Unlike pituitary micro- and macroadenomas, there are no well-established guidelines for radiographic surveillance. If ascribed to puberty in a young female, follow-up imaging is not indicated. Though exceedingly rare, pituitary apoplexy

Table 21.1 Medications that most commonly cause hyperprolactinemia

Medication	Prevalence of hyperprolactinemia
Typical antipsychotics (e.g., phenothiazines, butyrophenones)	38–47%[14,15]
Atypical antipsychotics	
• Risperidone	81–97%[14,15]
• Olanzapine	35%[15]
• Ziprasidone	29%[15]
• Clozapine	19%[14]
Metoclopramide	>50%[16,17]
Verapamil	8.5%[18]
Tricyclic antidepressants	
• Clomipramine	60–87.5%[17]
• Amitriptyline	14%[17]
• Desipramine	Rare[17]
Selective serotonin reuptake inhibitors (SSRI)	Rare[17]
Monoamine oxidase (MAO) inhibitors	Rare[17]

may occur during pregnancy due to physiologic hyperplasia. Urgent MR without gadolinium and hormonal evaluation is recommended during pregnancy if the patient develops neurologic symptoms.[22] If the gland is truly enlarged and no focal lesion is seen and yet there is no obvious etiology for the enlargement, neither physiologic nor pathologic, a follow-up MR should be obtained in 6 months with dynamic contrast administration to evaluate for the possibility of an isointense pituitary macroadenoma.

6. **In patients with pituitary hyperplasia, what is the risk of transformation to pituitary adenoma? If there is such a risk, are nulliparous women at lower risk of developing a pituitary adenoma than multiparous ones?**
Pituitary adenomas are unlikely to form in patients with pituitary hyperplasia as there is no increased incidence of prolactinomas in multiparous women.[23] Nevertheless, pituitary adenomas have been identified in a small number of patients with pituitary hyperplasia due to both hormonal hyposecretion (e.g., primary hypogonadism) and hypersecretion (e.g., ectopic corticotropin-releasing hormone).[7,24]

7. **Lymphocytic hypophysitis is a well-known cause of diffuse, symmetric enlargement of the pituitary gland that most often occurs in post-/peripartum patients. What is the range of clinical presentations? How is this entity pathologically distinct from the normal physiologic hyperplasia of the pituitary that routinely occurs in post-/peripartum women?**
Lymphocytic hypophysitis is characterized by autoimmune infiltration of the pituitary gland and has been classified based on the area affected, including lymphocytic adenohypophysitis (LAH), lymphocytic infundibulneurohypophysitis (LINH) and lymphocytic panhypophysitis (LPH). Clinical presentation is variable and includes symptoms related to mass effect, hypopituitarism, diabetes insipidus, and hyperprolactinemia. LAH commonly occurs during pregnancy or postpartum. The most common presenting symptoms are headache, visual disturbances, and hypopituitarism. Hypopituitarism is often disproportionate to the degree of pituitary enlargement. ACTH dysfunction is most common, followed by TSH, gonadotropin, and PRL deficiency. In contrast, polydipsia and polyuria are the most common presenting symptoms in patients with LINH and LPH.[10]

Although lymphocytic hypophysitis is in the neuroradiologist's differential diagnosis for diffuse enlargement of the pituitary gland, especially in the peripartum period, it does not present as an incidental finding. Typical MRI findings described in patients diagnosed with lymphocytic hypophysitis include loss of the posterior pituitary bright spot as well as diffuse, symmetric enlargement of the gland and a thickened pituitary stalk, both of which are enhancing prominently relative to the cavernous sinus.[25] On the T2W images, a rim of decreased signal about the periphery of the enlarged gland and within the cavernous sinus has also been described.[26]

Immunotherapeutic agents are an increasingly recognized cause of hypophysitis. Hypophysitis occurs in 10 to 15% of patients treated with ipilimumab, the first of these agents to be approved for the treatment of metastatic melanoma.[13,27,28] Hypophysitis appears to be a rare event in patients treated

with newer agents, including pembrolizumab, nivolumab, and atezolizumab. Patients typically present with headache and symptoms related to anterior pituitary deficiencies. Pituitary enlargement is typically mild, resulting in a lower rate of visual abnormalities compared to lymphocytic hypophysitis.[12] Glucocorticoids are recommended as initial therapy if hypophysitis is suspected based on clinical and radiographic evaluation.[10,12] Other immunosuppressive medications (e.g., azathioprine and methotrexate) have been used in patients with lymphocytic hypophysitis who did not respond to glucocorticoids.[29,30] Transsphenoidal surgery should be pursued in the setting of severe visual abnormalities and if symptoms persist despite medical management.[10]

21.9 Key Point Summary

- The most common cause of diffuse enlargement of the pituitary gland is physiologic hypertrophy: pregnancy, peripubescence in a young female, and perimenopause are most common.
- A diffusely enlarged gland in a male patient is not normal. End organ failure, most commonly hypothyroidism, should be considered.

References

[1] Elster AD, Sanders TG, Vines FS, Chen MY. Size and shape of the pituitary gland during pregnancy and post partum: measurement with MR imaging. Radiology. 1991; 181(2):531–535
[2] Dinç H, Esen F, Demirci A, Sari A, Resit Gümele H. Pituitary dimensions and volume measurements in pregnancy and post partum. MR assessment. Acta Radiol. 1998; 39(1):64–69
[3] Osborn AG. Osborn's Brain: Imaging, Pathology, and anatomy. 1st ed. Salt Lake City, UT: Amirsys Pub.; 2013
[4] Elster AD, Chen MY, Williams DW, III, Key LL. Pituitary gland: MR imaging of physiologic hypertrophy in adolescence. Radiology. 1990; 174(3 Pt 1):681–685
[5] Tsunoda A, Okuda O, Sato K. MR height of the pituitary gland as a function of age and sex: especially physiological hypertrophy in adolescence and in climacterium. AJNR Am J Neuroradiol. 1997; 18(3):551–554
[6] Joshi AS, Woolf PD. Pituitary hyperplasia secondary to primary hypothyroidism: a case report and review of the literature. Pituitary. 2005; 8(2):99–103
[7] Scheithauer BW, Moschopulos M, Kovacs K, Jhaveri BS, Percek T, Lloyd RV. The pituitary in klinefelter syndrome. Endocr Pathol. 2005; 16(2):133–138
[8] Zhou J, Ruan L, Li H, Wang Q, Zheng F, Wu F. Addison's disease with pituitary hyperplasia: a case report and review of the literature. Endocrine. 2009; 35(3): 285–289
[9] Wingrave SJ, Kay CR, Vessey MP. Oral contraceptives and pituitary adenomas. BMJ. 1980; 280(6215):685–686
[10] Caturegli P, Newschaffer C, Olivi A, Pomper MG, Burger PC, Rose NR. Autoimmune hypophysitis. Endocr Rev. 2005; 26(5):599–614
[11] Neves CP, Massolt ET, Peeters RP, Neggers SJ, de Herder WW. Pituitary hyperplasia: an uncommon presentation of a common disease. Endocrinol Diabetes Metab Case Rep. 2015; 2015:150056
[12] Faje A. Immunotherapy and hypophysitis: clinical presentation, treatment, and biologic insights. Pituitary. 2016; 19(1):82–92
[13] Faje AT, Sullivan R, Lawrence D, et al. Ipilimumab-induced hypophysitis: a detailed longitudinal analysis in a large cohort of patients with metastatic melanoma. J Clin Endocrinol Metab. 2014; 99(11):4078–4085
[14] Kearns AE, Goff DC, Hayden DL, Daniels GH. Risperidone-associated hyperprolactinemia. Endocr Pract. 2000; 6(6):425–429
[15] Johnsen E, Kroken RA, Abaza M, Olberg H, Jørgensen HA. Antipsychotic-induced hyperprolactinemia: a cross-sectional survey. J Clin Psychopharmacol. 2008; 28(6):686–690
[16] Aono T, Shioji T, Kinugasa T, Onishi T, Kurachi K. Clinical and endocrinological analyses of patients with galactorrhea and menstrual disorders due to sulpiride or metoclopramide. J Clin Endocrinol Metab. 1978; 47(3):675–680
[17] Molitch ME. Drugs and prolactin. Pituitary. 2008; 11(2):209–218

[18] Romeo JH, Dombrowski R, Kwak YS, Fuehrer S, Aron DC. Hyperprolactinaemia and verapamil: prevalence and potential association with hypogonadism in men. Clin Endocrinol (Oxf). 1996; 45(5):571–575

[19] Melmed S, Casanueva FF, Hoffman AR, et al. Endocrine Society. Diagnosis and treatment of hyperprolactinemia: an Endocrine Society clinical practice guideline. J Clin Endocrinol Metab. 2011; 96(2):273–288

[20] Pollock A, McLaren EH. Serum prolactin concentration in patients taking neuroleptic drugs. Clin Endocrinol (Oxf). 1998; 49(4):513–516

[21] Pariante CM, Dazzan P, Danese A, et al. Increased pituitary volume in antipsychotic-free and antipsychotic-treated patients of the AEsop first-onset psychosis study. Neuropsychopharmacology. 2005; 30(10):1923–1931

[22] Grand'Maison S, Weber F, Bédard MJ, Mahone M, Godbout A. Pituitary apoplexy in pregnancy: a case series and literature review. Obstet Med. 2015; 8(4):177–183

[23] Coogan PF, Baron JA, Lambe M. Parity and pituitary adenoma risk. J Natl Cancer Inst. 1995; 87(18):1410–1411

[24] Puchner MJ, Lüdecke DK, Valdueza JM, et al. Cushing's disease in a child caused by a corticotropin-releasing hormone-secreting intrasellar gangliocytoma associated with an adrenocorticotropic hormone-secreting pituitary adenoma. Neurosurgery. 1993; 33(5):920–924, discussion 924–925

[25] Gutenberg A, Larsen J, Lupi I, Rohde V, Caturegli P. A radiologic score to distinguish autoimmune hypophysitis from nonsecreting pituitary adenoma preoperatively. AJNR Am J Neuroradiol. 2009; 30(9):1766–1772

[26] Nakata Y, Sato N, Masumoto T, et al. Parasellar T2 dark sign on MR imaging in patients with lymphocytic hypophysitis. AJNR Am J Neuroradiol. 2010; 31(10):1944–1950

[27] Albarel F, Gaudy C, Castinetti F, et al. Long-term follow-up of ipilimumab-induced hypophysitis, a common adverse event of the anti-CTLA-4 antibody in melanoma. Eur J Endocrinol. 2015; 172(2):195–204

[28] Min L, Hodi FS, Giobbie-Hurder A, et al. Systemic high-dose corticosteroid treatment does not improve the outcome of ipilimumab-related hypophysitis: a retrospective cohort study. Clin Cancer Res. 2015; 21(4):749–755

[29] Lecube A, Francisco G, Rodríguez D, et al. Lymphocytic hypophysitis successfully treated with azathioprine: first case report. J Neurol Neurosurg Psychiatry. 2003; 74(11):1581–1583

[30] Tubridy N, Saunders D, Thom M, et al. Infundibulohypophysitis in a man presenting with diabetes insipidus and cavernous sinus involvement. J Neurol Neurosurg Psychiatry. 2001; 71(6):798–801

22 Incidental Glial Neoplasms

Keith Kerr, Nitin Tandon, Raul F. Valenzuela, and Yoshua Esquenazi

22.1 Introduction

The widespread availability of MR imaging has led to an increase in discovery of incidental gliomas. Historically, the "watch-and-wait" approach was used for incidentally detected lesions suspected to be low-grade gliomas (LGGs). It is now known that, although slow growing, these tumors often progress to high-grade malignancies. Improved microsurgical techniques for tumor resection coupled with multiple techniques for functional preservation, and a better understanding of how tumor genotype influences the natural history, have led to a paradigm shift in the management of these incidental lesions. The evidence strongly favors an early, more aggressive, function-preserving resection coupled with adjuvant chemoradiation.

In this chapter, we present the radiographic findings and management of two cases of diffuse gliomas that presented incidentally. We start with the radiographic analysis and include conventional imaging pearls that help distinguish among the different entities within the differential diagnosis. We discuss advanced brain tumor imaging techniques like diffusion tensor imaging (DTI)/tractography, perfusion and arterial spin label imaging, and MR spectroscopy, and show how they assist with preoperative diagnosis and surgical planning. Finally, we review clinical and imaging correlates of the 2016 WHO update on brain tumors, which has fundamentally altered the classification of infiltrating gliomas in adults.

22.2 Case Presentation

22.2.1 History and Physical Examination

A 54-year-old man presents to the emergency room (ER) after a fall with minor superficial facial lacerations but no loss of consciousness (▶ Fig. 22.1). The ER physician found the patient was afebrile and the neurologic examination was unremarkable. A noncontrast head CT was performed.

22.2.2 Imaging Findings and Impression

There is an area of mass effect and low attenuation in the white matter of the inferior frontal gyrus (*arrow* in ▶ Fig. 22.1) and the anterior aspect of the insula (*arrowhead* in ▶ Fig. 22.1). Notably, the cortical gray matter remains normal in attenuation. This pattern of attenuation, which involves the white matter and spares the cortex, is compatible with vasogenic edema which is more suggestive of a tumor than a stroke, contusion, or encephalitis. Furthermore, the history of lack of symptoms and fever is helpful in clinically excluding an encephalitis or an acute cerebrovascular event.

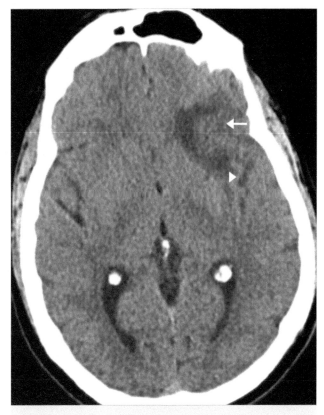

Fig. 22.1

22.2.3 Additional Imaging

MRI of the brain with and without contrast. The fluid-attenuated inversion recovery (FLAIR) sequence (▶ Fig. 22.2a) reveals a hyperintense mass involving primarily the cortex of the pars opercularis of the frontal operculum of the inferior frontal gyrus and the anterior most aspect of the insular cortex, the short gyrus, that is fairly well defined. There is minimal mass effect upon the left basal ganglia, which otherwise appears normal. Postcontrast (▶ Fig. 22.2b), there is minimal enhancement in the region of the insula (*arrow*). There was no evidence of restriction on diffusion-weighted images or of susceptibility on the susceptibility-weighted image (not shown).

22.3 Clinical Evaluation

Neurosurgery was consulted while the patient was in the ER. Given the patient's lack of fever or any other significant symptoms, contusion, an infectious process, or acute venous infarction were considered unlikely.

Additional testing needed and results: None.

22.3.1 Clinical Impression and Management

Incidentally detected mass is most likely a primary brain tumor. The patient underwent an awake craniotomy for resection with speech mapping.

Final pathology revealed *anaplastic oligodendroglioma, isocitrate dehydrogenase (IDH) mutant, 1p/19q-codeleted, WHO grade III.*

22.4 Differential Diagnosis (▶ Table 22.1)

- **Primary brain tumor, diffuse "low-grade" glioma**:
  - Abnormal signal and subtle mass effect involving cortical gray matter and underlying white matter with neither significant enhancement nor restriction of diffusion.
- Congenital: focal cortical dysplasia (FCD):
  - Difficult to distinguish from LGG.
  - The transmantle sign, a linear area of increased signal on T2-weighted imaging (T2WI) extending from the abnormally thickening, dysplastic cortex toward the ventricle, may be present.
  - Congenital abnormality that presents with seizures.
  - No significant restriction of diffusion.
- Infection: encephalitis:
  - Restriction of diffusion.
  - The most common, herpes simplex encephalitis, affects medial temporal lobes, usually bilaterally, as well as insular cortex and cingulate gyri.
- Vascular: venous infarction:
  - Restriction of diffusion, often parasagittal high convexities.
  - Usually hemorrhagic and associated with venous sinus and cortical vein thrombosis.
- Traumatic: contusion:
  - Inferior aspect of frontal lobes and anterior aspect of temporal lobes, history of trauma and hemorrhagic.

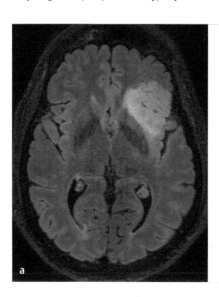 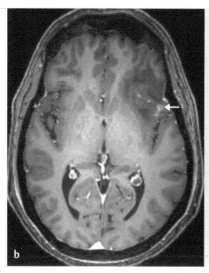

Fig. 22.2 (a, b)

Table 22.1 Characteristics of conventional imaging findings of diagnoses

Differential diagnosis	CE+	Ca^{2+}	Multifocal multilobar	White matter edema	Restricted diffusion	Comments
Diffuse glioma: oligodendroglioma IDH mutant, 1p/19q codeleted	+/–	++	–	+/–	–	More often in frontal lobe; Ca^{2+} common and may be ribbonlike; T2-weighted heterogeneous; margins almost always indistinct
Diffuse glioma: diffuse astrocytoma IDH mutant, 1p/19q intact	+/–	+/–	+/–	+/–	–	Often temporal-insular; T2-FLAIR mismatch (signal intensity on FLAIR < T2); distinct margin suggests 1p/19q-intact tumor
DNET	+/–	+/–	–	–	–	"Bubbly" cortical temporal lobe mass; associated focal cortical dysplasia (FCD); bright rim on FLAIR; inner table skull remodeling; young patient with seizures
PXA	++	Rare	–	+/–	–	Temporal lobe common; enhancing nodule with dural tail; 70% present as a cyst + nodule; more common in children
Ganglioglioma	+	++	–	+/–	–	Temporal lobe cyst + nodule appearance; more common in older child/young adult
Encephalitis	+/–	–	+	+	++	HSV—medial temporal lobes
Venous infarction	+/–	–	+	+	++	Hemorrhagic foci and dural sinus clot
Arterial infarction	+/–	–	+/–	+	++	Wedge-shaped gray and white matter edema in vascular territory
FCD	–	+/–	–	–	–	May have transmantle sign; blurring of gray–white junction; C + overlying primitive veins
Cortical tuber of tuberous sclerosis	–	+/–	+	–	–	Subependymal nodules; SEGA
Nonspecific gliosis	–	+/–	+/–	+/–	–	Lack of interval change; volume loss

Abbreviations: DNET, dysembryoplastic neuroepithelial tumor; FLAIR, fluid-attenuated inversion recovery; HSV, herpes simplex virus; PXA, pleomorphic xanthoastrocytoma; SEGA, subependymal giant cell astrocytoma.

22.5 Clinical and Diagnostic Imaging Pearls and Pitfalls

- Diffuse gliomas may present with seizures or other neurological abnormalities, but may also be completely asymptomatic, incidental findings as opposed to infection, contusion and venous/arterial infarction that are virtually always symptomatic with an appropriately "nonincidental" clinical history.
- Diffuse, LGGs do not show significant restriction on diffusion as opposed to arterial or venous infarctions and encephalitis.
- Differentiating diffuse, LGGs from FCD can be challenging as both typically present with a thickened, hyperintense cortex and varying degrees of underlying white matter signal abnormality and may also present with seizures.
- The transmantle sign, inconsistently seen but highly characteristic of type IIb FCD, is a linear area of increased signal on T2WI extending from the abnormally thickening, dysplastic cortex toward the ventricle.
- Magnetic resonance spectroscopy (MRS) has been shown to be of possible value as LGGs had marked increase in Cho and a decrease in N-acetylaspartate (NAA), whereas the FCDMs

(focal cortical developmental malformations) had milder Cho increase and NAA decrease.

22.6 Essential Facts about Gliomas

- Gliomas are the most common type of primary adult brain tumor and have traditionally been classified and graded by histopathology according to the WHO classification system.
- "LGGs" refers to WHO grade II astrocytomas and oligodendrogliomas, which are now grouped together due to similarities in their growth pattern, behavior and IDH mutation status.
- The latest WHO classification of central nervous system tumors, 2016, utilizes molecular parameters in addition to histology to define tumor entities.[1] The most important of these has been identification of *IDH* mutations in most diffuse grade II and III gliomas and *1p19q* codeletion, which is now definitional for oligodendroglial tumors.
- *IDH* mutations occur early in pathogenesis of gliomas and are therefore often associated with TP53 and ATRX mutations in astrocytomas and 1p/19q codeletion in oligodendrogliomas.[2,3]

22.7 Clinical Relevance of Genomic Alterations and Correlation with Conventional and Advanced Imaging Techniques

22.7.1 Isocitrate Dehydrogenase Mutations in Gliomas

- Clinical relevance:
  - *IDH* mutant gliomas are more common in younger patients.
  - *IDH* mutant gliomas have a better prognosis (8.0–8.4 years median survival) compared with *IDH* wild type (*IDHwt*) (1.4–1.7 years).[4,5,6]
  - Grade II and III *IDHwt* behave similarly to primary glioblastomas (GBMs)—they have a very poor prognosis. All *IDHwt* tumors should be evaluated for GBM features.[1]
  - Aggressive surgical resection beyond enhancing margins benefits *IDH* mutant tumors.[7]
- Conventional imaging:
  - *IDH*-mutated LGGs are found to have a significant preferential localization in the frontal lobe and in the limbic structures.[8]
  - *IDH*-mutated grade II and III astrocytomas are more likely to be confined to a single lobe as compared to *IDHwt* tumors, which are more likely multifocal.
  - *IDH*-mutated gliomas often have a well-defined boundary on MRI, they may have a larger nonenhancing component than *IDHwt* tumors, and are more likely to have tumor-related cystic components.
- Advanced imaging:
  - Diffusion: A lower apparent diffusion coefficient (ADC) reflects greater restriction of water molecule movement within higher grade tumors due to their increased cellularity.
    - Lower ADC values are found in *IDHwt* GBMs and grade III gliomas.[9,10,11,12,13] Low ADC values, independent of tumor grade, correlate with poor survival in grade III and IV gliomas.[14]
    - Minimum ADC (ADCmin) and rADC (relative ADC) are significantly higher in grade II and III astrocytomas with the *IDH* mutation.[15]
    - Diffusion restriction has been found to be an independent predictor of *IDH* mutation status in grade II gliomas and has independent prognostic value. ADCmin, threshold < 0.9 × 10 to 3 mm^2/s, had 91% sensitivity and 76% specificity for *IDHwt* and when combined with *IDH* status was better in predicting progression-free and overall survival better than mutation status alone.[16]
  - MRS:
    - MRS has been used to directly detect 2-HG (2-hydroxyglutarate), an oncometabolite produced in tumors with an *IDH* mutation; currently, however, it cannot replace pathological markers for determining the IDH mutation status.[17]

- Perfusion imaging provides a measure of tumor neovascularity that has been used to index malignant potential.
  - However, the data are conflicting—some studies show no definite distinction between *IDHwt* and *IDH*-mutated tumors using relative cerebral blood volume (rCBV) mean or maximum rCBV,[16] while others show a lower rCBV max in mutant tumors.[10,15]

22.7.2 1p19q Codeletion, IDH Mutated ("Oligodendroglioma Phenotype")

- Clinical relevance:
  - Much more favorable outcome; median survival of 12 to 14 years.
  - Radiotherapy (RT) with early adjuvant procarbazine, lomustine, and vincristine greatly improves survival compared with RT alone.[4,18,19,20]
- Conventional imaging:
  - Location most common in frontal lobes.
  - Heterogeneous on T2 W images.
  - Calcifications common; best detected by CT. Ribbonlike calcifications are characteristic.[21]
  - Large, nonenhancing portion of tumor associated with *IDH* mutation.
- Advanced imaging:
  - Perfusion imaging: elevated rCBV > 1.6, consistent with codeleted tumor, 92% sensitivity, and 76% specificity in grade II tumors.[22]
  - MRS: MRS Cho/Cr in area of maximum rCBV had accuracy of 69% in distinguishing codeleted from intact grade II and III tumors.[23]

22.7.3 ATRX Mutated,1p19q Intact, IDH Mutated ("Diffuse Astrocytoma Phenotype")

- Clinical relevance:
  - Worse prognosis than codeleted tumor; median survival of 3 to 8 years.
  - Much better prognosis than *IDHwt*.
  - Intact, IDH-mutated grade III tumors have improved survival after combined alkylating chemotherapy and RT.
- Conventional imaging features:
  - Compared with codeleted tumors, location more commonly in temporal, insular, or temporoinsular region.
  - Although the majority have an indistinct border, a sharp border makes the tumor much more likely to have an ATRX mutation than a 1p19q codeletion.
  - A T2-FLAIR mismatch is highly specific for 1p19q-intact, *IDH*-mutant tumors. This is T2 W imaging hyperintensity throughout the lesion with relatively FLAIR hypointensity except for a peripheral rim of high signal.[13,24]

22.7.4 IDH-Mutated GBM ("Secondary GBM Phenotype")

- Clinical relevance:
  - Commonly a secondary GBM, arising from a grade II or III diffuse glioma.
  - Younger patients relative to *IDHwt* tumors.
  - Ten percent of GBMs.
  - Commonly of the proneural gene expression subtype of GBM.
  - Better prognosis than nonmutated *IDHwt* tumors.
- Conventional imaging:
  - Found most frequently around the frontal horns of the lateral ventricles.
  - Large nonenhancing portion of the tumor.

22.7.5 IDHwt GBM ("Primary GBM Phenotype")

- Clinical relevance:
  - Older patients.
  - Ninety percent of GBMs.
  - Primary GBM.
  - Classic gene expression subtype of GBM.
  - EGFR (epidermal growth factor receptor) overexpression.

- Conventional imaging:
  - Often multilobar location.
  - Heterogeneous, central necrosis and cystic areas.
  - Multifocal enhancement.

22.7.6 MGMT promoter methylation

- Clinical relevance:
  - In grade III and IV tumors, MGMT promoter methylation predicts a better response to temozolomide and is associated with better outcomes.
- Conventional imaging features:
  - Conflicting, inconsistent results with no definite distinction between methylated and nonmethylated tumors by conventional imaging.
- Advanced imaging:
  - Diffusion imaging: data have been inconsistent and therefore clinical value has not been established. However, measurement of minimal ADC using histogram analysis, which is not widely available, may be more promising.[25]
  - Perfusion imaging: multiple study results have been inconsistent but suggest that a lower rCBV may be associated with methylated status. K-trans, thought to be a marker of blood vessel permeability, has been found to be increased in methylated compared with unmethylated GBM.[26]

22.8 Companion Case

22.8.1 History and Physical Examination

A 24-year-old woman presented to the ER after experiencing headaches and syncope. The physical examination was unremarkable. An MRI was performed for further evaluation.

22.8.2 Imaging Analysis

Imaging Findings and Impression

The MRI reveals a left frontal mass involving the orbital gyrus (▶ Fig. 22.3; *arrow*). On the T1-weighted sequence (▶ Fig. 22.3a),

a "**V**"-shaped, hypointense cortical and subcortical lesion of the orbital gyrus is noted. On the T2-weighted sequences (▶ Fig. 22.3c,d), the lesion is mildly hyperintense without perilesional vasogenic edema. On the postgadolinium T1 W image sequence (▶ Fig. 22.3b), there is no evidence of enhancement. Similar to the opening case of this chapter, this focal area of abnormal signal intensity with subtle mass effect involving both the cortex and underlying white matter in an asymptomatic patient is most likely an LGG. The differential diagnosis in this first companion case is identical to that of the opening case.

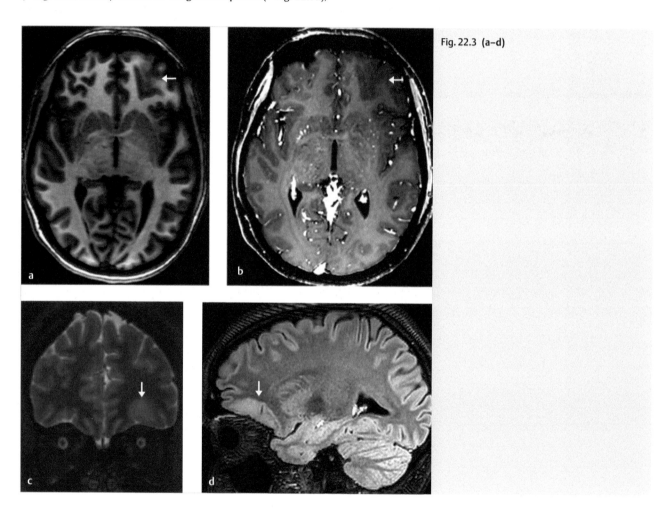

Fig. 22.3 (a–d)

Additional Imaging

Advanced brain tumor imaging was performed in this case, as discussed below.

- DTI and tractography: Visualization of white matter tract displacement may be helpful in preoperative surgical planning. Note displacement of the inferior frontal-occipital fasciculus (IFOF; *long arrow*; ▶ Fig. 22.4a) above the tumor (*short arrow*; ▶ Fig. 22.4a).

- Perfusion imaging: Arterial spin labeling (ASL) revealed increased blood flow in the region of the tumor (▶ Fig. 22.4b). Dynamic susceptibility contrast (DSC) imaging indicated increased rCBV (▶ Fig. 22.4c) in the orbital gyrus.

- MRS: MRS performed with a single voxel, low TE (TE = 35 ms) technique revealed a decrease in NAA (*short arrow*; ▶ Fig. 22.4d) at 2.0 pmm and relative increase in myoinositol (mI.; *long arrow*; ▶ Fig. 22.4d).

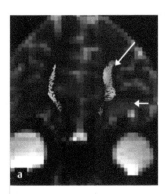
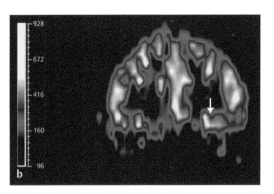
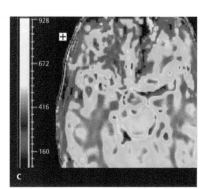

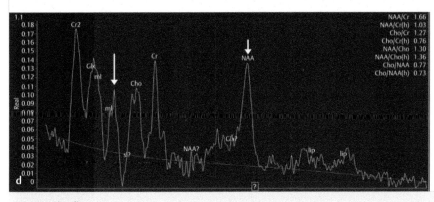

Fig. 22.4 (a–d)

Advanced Imaging Interpretation

The combination of a nonenhancing lesion with mildly increased rCBV on DSC, CBF (cerebral blood flow) on ASL, and MI on MRS led to the diagnosis of a low-grade diffuse glioma.

22.8.3 Clinical Evaluation

The patient underwent surgical resection and pathology revealed *diffuse astrocytoma, IDH-mutant, WHO grade II.*

22.9 Neurosurgery Questions and Answers

1. **Given the presentation and imaging findings, what specific findings on physical examination and/or elements of the history are important in your determination of the diagnosis? If symptomatic, what are the typical presentations of patients with LGGs?**

   The typical patient with an LGG is younger than 40 years of age presenting with a seizure(s). Other presenting signs and symptoms for LGGs include headaches, unilateral weakness or sensory changes, and speech difficulties. Patients may also be asymptomatic.[34] They rarely have focal deficits on neurological examination.[35] Key diagnoses in the differential of an LGG include infection (abscess, herpes encephalitis), multiple sclerosis (MS), vascular pathologies, and cortical dysplasia.[36,37] Many key differentiating factors of these diagnoses can be found in a detailed history and physical examination.

   As with any patient encounter, the beginning of the interaction with an LGG patient begins by taking a chief complaint and history of presenting symptoms. Differentiating symptoms in the history that would favor an infection would be the presence of fever, altered mental status, chills, nausea or vomiting, none of which are attributable to an LGG.[38] Patients with immunocompromising conditions are more susceptible to infections, so past histories of HIV, organ transplant, or immune-modulating medications are important to inquire about. MS patients can present with bilateral weakness or sensory complaints that correspond to multiple, noncontiguous locations in the brain. LGGs do not typically occur in a multifocal fashion, so they are extremely unlikely to present with bilateral symptoms. MS can cause ocular pain related to optic neuritis, which does not occur in patients with a glioma. Certain forms of MS also present with a relapsing–remitting pattern of symptoms that would not occur with a glioma, a primarily progressive disease.[39] Both LGGs and strokes can present with hypodense lesions on an initial CT scan of the brain. However, stroke patients present with an acute onset of their symptoms, while the symptoms of an LGG will be more insidious. Strokes are more typical in older individuals who may have other comorbidities described in their past medical problems such as dementia, hypertension, diabetes, coronary artery disease, and systemic vascular disease.[40] Patients with vasculitis may describe a previously diagnosed systemic syndrome or disease associated with intracranial lesions in their history such as Behcet's syndrome, Wegener's granulomatosis, or systemic lupus erythematosus.[36] FCD often presents with seizures in a similar manner to patients with an LGG. However, a patient with an FCD more often presents in childhood, or adult patients with a history of febrile seizures, CNS infection, status epilepticus, traumatic brain injury, or perinatal complications.[41]

   On physical examination, it is important to be aware that patients with LGG uncommonly have focal deficits on examination.[42] The presence of fever, tachycardia, and loss of orientation are more common in infection than in LGGs. MS patients can have bilateral weakness or sensory deficits on examination due to multiple lesions, something that would be exceedingly rare for an LGG patient to have. If an MS patient is presenting with optic neuritis, then they can have visual field deficits in addition to complaining of pain in that eye. While an LGG patient could have a visual field deficit, it would not occur in combination with pain. Patients presenting with a stroke typically have dense motor and sensory deficits on examination that are slow to recover, while LGGs cause mild, subtle weakness and sensory deficits.

2. **What additional testing, if any, is required or recommended in the workup?**

   With respect to imaging studies, advanced brain tumor imaging can be helpful to distinguish an LGG from nonneoplastic processes such as a cortical dysplasia or MS. In addition, specific sequences such as diffusion-weighted MRI can assist in differentiating an abscess from a glioma or other malignancies such as a lymphoma and must be included in the original imaging workup.[32]

   In the cases where the diagnosis is not clear, a lumbar puncture should be performed. It should be sent for gram stain and culture, cell count with a differential, glucose, and protein to identify an infectious process. Additional studies that should be sent include cytology and oligoclonal bands.[43] Infections and MS will have distinct cerebrospinal fluid profiles or findings that will confirm the diagnosis, whereas an LGG would be expected to have a normal cerebrospinal fluid profile.

3. **What is the natural history of the condition and how would that assist in decision-making?**

   The natural history and proper management of LGGs is still a highly debated subject. According to a 2017 Cochrane Library review, there are currently no randomized, controlled trials that examine biopsy versus resection for the management of these lesions.[44] Previous retrospective studies have demonstrated that these tumors have linear growth rates of around 4 mm/y and that the natural history is to progress to malignant tumors.[45,46] So while the immediate prognosis after discovery of these lesions is positive, they eventually will become malignant, symptomatic tumors. Given this information, many studies have examined the effects of resection on survival and symptom control. Current literature indicates that maximal safe resection of LGGs may improve progression-free survival, overall survival, and seizure control, and reduce the risk of malignant transformation.[47,48,49,50,51] In addition, one study looking specifically at incidentally found LGGs found that they tend to be smaller and less likely to occur in eloquent locations, allowing for a greater extent of resection and better subsequent overall survival.[45] The only prospective study investigating early resection versus a wait-and-watch strategy in LGG favored early resection. In this study, a significant survival advantage and a significant reduction in malignant transformation were found for patients undergoing early resection.[51]

4. **If electing to follow, what is the suggested time interval and modality? Are there any American Association of Neurological Surgeons (AANS)/Congress of Neurological Surgeons (CNS) published guidelines for the management of this condition?**

There are published guidelines from the CNS on the management of LGGs, most recently published in 2015.[52] They include guidance on the diagnostic workup, surgical management, role of RT and chemotherapy in the initial management of these tumors, and recommendations on recurrent tumors. The following summarizes the guidelines.

An MRI with and without gadolinium-based contrast should be included in the initial workup of patients with a suspected LGG and include T1 W and FLAIR sequences. Diffusion- and perfusion-weighted MRI, MRS, and PET scans can also add diagnostic specificity and should be considered to differentiate these tumors from other pathologies.[53] Stereotactic biopsy is recommended to obtain a tissue diagnosis to guide further therapy for lesions that are deep seated, not resectable, located within eloquent cortex, or in patients that are not surgical candidates due to medical comorbidities.[54] Surgical resection is recommended over observation for patients to improve overall survival. A gross total or subtotal resection is recommended over biopsy alone when feasible to decrease the frequency of tumor progression and to improve overall survival. The use of intraoperative MRI should be considered in order to maximize the extent of resection, and intraoperative mapping of tumors in eloquent areas is recommended to preserve function.[55] Postoperative RT at lower doses (45–50.4 Gy) extends progression-free survival with less overall toxicity. Limited field radiation should be used over whole brain radiation. It can be initiated in the immediate postoperative period or in a delayed fashion when recurrence or progression occurs.

Stereotactic radiosurgery and brachytherapy are recommended as acceptable alternatives to external RT.[56] Chemotherapy is recommended as a potential treatment to postpone the use of RT and has been shown to slow growth and improve progression-free survival and overall survival. It is recommended specifically for patients who cannot undergo a gross total resection (GTR) and those with IDH mutations. If a patient harbors the 1p/19q codeletion, then temozolomide is recommended. These therapies should be started no later than 12 weeks from surgery or diagnosis. At this time, there is insufficient evidence to recommend duration or dosing of chemotherapy. Chemotherapy should be added to RT in patients with unfavorable characteristics (younger than 40 years and a less than GTR or any patient older than 40 years) to improve progression-free survival.[57]

5. **Why are the indications for surgery? What are the surgical options/risks?**

The above guidelines and other studies indicate that suspected LGGs should be offered surgical resection to improve overall survival.[45,46,47,51] The inability of current imaging modalities to confirm that the glioma is low grade is another reason to argue against a wait-and-observe approach. Up to 30 to 40% of nonenhancing, so-called LGGs may have anaplastic components.[58] The options for surgery are largely determined by the location of the lesion and the surgical candidacy of the patient. For patients that are not candidates for a full resection, or their lesions are in deep-seated locations that do not permit a significant resection with acceptable risk, stereotactic biopsy is offered. In patients with lesions in noneloquent cortex, a standard resection is offered with the goal of a GTR. For lesions located near primary sensory, motor, or language cortex, surgical resection with varying combinations of awake or asleep motor mapping, awake language mapping, and somatosensory evoked potentials is recommended to maximize the extent of resection and to decrease morbidity.[59,60,61,62] The exact combination of these techniques is determined by the location of the tumor.

A decision tree algorithm for incidental LGGs is shown in ▶ Fig. 22.5.

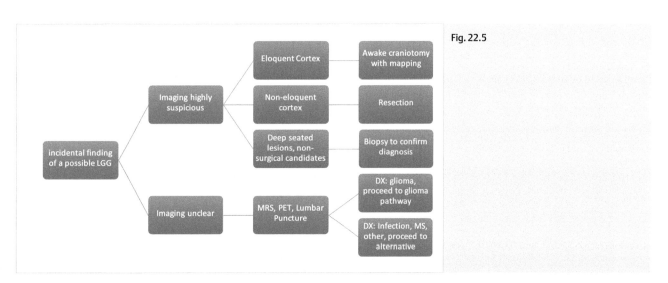

Fig. 22.5

22.10 Key Point Summary

- Incidentally discovered diffuse gliomas are becoming more common during the age of surveillance scans completed for various symptoms or signs not related to the incidental lesion.
- The advantages significantly outweigh the risks with regard to an early, more aggressive resection with gliomas.
- These tumors should no longer be observed when incidentally discovered—early intervention is generally indicated.
- Intraoperative mapping techniques should be incorporated when the tumor is located in or around eloquent structures to allow a more aggressive resection while preserving function.

References

[1] Louis DN, Perry A, Reifenberger G, et al. The 2016 World Health Organization Classification of Tumors of the Central Nervous System: a summary. Acta Neuropathol. 2016; 131(6):803–820

[2] Larsen J, Wharton SB, McKevitt F, et al. "Low grade glioma": an update for radiologists. Br J Radiol. 2017; 90(1070):20160600

[3] Arevalo OJ, Valenzuela R, Esquenazi Y, et al. The 2016 World Health Organization Classification of Tumors of the Central Nervous System: A Practical Approach for Gliomas, Part 1. Basic Tumor Genetics. Neurographics.. 2017; 7:334–343

[4] Brat DJ, Verhaak RG, Aldape KD, et al. Cancer Genome Atlas Research Network. Comprehensive, integrative genomic analysis of diffuse lowergrade gliomas. N Engl J Med. 2015; 372(26):2481–2498

[5] van den Bent MJ, Brandes AA, Taphoorn MJ, et al. Adjuvant procarbazine, lomustine, and vincristine chemotherapy in newly diagnosed anaplastic oligodendroglioma: long-term follow-up of EORTC brain tumor group study 26951. J Clin Oncol. 2013; 31(3):344–350

[6] Olar A, Wani KM, Alfaro-Munoz KD, et al. IDH mutation status and role of WHO grade and mitotic index in overall survival in grade II-III diffuse gliomas. Acta Neuropathol. 2015; 129(4):585–596

[7] Beiko J, Suki D, Hess KR, et al. IDH1 mutant malignant astrocytomas are more amenable to surgical resection and have a survival benefit associated with maximal surgical resection. Neuro-oncol. 2014; 16(1):81–91

[8] Wang Y, Zhang T, Li S, et al. Anatomical localization of isocitrate dehydrogenase 1 mutation: a voxel-based radiographic study of 146 low-grade gliomas. Eur J Neurol. 2015; 22(2):348–354

[9] Yamashita K, Hiwatashi A, Togao O, et al. MR imaging-based analysis of glioblastoma multiforme: estimation of IDH1 mutation status. AJNR Am J Neuroradiol. 2016; 37(1):58–65

[10] Lee S, Choi SH, Ryoo I, et al. Evaluation of the microenvironmental heterogeneity in high-grade gliomas with IDH1/2 gene mutation using histogram analysis of diffusion-weighted imaging and dynamic-susceptibility contrast perfusion imaging. J Neurooncol. 2015; 121(1):141–150

[11] Tan WL, Huang WY, Yin B, Xiong J, Wu JS, Geng DY. Can diffusion tensor imaging noninvasively detect IDH1 gene mutations in astrogliomas? A retrospective study of 112 cases. AJNR Am J Neuroradiol. 2014; 35(5):920–927

[12] Hempel JM, Bisdas S, Schittenhelm J, et al. In vivo molecular profiling of human glioma using diffusion kurtosis imaging. J Neurooncol. 2017; 131(1):93–101

[13] Lasocki A, Gaillard F, Gorelik A, Gonzales M. MRI features can predict 1p/19q status in intracranial gliomas. AJNR Am J Neuroradiol. 2018; 39(4):687–692

[14] Zulfiqar M, Yousem DM, Lai H. ADC values and prognosis of malignant astrocytomas: does lower ADC predict a worse prognosis independent of grade of tumor?: a meta-analysis. AJR Am J Roentgenol. 2013; 200(3):624–629

[15] Xing Z, Yang X, She D, Lin Y, Zhang Y, Cao D. Noninvasive assessment of IDH mutational status in WHO grade II and III astrocytomas using DWI and DSC-PWI combined with conventional MR imaging. AJNR Am J Neuroradiol. 2017; 38:1138–1144

[16] Villanueva-Meyer JE, Wood MD, Choi BS, et al. MRI features and IDH mutational status of grade II diffuse gliomas: impact on diagnosis and prognosis. AJR Am J Roentgenol. 2018; 210(3):621–628

[17] Choi C, Ganji SK, DeBerardinis RJ, et al. 2-hydroxyglutarate detection by magnetic resonance spectroscopy in IDH-mutated patients with gliomas. Nat Med. 2012; 18(4):624–629

[18] Wick W, Hartmann C, Engel C, et al. NOA-04 randomized phase III trial of sequential radiochemotherapy of anaplastic glioma with procarbazine, lomustine, and vincristine or temozolomide. J Clin Oncol. 2009; 27(35):5874–5880

[19] van den Bent MJ. Chemotherapy for low-grade glioma: when, for whom, which regimen? Curr Opin Neurol. 2015; 28(6):633–938

[20] Cairncross G, Wang M, Shaw E, et al. Phase III trial of chemoradiotherapy for anaplastic oligodendroglioma: long-term results of RTOG 9402. J Clin Oncol. 2013; 31(3):337–343

[21] Saito T, Muragaki Y, Maruyama T, et al. Calcification on CT is a simple and valuable preoperative indicator of 1p/19q loss of heterozygosity in supratentorial brain tumors that are suspected grade II and III gliomas. Brain Tumor Pathol. 2016; 33(3):175–182

[22] Jenkinson MD, Smith TS, Brodbelt AR, Joyce KA, Warnke PC, Walker C. Apparent diffusion coefficients in oligodendroglial tumors characterized by genotype. J Magn Reson Imaging. 2007; 26(6):1405–1412

[23] Chawla S, Krejza J, Vossough A, et al. Differentiation between oligodendroglioma genotypes using dynamic susceptibility contrast perfusion-weighted imaging and proton MR spectroscopy. AJNR Am J Neuroradiol. 2013; 34(8):1542–1549

[24] Patel SH, Poisson LM, Brat DJ, et al. T2-FLAIR mismatch, an imaging biomarker for IDH and 1p/19q status in lower-grade gliomas: a TCGA/TCIA project. Clin Cancer Res. 2017; 23(20):6078–6085

[25] Rundle-Thiele D, Day B, Stringer B, et al. Using the apparent diffusion coefficient to identifying MGMT promoter methylation status early in glioblastoma: importance of analytical method. J Med Radiat Sci. 2015; 62(2):92–98

[26] Ahn SS, Shin NY, Chang JH, et al. Prediction of methylguanine methyltransferase promoter methylation in glioblastoma using dynamic contrast-enhanced magnetic resonance and diffusion tensor imaging. J Neurosurg. 2014; 121(2):367–373

[27] Burger PC. Malignant astrocytic neoplasms: classification, pathologic anatomy, and response to treatment. Semin Oncol. 1986; 13(1):16–26

[28] Boxerman JL, Shiroishi MS, Ellingson BM, Pope WB. Dynamic susceptibility contrast MR imaging in glioma: review of current clinical practice. Magn Reson Imaging Clin N Am. 2016; 24(4):649–670

[29] Noguchi T, Yoshiura T, Hiwatashi A, et al. Perfusion imaging of brain tumors using arterial spin-labeling: correlation with histopathologic vascular density. AJNR Am J Neuroradiol. 2008; 29(4):688–693

[30] Vuori K, Kankaanranta L, Häkkinen AM, et al. Low-grade gliomas and focal cortical developmental malformations: differentiation with proton MR spectroscopy. Radiology. 2004; 230(3):703–708

[31] Castillo M, Smith JK, Kwock L. Correlation of myo-inositol levels and grading of cerebral astrocytomas. AJNR Am J Neuroradiol. 2000; 21(9):1645–1649

[32] Cha S, Pierce S, Knopp EA, et al. Dynamic contrast-enhanced T2*-weighted MR imaging of tumefactive demyelinating lesions. AJNR Am J Neuroradiol. 2001; 22(6):1109–1116

[33] Miller TR, Mohan S, Choudhri AF, Gandhi D, Jindal G. Advances in multiple sclerosis and its variants: conventional and newer imaging techniques. Radiol Clin North Am. 2014; 52(2):321–336

[34] Shah AH, Madhavan K, Heros D, et al. The management of incidental low-grade gliomas using magnetic resonance imaging: systematic review and optimal treatment paradigm. Neurosurg Focus. 2011; 31(6):E12

[35] Chang EF, Potts MB, Keles GE, et al. Seizure characteristics and control following resection in 332 patients with low-grade gliomas. J Neurosurg. 2008; 108(2):227–235

[36] Rapalino O, Mullins ME. Intracranial infectious and inflammatory diseases presenting as neurosurgical pathologies. Neurosurgery. 2017; 81(1):10–28

[37] Upadhyay N, Waldman AD. Conventional MRI evaluation of gliomas. Br J Radiol. 2011; 84(Spec No 2):S107–S111

[38] Udoh DO, Ibadin E, Udoh MO. Intracranial abscesses: retrospective analysis of 32 patients and review of literature. Asian J Neurosurg. 2016; 11(4):384–391

[39] Confavreux C, Vukusic S. The clinical course of multiple sclerosis. Handb Clin Neurol. 2014; 122:343–369

[40] Gupta A, Nair S, Schweitzer AD, et al. Neuroimaging of cerebrovascular disease in the aging brain. Aging Dis. 2012; 3(5):414–425

[41] Bast T, Ramantani G, Seitz A, Rating D. Focal cortical dysplasia: prevalence, clinical presentation and epilepsy in children and adults. Acta Neurol Scand. 2006; 113(2):72–81

[42] Masdeu JC, Moreira J, Trasi S, Visintainer P, Cavaliere R, Grundman M. The open ring. A new imaging sign in demyelinating disease. J Neuroimaging. 1996; 6(2):104–107

[43] Ikeguchi R, Shimizu Y, Shimizu S, Kitagawa K. CSF and clinical data are useful in differentiating CNS inflammatory demyelinating disease from CNS lymphoma. Mult Scler. 2018; 24(9):1212–1223

[44] Jiang B, Chaichana K, Veeravagu A, Chang SD, Black KL, Patil CG. Biopsy versus resection for the management of low-grade gliomas. Cochrane Database Syst Rev. 2017; 4:CD009319

[45] Potts MB, Smith JS, Molinaro AM, Berger MS. Natural history and surgical management of incidentally discovered low-grade gliomas. J Neurosurg. 2012; 116(2):365–372

[46] Pallud J, Fontaine D, Duffau H, et al. Natural history of incidental World Health Organization grade II gliomas. Ann Neurol. 2010; 68(5):727–733

[47] Ius T, Isola M, Budai R, et al. Low-grade glioma surgery in eloquent areas: volumetric analysis of extent of resection and its impact on overall survival. A single-institution experience in 190 patients: clinical article. J Neurosurg. 2012; 117(6):1039–1052

[48] Smith JS, Chang EF, Lamborn KR, et al. Role of extent of resection in the long-term outcome of low-grade hemispheric gliomas. J Clin Oncol. 2008; 26(8):1338–1345

[49] Soffietti R, Baumert BG, Bello L, et al. European Federation of Neurological Societies. Guidelines on management of low-grade gliomas: report of an EFNS-EANO task force. Eur J Neurol. 2010; 17(9):1124–1133

[50] Keles GE, Lamborn KR, Berger MS. Low-grade hemispheric gliomas in adults: a critical review of extent of resection as a factor influencing outcome. J Neurosurg. 2001; 95(5):735–745

[51] Jakola AS, Myrmel KS, Kloster R, et al. Comparison of a strategy favoring early surgical resection vs a strategy favoring watchful waiting in low-grade gliomas. JAMA. 2012; 308(18):1881–1888

[52] Rock J. Low grade glioma guidelines: foreword. J Neurooncol. 2015; 125(3):447–448

[53] Fouke SJ, Benzinger T, Gibson D, Ryken TC, Kalkanis SN, Olson JJ. The role of imaging in the management of adults with diffuse low grade glioma: a systematic review and evidence-based clinical practice guideline. J Neurooncol. 2015; 125(3):457–479

[54] Ragel BT, Ryken TC, Kalkanis SN, Ziu M, Cahill D, Olson JJ. The role of biopsy in the management of patients with presumed diffuse low grade glioma: a systematic review and evidence-based clinical practice guideline. J Neurooncol. 2015; 125(3):481–501

[55] Aghi MK, Nahed BV, Sloan AE, Ryken TC, Kalkanis SN, Olson JJ. The role of surgery in the management of patients with diffuse low grade glioma: a systematic review and evidence-based clinical practice guideline. J Neurooncol. 2015; 125(3):503–530

[56] Ryken TC, Parney I, Buatti J, Kalkanis SN, Olson JJ. The role of radiotherapy in the management of patients with diffuse low grade glioma: a systematic review and evidence-based clinical practice guideline. J Neurooncol. 2015; 125(3):551–583

[57] Ziu M, Olson JJ. Update on the evidence-based clinical practice parameter guidelines for the treatment of adults with diffuse low grade glioma: the role of initial chemotherapy. J Neurooncol. 2016; 128(3):487–489

[58] Scott JN, Brasher PM, Sevick RJ, Rewcastle NB, Forsyth PA. How often are non-enhancing supratentorial gliomas malignant? A population study. Neurology. 2002; 59(6):947–949

[59] Hervey-Jumper SL, Berger MS. Maximizing safe resection of low- and high-grade glioma. J Neurooncol. 2016; 130(2):269–282

[60] De Witt Hamer PC, Robles SG, Zwinderman AH, Duffau H, Berger MS. Impact of intraoperative stimulation brain mapping on glioma surgery outcome: a meta-analysis. J Clin Oncol. 2012; 30(20):2559–2565

[61] Esquenazi Y, Friedman E, Liu Z, Zhu JJ, Hsu S, Tandon N. The survival advantage of "supratotal" resection of glioblastoma using selective cortical mapping and subpial technique. Neurosurgery. 2017; 81(2):275–288

[62] Tandon N, Esquenazi Y. Resection strategies in tumoral epilepsy: is a lesionectomy enough? Epilepsia. 2013; 54(9) Suppl 9:72–78

23 Incidental Meningioma

Phillip A. Choi, Pejman Rabiei, Shekhar D. Khanpara, Mohamed Elgendy, Roy F. Riascos, and Dong H. Kim

23.1 Introduction

As the quality and accessibility of diagnostic imaging has increased, so has the number of incidental findings that require management. Incidental findings are unrelated to the original purpose of the examination. Meningiomas are one of the most common brain tumors to be detected incidentally because they can be small in size and asymptomatic. Management of these tumors may include observation, radiation, or surgery. Many of these tumors can be managed conservatively. However, a small proportion of meningiomas with high growth rate or concerning location and patient demographics are best treated with early surgical resection.

In this chapter, we present the radiographic findings and management of two cases of meningioma that presented incidentally. We start with the radiographic analysis and include conventional imaging pearls that help distinguish between the different entities within the differential diagnosis. We include a companion case of meningioma that was followed up with imaging to explore the factors affecting growth potential and ultimate follow-up time frame for incidentally found meningiomas.

23.2 Case Presentation

23.2.1 History and Physical Examination

A 37-year-old with history of motor vehicle accident has head CT for scalp laceration. MRI was done afterward for incidental finding on head CT.

The neurological examination was normal.

23.2.2 Imaging Findings

Contrast MRI brain shows a large extra-axial mass of an approximate size of 4.5 × 5.2 cm in the right parieto-occipital region. The mass is isointense on T2-weighted imaging (T2WI; ▶ Fig. 23.1a), hypointense on T1WI (▶ Fig. 23.1b), and hyperintense on fluid-attenuated inversion recovery (FLAIR; ▶ Fig. 23.1c), and enhances homogeneously with a dural tail (*white arrow* in ▶ Fig. 23.1e, f).

Diagnosis: Right parieto-occipital meningioma.

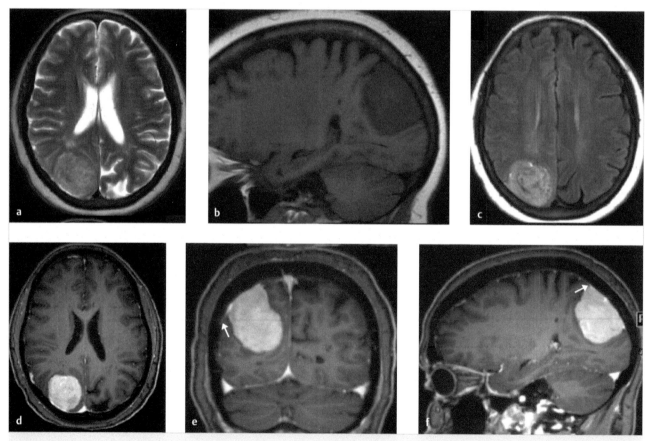

Fig. 23.1 (a–f)

23.2.3 Additional Tests to Consider

No additional tests are recommended.

23.3 Neurosurgical Consultation

There is a large right parieto-occipital convexity meningioma in a relatively young and healthy woman, so surgical intervention was offered. The lesion is in a very surgically accessible region and does not yet involve any key vascular or neuronal structures. The risk of growth is moderately high with this tumor. Surgical resection at this time would allow for operating on the tumor while the risk is relatively low as well as provide a tissue diagnosis to guide further treatment. Stereotactic radiosurgery would not be offered for this lesion because it is larger than 3 cm and there is an increased risk of posttreatment edema and radiation necrosis.

23.4 Differential Diagnosis of Dural Based Masses

- **Meningioma:**
  - On CT often hyperdense, may calcify, and often associated with hyperostosis and dilatation of the adjacent paranasal sinuses.
  - On MRI, homogeneous enhancement, usually isointense T1/T2, and dural tail may be seen but not pathognomonic.
- Metastatic disease to dura:
  - Frequently multiple with infiltrating behavior and extensive adjacent dural thickening rather than a well-defined globular mass.
- Sarcoid:
  - Associated leptomeningeal enhancement, thickened pituitary stalk, clinical features present including elevated angiotensin-converting enzyme (ACE) and abnormal chest X-ray.
- Hemangiopericytoma/solitary fibrous tumor:
  - Often invades bone and appears more aggressive.

- Demonstrates microlobulation and extensive peripheral vascularity.
- Primary dural lymphoma:
  - Often multifocal without calvarial invasion.
  - Demonstrates restricted diffusion and T2 low signal due to hypercellularity.

23.5 Diagnostic Pearls and Pitfalls

- Meningioma is one of few tumors that have distinct female predominance.
- Association with prior radiation.
- The dural tail is NOT pathognomonic and may be seen in PXA, lymphoma, and pituitary adenoma, as well as granulomatous/inflammatory conditions such as sarcoidosis.
- No reliable way to distinguish between malignant and typical meningiomas; however, factors associated with increased growth potential include increased signal on T2WI, extensive surrounding edema, younger-age patient, absence of calcification, and recurrent lesions. Features suggesting less growth potential include smaller size, highly calcified lesion, and older-age patient.
- Close inspection of dural venous sinus when meningioma is in close proximity is important as meningiomas may occlude the sinus. Determination as to the patency of the sinus is important for surgical planning.
- Consider neurofibromatosis type 2 (NF2) if the patient presents with meningioma and any of the following: cataract, schwannoma, glioma, and a parent, sibling, or child with NF2; or if the patient had vestibular schwannoma diagnosed at younger 30 years of age; or if the patient had multiple meningiomas and any of the following: vestibular schwannoma diagnosed before the age of 30 years, cataract, or glioma.

23.6 Companion Case

23.6.1 History

A 46-year-old woman presented with an incidentally found meningioma.

23.6.2 Imaging Description and Impression

Contrast MRI of the brain shows an extra-axial mass of approximate size 1.26 × 1.22 cm arising from the lesser wing of the sphenoid bone with dural tail (*white arrow* in ▶ Fig. 23.2b) and partially encasing the right middle cerebral artery (MCA). The mass has intermediate signal on T1WI (▶ Fig. 23.2a) and T2WI (▶ Fig. 23.2e) and enhances homogenously (▶ Fig. 23.2c,d), most likely representing a meningioma.

23.6.3 Neurosurgery Consultation

A relatively healthy 46-year-old woman found to have a small incidental meningioma arising from the medial lesser wing of the sphenoid. Surgical intervention is offered to this patient because she is young and the tumor is in close proximity to the MCA and the superior orbital fissure. This tumor is ideally treated before it encases these vital structures and becomes symptomatic. The patient elected against surgical intervention, so the recommendation for follow-up MRI in 3 months was made. If no growth were seen, the next follow-up MRI would be 1 year after. If there were any interval growth, surgical resection would again be recommended.

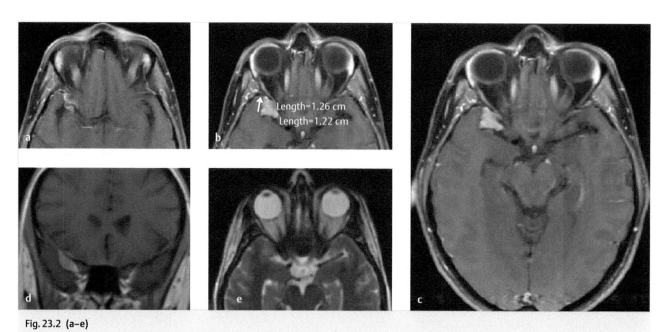

Fig. 23.2 (a–e)

23.7 Neurosurgery Questions and Answers

1. **What is the etiology and natural history of meningioma that may assist in clinical decision-making?**

   Meningiomas are typically benign, extra-axial tumors that originate from arachnoid cap cells.[1] They are associated with venous sinuses in the intracranial space and are fed by branches of the external carotid artery. The most common locations for incidentally found meningiomas are skull base and convexity, followed by falcine, parasagittal, intraventricular, and other locations.[2] The incidence of meningioma increases dramatically with age and female sex.[3,4]

   Meningiomas are broadly categorized into grade I, II, and III pathologies.[5] Grade I meningiomas are benign, while grade II and III meningiomas are atypical and malignant/anaplastic, respectively. Grade II and III meningiomas are thought to comprise approximately 5% of all meningiomas.[6] Higher grade has been associated with increased growth rate, recurrence after treatment, and mortality.[1,7,8,9]

   The growth rate of meningiomas is complex and dependent on multiple imaging and pathological factors. Nakasu et al proposed that meningiomas can follow one of three different patterns of growth: no growth, linear growth, or exponential growth.[7] A volumetric growth analysis of tumor size by Hashiba et al found that 70% of tumors had growth on follow-up.[10] The annual growth rate for those with a linear pattern was 15% per year, while tumors with an exponential growth rate increased by 25% per year. A systematic review by Sughrue et al demonstrated that most small meningiomas (< 2.5 cm in diameter) do not become symptomatic over 5 years of follow-up and can be observed.[11]

   Multiple radiographic parameters of meningiomas have been associated with increased growth potential. Oya et al observed that age younger than 60 years, lack of calcification, intrinsic T2 hyperintensity, size greater than 25 mm, and surrounding edema were associated with tumor growth.[12] Multiple other studies have variably reported these factors to be associated with tumor growth.[13] Presence of calcifications within the lesion has consistently been associated with no growth.[13]

   Meningiomas are usually sporadic but can be associated with NF2. Mutation of the NF2 on chromosome 22 leads to changes in the protein known as schwannomin or merlin.[1] Patients with NF2 can have multiple meningiomas that require surveillance. In addition to exponential and linear growth patterns, meningiomas in patients with NF2 may also show a saltatory growth pattern (alternating periods of growth and quiescence).[14] Patients with NF2 have a high rate of de novo meningioma formation compared to the general public.[14,15] Management of these meningiomas is usually determined by which lesions are symptomatic since it is expected that patients will continue to have growth and de novo formation of multiple lesions throughout their lifetime.

2. **In patients in whom a meningioma has been detected, what specific findings on physical examination and/or elements of the history are important in your determination that this problematic incidental finding is truly asymptomatic?**

   Signs and symptoms indicative of a symptomatic meningioma are dependent on the location of the lesion. Convexity or parasagittal lesions can cause neurological dysfunction of nearby cortex. Skull base meningiomas can cause symptoms when they encase or compress adjacent cranial nerves. Patients may also have symptoms of increased intracranial pressure when meningiomas are large such as progressively worsening headaches, nausea, and vomiting.

3. **What additional testing, if any, is required or recommended in the workup?**

   No additional evaluation is needed after MRI brain with and without gadolinium for lesions with typical appearance on MRI. Diagnostic cerebral angiography is helpful for assessing venous anatomy in meningiomas abutting or invading venous sinuses.

4. **Are there any AANS (American Association of Neurological Surgeons)/CNS (Congress of Neurological Surgeons) published guidelines for the management of this condition?**

   No published guidelines are available.

5. **If electing to follow, what is the suggested time interval and modality?**

   Initial follow-up imaging in 3 months with an MRI brain with and without gadolinium is recommended to assess for rapid growth. If initial follow-up imaging is stable, then the intervals for surveillance imaging can be increased to 6 months and then yearly afterward.

6. **What are the treatment options for meningiomas?**

   Meningiomas can be treated with open surgical resection and/or Gamma Knife radiosurgery. Open resection of meningiomas is a good choice when the lesion is easily accessible, larger in size, and the patient is healthy enough to tolerate general anesthesia. Goals of surgery include maximal safe resection and obtaining tissue for pathological diagnosis. Residual tumor attached to sensitive structures can be left during surgery and later treated with radiosurgery. Gamma Knife radiosurgery can be used safely in lesions less than 3 cm in diameter or lesions in locations that are difficult to access surgically. Radiosurgery is also preferred in patients who are too unhealthy to undergo general anesthesia.

23.8 Key Point Summary

- Incidental meningiomas are more commonly detected due to increased utilization of MRI cranial imaging.
- These patients often have no symptoms or findings on examination.
- MRI is the mainstay of diagnosis to characterize and evaluate the extent of a meningioma.
- Size, patient demographics, growth rate and proximity to dural sinuses, and other critical structures determine if an incidental meningioma will be offered surgical treatment or radiation.

References

[1] Mawrin C, Perry A. Pathological classification and molecular genetics of meningiomas. J Neurooncol. 2010; 99(3):379–391

[2] Spasic M, Pelargos PE, Barnette N, et al. Incidental meningiomas: management in the neuroimaging era. Neurosurg Clin N Am. 2016; 27(2):229–238

[3] Claus EB, Bondy ML, Schildkraut JM, Wiemels JL, Wrensch M, Black PM. Epidemiology of intracranial meningioma. Neurosurgery. 2005; 57(6):1088–1095, discussion 1088–1095

[4] Staneczek W, Jänisch W. Epidemiologic data on meningiomas in East Germany 1961–1986: incidence, localization, age and sex distribution. Clin Neuropathol. 1992; 11(3):135–141

[5] Louis DN, Perry A, Reifenberger G, et al. The 2016 World Health Organization Classification of Tumors of the Central Nervous System: a summary. Acta Neuropathol. 2016; 131(6):803–820

[6] Wiemels J, Wrensch M, Claus EB. Epidemiology and etiology of meningioma. J Neurooncol. 2010; 99(3):307–314

[7] Nakasu S, Fukami T, Nakajima M, Watanabe K, Ichikawa M, Matsuda M. Growth pattern changes of meningiomas: long-term analysis. Neurosurgery. 2005; 56(5):946–955, discussion 946–955

[8] Durand A, Labrousse F, Jouvet A, et al. WHO grade II and III meningiomas: a study of prognostic factors. J Neurooncol. 2009; 95(3):367–375

[9] Perry A, Stafford SL, Scheithauer BW, Suman VJ, Lohse CM. Meningioma grading: an analysis of histologic parameters. Am J Surg Pathol. 1997; 21(12):1455–1465

[10] Hashiba T, Hashimoto N, Izumoto S, et al. Serial volumetric assessment of the natural history and growth pattern of incidentally discovered meningiomas. J Neurosurg. 2009; 110(4):675–684

[11] Sughrue ME, Rutkowski MJ, Aranda D, Barani IJ, McDermott MW, Parsa AT. Treatment decision making based on the published natural history and growth rate of small meningiomas. J Neurosurg. 2010; 113(5):1036–1042

[12] Oya S, Kim S-H, Sade B, Lee JH. The natural history of intracranial meningiomas. J Neurosurg. 2011; 114(5):1250–1256

[13] Chamoun R, Krisht KM, Couldwell WT. Incidental meningiomas. Neurosurg Focus. 2011; 31(6):E19

[14] Dirks MS, Butman JA, Kim HJ, et al. Long-term natural history of neurofibromatosis type 2-associated intracranial tumors. J Neurosurg. 2012; 117(1):109–117

[15] Goutagny S, Bah AB, Henin D, et al. Long-term follow-up of 287 meningiomas in neurofibromatosis type 2 patients: clinical, radiological, and molecular features. Neuro-oncol. 2012; 14(8):1090–1096

Section III

Head and Neck–Associated Incidental Findings

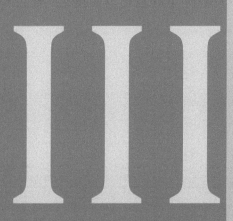

Introduction

The radiologist is responsible not only to thoroughly study the region of interest and address the clinical concern but also to detect incidental findings, which may range from benign lesions that are clinically irrelevant to lesions with significant clinical impact, where the expertise of the head and neck radiologist and otolaryngologist becomes crucial. In this section, we will show several examples of pathology found incidentally on neuroimaging studies that were performed for other indications. Key imaging features and the differential diagnosis of each entity will be discussed. The otolaryngologist's clinical evaluation and management of each patient will be described. Each case concludes with essential facts about the clinical and pathological final diagnosis.

24 Head and Neck–Related Incidental Findings

Mumtaz B. Syed, Maria O. Patino, Jeanie M. Choi, and Ron J. Karni

24.1 Parotid Mass

24.1.1 Case Presentation

History

A 44-year-old man presents with hoarseness. A CT scan of the neck with contrast was performed.

Imaging Findings and Impression

Axial contrast-enhanced CT images of the neck shows a well-circumscribed mass in the superficial lobe of the right parotid gland (*arrow* in ▶ Fig. 24.1a). There is an area of calcification within the mass (*arrow* in ▶ Fig. 24.1b). There is no evidence of infiltration into the superficial or deep soft tissues. This is a solitary, solid mass in the parotid gland. The differential diagnosis is given below; however, clinical evaluation by an otolaryngologist will be needed to make the definitive tissue diagnosis.

24.1.2 Clinical Evaluation

History

A 44-year-old man presents to otolaryngology clinic for evaluation of hoarseness. An incidental parotid mass is identified on neck CT with contrast. He denies any recent illness, pain, or swelling in the region of the parotid gland.

Physical Examination

A small, firm mass detected in the right parotid gland was non-tender and slightly mobile. There was no adenopathy or overlying skin lesions. Sensation was intact and there was no evidence of trismus or facial nerve palsy. Examination of the airway revealed an incidental polyp of the right vocal cord.

Impression

Incidentally detected solid mass of the superficial lobe of the right parotid gland.

Management

Fine needle aspirate was performed and pathology suggested acinic cell carcinoma. Superficial parotidectomy with identification and preservation of the facial nerve was performed. Clear margins were reported by the pathologist and the patient was referred to a head and neck surveillance clinic for monitoring.

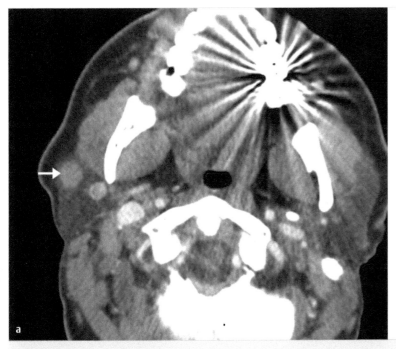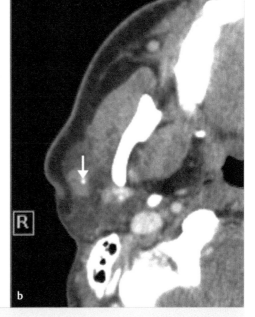

Fig. 24.1 (a, b)

24.1.3 Differential Diagnosis

- **Parotid acinic cell carcinoma:**
  - The majority arise in the parotid gland.
  - A rare, slow-growing variant of adenocarcinoma.
  - On CT, it is well defined, usually homogenously enhancing, and may have cystic areas.
  - Important to evaluate for extent of tumor and CN VII perineural invasion.
- Parotid benign mixed tumor (pleomorphic adenoma):
  - Most common benign parotid neoplasm.
  - Most often demonstrates homogeneous enhancement with contrast.
  - Well defined, typically marked T2 hyperintense on MRI.
  - Calcifications may be present.
- Warthin's tumor (lymphomatous papillary cystadenomas):
  - Second most common benign parotid tumor.
  - Most common cause of bilateral or multifocal solid parotid masses.
  - Propensity to be located within the parotid tail.
  - Mural nodule in a cyst is a common appearance.
  - Calcification is rare.
  - Usually does not enhance with contrast.
  - Low incidence of malignant transformation.
  - Tumor of the elderly with a male predominance. Extremely rare in patients younger than 40 years.
  - A Warthin Tumor Score, which incorporated low mean and standard deviation ADC in addition to age older than 49 years and male sex, has been found to have a 100% specificity and 85.7% sensitivity for distinguishing Warthin's tumor from pleomorphic adenomas and carcinomas.
- Mucoepidermoid carcinoma:
  - Most common malignant parotid neoplasm.
  - Imaging appearance depends upon the tumor grade:
    - Low-grade tumors: similar to benign mixed tumors, well defined, T2 hyperintense.
    - High-grade tumors: poorly defined margins, low signal intensity on T2-weighted imaging.
- Adenoid cystic carcinoma:
  - Most common malignancy involving the MINOR salivary glands but relatively rare in the parotid gland.
  - Locally aggressive tumor with tendency for perineural spread, local infiltration, recurrence postresection, and distant, late metastasis.

24.1.4 Clinical and Diagnostic Imaging Pearls and Pitfalls

- CT is the imaging modality of choice to evaluate extent of lesion within the gland and to evaluate for cervical adenopathy
- MRI is superior for evaluation of perineural tumor spread.
- In the absence of infiltrating tumor or perineural tumor spread, imaging alone lacks the specificity to differentiate malignant tumors from benign etiologies.
- Tissue diagnoses remain the standard of care for most parotid lesions.
- Clinical findings that suggest malignancy include the following:
  - Lymphadenopathy.
  - Rapid increase in size.
  - History of new onset of pain.

24.1.5 Essential Facts

- Nonspecific imaging appearance. Tissue diagnosis is required.
- Considered a low-grade malignancy.
- Good prognosis with surgical resection alone.
- Post-op XRT (radiotherapy) is performed if there is concern for margins or perineural invasion.
- Poorer prognosis if perineural or vascular invasion.

24.2 Thyroglossal Duct Cyst

24.2.1 Case Presentation

History

A 69-year-old woman presents with neck pain. A CT scan of the neck without contrast was performed.

Imaging Findings and Impression

CT of the cervical spine without contrast shows a well-circumscribed, lobular hypodense mass in the right paramidline anterior infrahyoid neck (*arrows* in ▶ Fig. 24.2a–c). The mass is embedded with the strap muscles (*arrowheads* in ▶ Fig. 24.2b). There is no solid nodule associated with the hypodense mass. This is an incidentally detected cystic, midline mass with no evidence of inflammation about the cyst or solid component. It most likely is an uncomplicated thyroglossal duct cyst (TDC).

24.2.2 Clinical Evaluation

This 69-year-old woman was referred to otolaryngology clinic for an incidentally detected midline cystic lesion in the infrahyoid neck. The lesion was nontender, soft, and slightly mobile. There was no evidence of adenopathy. The airway examination was unremarkable. The mass elevated upon tongue protrusion.

Recommended Management

The patient was offered a Sistrunk procedure (removal of the cyst and midline portion of the hyoid bone). Pathology revealed a benign thyroglossal duct cyst.

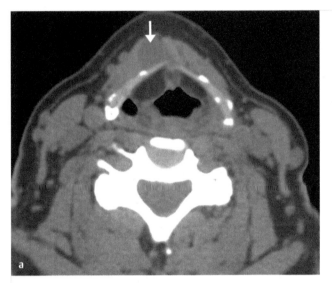
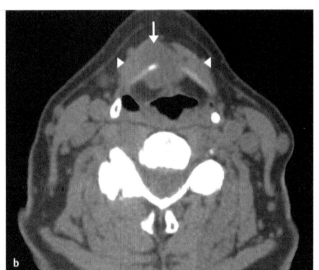
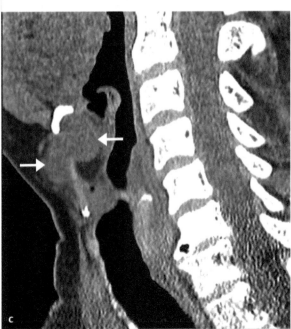

Fig. 24.2 (a–c)

24.2.3 Differential Diagnosis

- **TDC:**
  - Remnant of thyroglossal duct, between the foramen cecum at the tongue base and the thyroid bed in the infrahyoid neck.
  - Midline suprahyoid or midline/paramidline infrahyoid cystic neck mass.
  - In the infrahyoid neck, they are embedded in the strap muscles with a "claw sign."
- Lymphatic malformation:
  - Unilocular or multilocular.
  - Focal or trans-spatial.
  - Fluid–fluid levels common; secondary to hemorrhage.
  - Nonenhancing unless infected or part of combined veno-lymphatic vascular malformation.
- Dermoid and epidermoid:
  - Dermoid contains fat, fluid, or mixed.
  - Epidermoid contains fluid.
  - Neither directly involves the hyoid bone.
  - Submandibular, sublingual spaces or root of tongue
- Tongue base squamous cell carcinoma.

24.2.4 Imaging Pearls and Pitfalls

- Ultrasound of the neck is the first line of imaging to evaluate a midline neck mass and to confirm normal thyroid tissue in the lower neck.
- CT or MRI may be obtained if infection is suspected or the diagnosis is uncertain.
- Nuclear scintigraphy may be indicated if ectopic thyroid is suspected.

24.2.5 Essential Facts

- The most common congenital neck cyst, typically midline in location.
- Arises from remnants of the thyroglossal duct, so may arise anywhere along the course of the duct, with the infrahyoid location being most common.
- The wall of thyroglossal duct cyst may enhance if infected.
- Less than 1% contain associated papillary thyroid carcinoma, which is solid eccentric mass often with calcification within cyst.

24.3 Prominent Nasopharyngeal Soft Tissue

24.3.1 Case Presentation

History

A 36-year-old man with dizziness. An MRI of the brain without contrast was ordered.

Imaging Findings and Impression

Sagittal T1-weighted MRI of the brain shows prominent nasopharyngeal soft tissues (*arrow* in ▶ Fig. 24.3a). Axial T2-weighted MRI of the brain shows that the prominent nasopharyngeal soft tissues are symmetric (*arrow* in ▶ Fig. 24.3b). Multiple mucous retention cysts are present in the left maxillary sinus (*arrowhead* in ▶ Fig. 24.3b). Axial T2-weighted MRI shows a 10-mm right lateral retropharyngeal lymph node (*arrow* in ▶ Fig. 24.3c). The nasopharyngeal soft tissues are markedly prominent but symmetric for an adult patient. Although this is very likely reactive or HIV related, the possibility of malignancy cannot be excluded. Additional imaging will not be definitive in excluding lymphoma or nasopharyngeal carcinoma. Therefore, clinical evaluation by an otolaryngologist will be needed.

24.3.2 Clinical Management

This 36-year-old man was sent to the otolaryngology clinic for further evaluation of incidentally detected abnormal prominence of the nasopharyngeal soft tissues on brain MR.

Adenoidal tissue typically regresses in patients older than 16 years of age. Nasopharyngeal soft-tissue prominence in a 36-year-old is abnormal and the possibility of HIV infection should be investigated. Office nasopharyngoscopy was performed, demonstrating symmetric nonulcerative diffuse enlargement of the nasopharyngeal lymphoid tissue. An HIV test was negative. No biopsy was performed, but the patient was advised to return in 3 months for an interval examination.

24.3.3 Differential Diagnosis

- **Adenoidal benign lymphoid hyperplasia:**
  - Large adenoids seen in children, teenagers, and HIV patients.
  - Symmetric enlargement without infiltration of adjacent tissues.
  - Marrow signal changes associated with HIV can sometimes be used as an additional clue on imaging.
- Nasopharyngeal non-Hodgkin's lymphoma:
  - Midline symmetric mass with deep infiltration to prevertebral muscles.
  - Tends to be expansile in clivus rather than infiltrative.
- Nasopharyngeal carcinoma:
  - Mucosal tumor of the lateral nasopharyngeal recess.
  - More asymmetric with obstruction of the eustachian tube and subsequent unilateral mastoid effusion.
  - Nodal disease, especially involving the lateral retropharyngeal node at presentation 90% of the times.

24.3.4 Imaging Pearls and Pitfalls

- Size asymmetry was the best overall criterion in a recent study for differentiating benign lymphoid hyperplasia from nasopharyngeal carcinoma.
- ENT (ear, nose, and throat) referral and subsequent tissue diagnosis is the standard of care as lymphoma can present as a symmetric soft-tissue prominence on imaging.

24.3.5 Essential Facts

- Hypertrophy of the nasopharyngeal lymphoid tissue is reported in the first 4 years of life and its involution usually happens by the age of 6 to 16 years.
- The reported factors responsible for adenoid hypertrophy in adults include the following:
  - Persistence of childhood adenoids due to chronic inflammation.
  - Regrowth of involuted adenoidal tissue as a result of irritants, infections, or smoking.
- Studies also reported viral infection in immunocompromised patients, particularly HIV infection or after organ transplantation.

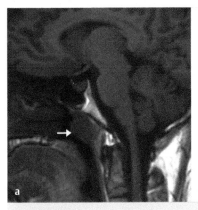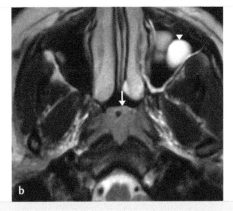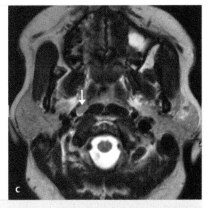

Fig. 24.3 (a–c)

24.4 Incidental Enlarged Lymph Node

24.4.1 Case Presentation

History

A 53-year-old man presents with MRI of brain obtained for meningioma follow-up.

An MRI of the brain with contrast was performed and, after identifying the incidental finding, additional sequences through the neck were obtained.

Imaging Findings and Impression

Coronal postcontrast T1-weighted (T1W) image of the brain shows enhancing extra-axial mass with a dural tail consistent with the patient's known meningioma. At the inferior most aspect of the image, a mass is present in the left side of the neck just lateral to the vessels (*arrow* in ▶ Fig. 24.4a).

Coronal postcontrast T1 W image of the neck (▶ Fig. 24.4b) shows enhancing mass in the left neck at level II. Axial T2 W image (▶ Fig. 24.4c) and axial T1 W image (▶ Fig. 24.4d) with contrast reveal a 2-cm mass that is on the left at level II.

This is a pathologically enlarged, level II lymph node. Further imaging and clinical evaluation will be necessary to determine possible primary site of malignancy.

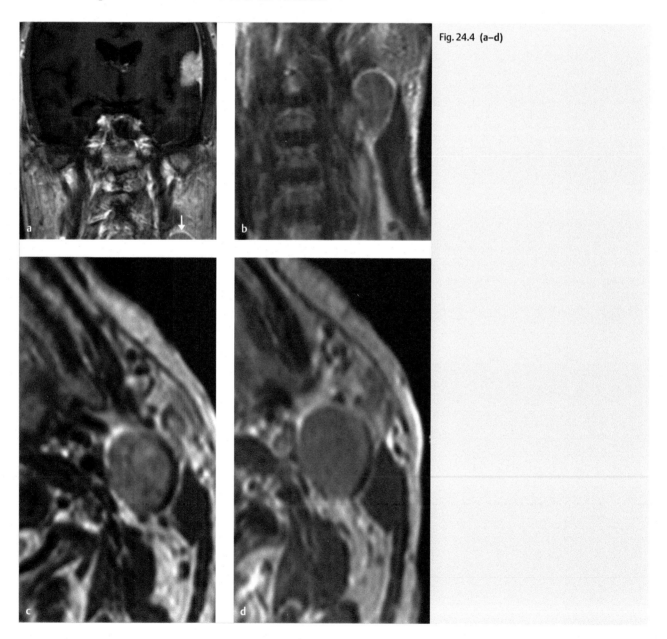

Fig. 24.4 (a–d)

24.4.2 Clinical Management

This 53-year-old man was referred to the otolaryngology clinic for further evaluation of an enlarged level II lymph node. The patient's history was remarkable for a 30 pack-year history of smoking. He denied any fever, sore throat, neck tenderness, or other constitutional symptoms.

Physical examination revealed a 1-cm nodular mass in the left palatine tonsil. Cytology of the neck lymph node revealed p16+squamous cell carcinoma (SCC). The patient underwent a transoral robotic radical tonsillectomy and left selective neck dissection, followed by unilateral radiation, and remained in 4 years of follow-up.

24.4.3 Differential Diagnosis

- **Metastatic node:**
  - Enlarged size greater than 1.0 cm. Level II lymph nodes tend to be larger and are considered enlarge if they are greater than 1.5 cm.
  - A round rather than oblong, oval shape, is worrisome for malignancy.
  - Presence of necrosis.
  - Signs of extracapsular invasion by imaging include irregular margins, stranding of the surrounding fat, and invasion into neighboring structures.
- Reactive lymphadenopathy:
  - Enlarged well-defined oval-shaped nodes. Viral illness including etiologies such as Epstein–Barr virus (EBV) and cytomegalovirus (CMV) can cause generalized lymphadenopathy and splenomegaly.
  - Bacterial infections such *Staphylococcus aureus* and group A *Streptococcus*. Lymph nodes associated with these infections can be fluctuant and suppurative if abscess is suspected clinically.
  - HIV, toxoplasmosis, *Bartonella henselae*, and *Mycobacterium tuberculosis*.
  - Also seen in rheumatological conditions such as Sjogren's disease.
- Lymphoproliferative process:
  - Lymphoma (Hodgkin's or non-Hodgkin's).
  - Round nodal masses with variable enhancement and variable central necrosis.
  - Single or multiple nodal stations.

24.4.4 Imaging Pearls and Pitfalls

- Single enlarged and necrotic cervical lymph node has to be further worked up with tissue sampling to evaluate for metastases from head and neck malignancy.
- A major pitfall of CT is that in a patient with known head and neck malignancy there is a 20% chance of metastases in a cervical lymph node, which is less than 10 mm in size.
- PET-CT imaging may identify an occult primary in the oropharynx and further define the extent of nodal metastatic disease.

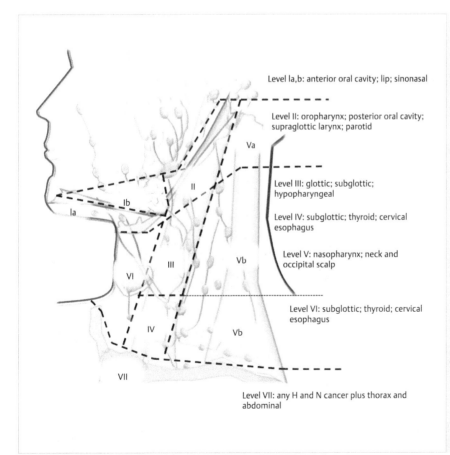

Fig. 24.5 Cervical lymph node levels. (Illustration courtesy of Dr. Roy F. Riascos.)

Level Ia,b: anterior oral cavity; lip; sinonasal

Level II: oropharynx; posterior oral cavity; supraglottic larynx; parotid

Level III: glottic; subglottic; hypopharyngeal

Level IV: subglottic; thyroid; cervical esophagus

Level V: nasopharynx; neck and occipital scalp

Level VI: subglottic; thyroid; cervical esophagus

Level VII: any H and N cancer plus thorax and abdominal

24.4.5 Essential Facts

- Level II metastatic lymphadenopathy is a very common presenting symptom of patients with SCC arising in the oropharynx.
- Level II lymph nodes normally drain the oropharynx, posterior oral cavity, supraglottic larynx, and the parotid gland.
- Pathologically enlarged level I to III lymph nodes are most often attributed to a presumable primary SCC located in the mucosa of the upper aerodigestive tract.
- Pathologically enlarged lymph nodes in levels IV and Vb may arise from proximal esophageal and thyroid carcinomas.
- Oropharyngeal cancers that contain human papillomavirus (HPV) DNA (p16 positive) have a better prognosis than those without HPV (p16 negative).

24.5 Key Point Summary

- In children, symmetric nasopharyngeal soft-tissue prominence is most often a normal incidental finding. In adults, especially if there is asymmetry, the differential diagnosis includes nasopharyngeal carcinoma, lymphoma, and HIV-associated disease. Referral to an otolaryngologist is necessary for definitive diagnosis.
- A midline infrahyoid cystic mass in an asymptomatic adult is most likely a thyroglossal duct cyst. Rarely, infection or tumor may develop.
- Solitary, solid parotid tumors are most commonly pleomorphic adenomas. However, tissue diagnosis is needed for definitive diagnosis and treatment.
- Carcinomas of the tonsillar fossa may be occult and come to attention due to a pathologically enlarged level II lymph node.
- Round shape and central necrosis are features of lymph nodes that may suggest metastatic disease in addition to an abnormal increase in size.

Suggested Readings

Bavle RM, Makarla S, Nadaf A, Narasimhamurthy S. Solid blue dot tumour: minor salivary gland acinic cell carcinoma. BMJ Case Rep. 2014; 2014:bcr2013200885

Christe A, Waldherr C, Hallett R, Zbaeren P, Thoeny H. MR imaging of parotid tumors: typical lesion characteristics in MR imaging improve discrimination between benign and malignant disease. AJNR Am J Neuroradiol. 2011; 32(7): 1202–1207

Hoang JK, Vanka J, Ludwig BJ, Glastonbury CM. Evaluation of cervical lymph nodes in head and neck cancer with CT and MRI: tips, traps, and a systematic approach. AJR Am J Roentgenol. 2013; 200:W17–W25

King AD, Wong LYS, Law BKH, et al. MR imaging criteria for the detection of nasopharyngeal carcinoma: discrimination of early-stage primary tumors from benign hyperplasia. AJNR Am J Neuroradiol. 2018; 39(3):515–523

Wang CW, Chu YH, Chiu DY, et al. JOURNAL CLUB: The Warthin tumor score: a simple and reliable method to distinguish warthin tumors from pleomorphic adenomas and carcinomas. AJR Am J Roentgenol. 2018; 210(6):1330–1337

Yildirim N, Sahan M, Karslioğlu Y. Adenoid hypertrophy in adults: clinical and morphological characteristics. J Int Med Res. 2008; 36(1):157–162

Zander DA, Smoker WR. Imaging of ectopic thyroid tissue and thyroglossal duct cysts. Radiographics. 2014; 34(1):37–50

Section IV

Spinal Incidental Findings

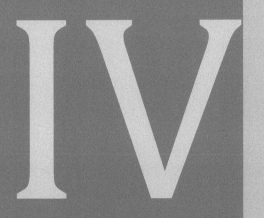

25 Os Odontoideum

Daniel R. Monsivais, Kaye D. Westmark, Susana Calle, and Daniel H. Kim

25.1 Introduction

The os odontoideum is a rare abnormality of the odontoid process that may present with neck pain and myelopathy but may also be detected as an incidental finding. In this chapter, the diagnostic workup, as it relates to management of the patient, will be discussed. In addition, the developmental anatomy of the craniocervical junction is presented as it provides the key to understanding the distinction between the os odontoideum and other entities in the differential diagnosis.

25.2 Case Presentation

25.2.1 History and Physical Examination

A 15-year-old boy status post a fall presents to the emergency room (ER) with a deep laceration present on his forehead but does not complain of neck pain. The head CT performed in the ER showed a possible abnormality of the craniocervical junction. Therefore, a cervical spine CT scan was performed. The physical examination was normal and his neck was not tender and had a full range of motion.

25.2.2 Imaging Findings and Impression

Sagittal reformatted CT image of the upper cervical spine reveals a well-corticated, prominent ossicle (*arrow* in ▶ Fig. 25.2) separate from and superior to a hypoplastic odontoid whose superior margin is also well corticated. The ossicle lies near the basion but is not fused to it or to the anterior arch of C1. The basion is normal. There is no evidence of soft-tissue swelling. These findings are typical of an os odontoideum.

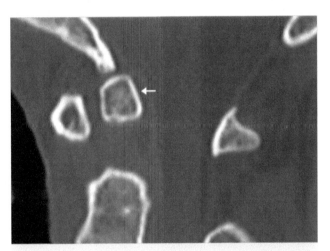

Fig. 25.2

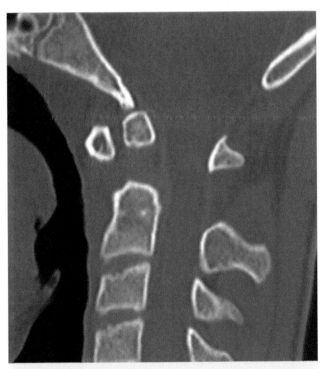

Fig. 25.1 Sagittal reformatted CT scan without contrast of the upper cervical spine.

25.2.3 Additional Imaging to Be Considered for Further Evaluation

- **Flexion–extension lateral cervical spine radiographs.**
  Flexion–extension lateral views of the cervical spine are the most important diagnostic test after detection of an os odontoideum. Abnormal motion between C1 and C2 is present in the vast majority of cases imaged (93%). Anterior instability is most common, occurring in 70%, with posterior instability (10%) and both posterior and anterior instability (13%) occurring less commonly. Lack of motion is uncommon and occurs in only 7%.[1] In the majority of cases, the ossicle will move with the anterior arch of C1.
  Lateral views in flexion and extension show significant anterior subluxation of C1 and of the ossicle relative to the body of C2 (▸ Fig. 25.3). The space available for the spinal cord between the posterior aspect of the body of C2 and the posterior arch of C1 is less than 13 mm in flexion.

- **CT of the cervical spine.** CT scan of the craniocervical junction is not needed for diagnosis but provides greater anatomic detail especially if the bony anatomy of C1–C2 is obscured on plain films. If surgery is contemplated, CT with multiplanar reconstruction is very helpful to define the bony anatomy. If a C1–C2 fusion is considered, close inspection of the posterior arch of C1 is important to be sure that the arch is not incomplete or assimilated into the skull base.

- **MRI of the cervical spine.** MRI may show associated soft-tissue/synovial hypertrophy not detected by plain film. MRI should be performed if there are subtle signs of myelopathy to look for intrinsic increased signal in the spinal cord on the T2-weighted images. An os odontoideum may be associated with an anomalous vertebral artery or persistent fetal circulation; therefore, MRI with or without MRA may be useful if surgery is contemplated. Flexion–extension MRI may be useful as well. Contrast administration for either MRI or CT is not indicated. The sagittal T2-weighted image of the cervical spine (▸ Fig. 25.4) reveals abnormal subluxation of C1 and of the ossicle (*asterisk*) relative to the base of the dens and the body of C2 as the patient's neck was in a relatively flexed position for the MRI. There is effacement of CSF signal anterior to the cord at the base of the odontoid, immediately superior to the subdental synchondrosis (SDS; *arrow*). The space available for cord (SAC, indicated by the *thick horizontal white line*) measures less than 13 mm. Most commonly, the os will move with the anterior arch of the atlas and SAC will be most compromised in flexion. On plain radiographs, the SAC is measured with a line drawn from the dorsum of the odontoid base/body of C2 to a perpendicular line tangential to the anterior cortical margin of the posterior arch of C1 (*vertical thin white line* as shown on ▸ Fig. 25.4). On this MRI, upon which these lines have been constructed, it is revealed that ligamentous tissue further decreases the SAC in comparison to that which would be suggested by plain radiographs.

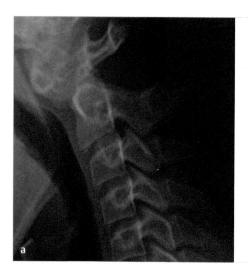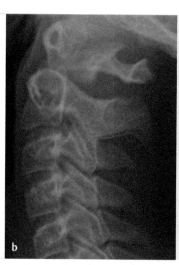

Fig. 25.3 Lateral radiographs in flexion **(a)** and extension **(b)** were obtained for further evaluation of the C1–C2 instability.

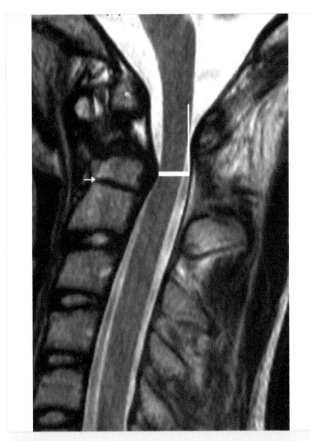

Fig. 25.4

25.3 Clinical Evaluation

This is a 15-year-old adolescent boy with an incidentally detected os odontoideum. There is significant motion of C1 on C2 and the space available for the spinal cord is less than 13 mm at C2, which has been associated with development of myelopathy.

Although the os odontoideum was incidentally detected and asymptomatic, the decision was made to perform C1–C2 posterior fusion (▶ Fig. 25.5) due to the patient's young age, and significant anterior subluxation and instability on the flexion/extension radiographs.

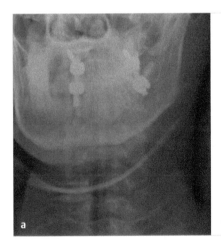
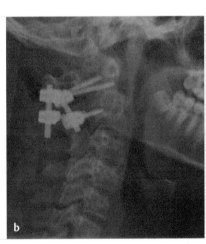

Fig. 25.5 Anteroposterior (a) and lateral (b) cervical spine radiographs status post C1–C2 posterior fusion.

25.4 Differential Diagnosis

- **Os odontoideum:**
  - Round or oval, well-corticated ossicle at the skull base between the smoothly corticated but hypoplastic odontoid process and the basion.
- Type 2 fracture of odontoid with nonunion (see companion Cases 1 and 2):
  - The plane of the separation in the os odontoideum is most often well above the superior articulating facets of C2, whereas a type 2 fracture, through the "neck of the odontoid," often extends below this level.[2]
  - The os odontoideum is round or oval in shape, whereas a type 2 odontoid process fracture fragment has a "peg-shaped" appearance.
  - Hypertrophy and rounding of the anterior arch of C1 rather than its usual half-moon shape has also been reported in patients with the os odontoideum and may distinguish it from a type 2 fracture fragment.[3]
  - Importantly, in chronic cases, it is often not possible or of importance clinically to distinguish the os odontoideum from a chronic nonunion of an odontoid process fracture as both may have a similar posttraumatic etiology and be functionally equivalent in terms of their potential for C1–C2 instability.[4]
- Os terminale/os terminale persistens (see companion Cases 3 and 4):
  - A secondary ossification center, the os terminale (ossiculum terminale of Bergmann) sometimes forms within the distal tip of the dens, an epiphysis called the chondrum terminale. It usually appears by 3 to 6 years of age and unites with the body of the odontoid around 11 to 12 years of age.[5,6,7] If it does not fuse with the base of the odontoid, and the **apicodental synchondrosis (ADS)** remains open in the adult, it is termed an os terminale persistens.[5,8]
  - An os terminale persistens is readily diagnosed when the ossicle is small, the proximal dens is virtually normal, and, on coronal imaging, the characteristic "**V**" shape of the unfused ADS is seen.
  - Importantly, the os terminale with minimal or no odontoid hypoplasia has very little potential for atlantoaxial instability (AAI), unlike a large os odontoideum with significant dens hypoplasia.[1,5,6]
  - Large os terminale versus small os odontoideum: The distinction between os terminale persistens and os odontoideum is semantic in many cases as a dislocated ossiculum terminale may aberrantly enlarge to "give rise" to an os

odontoideum and the proximal dens becomes increasingly hypoplastic over time.[5,6,9,10,11,12,13]

- Unfused SDS, also known as the dentocentral or lower dental synchondrosis:
  - The SDS is a wide cartilaginous epiphyseal plate, a remnant of the C1–C2 intervertebral disk, that is visualized in 100% of children ≤ 3 years of age and 50% of children 4 to 5 years of age and therefore may be mistaken for a fracture in children younger than 5 years of age. It may persist as a thin sclerotic line on CT and a dark line on T2 W MR images from 5 to 11 years of age.[7,14]
  - The SDS lies well caudal to the plane of the C2 superior articulating facets, deep within the body of C2.[5]
  - An unfused SDS should not show any motion with flexion and extension.[1]
  - In children younger than 7 years of age, the SDS is a site of relative weakness and the most common site of injury.[15,16]
  - If there are symptoms or a high clinical suspicion of injury, MRI is useful to look for associated edema in the vertebral body, adjacent to and through the SDS, and within ligaments of the craniocervical junction.
- Dystrophic calcification in ligaments due to old injury or arthritis (see companion Case 8):
  - The odontoid appears to have formed normally but may be sclerotic and/or eroded.
  - Dystrophic calcifications are not well rounded and corticated and their location is variable.
- Calcium pyrophosphate dihydrate crystal deposition disease (CPPD)/"pseudogout":
  - Dystrophic calcification and erosion of the odontoid process in patients with "pseudogout."
  - It may result in the "crowned dens syndrome" in which soft-tissue calcium deposits occur around the dens and result in neck pain.
- Condylus tertius (see companion Case 7):
  - Rare congenital abnormality that results from lack of integration of embryonic mesenchymal tissue ventral to the notochord.[4,17,18,19,20,21,22,23,24]
  - It appears as a small midline bony tubercle firmly attached to the basion and is essentially a third occipital condyle that may form a true synovial joint with the anterior arch of C1 and/or the odontoid process and limit the range of motion of the craniocervical junction.
  - If the odontoid process appears normal and the clivus hypoplastic, or dysmorphic with a comma-shaped basion, the diagnosis of condylus tertius is favored over an os odontoideum that has fused to the skull base (aka os avis).[8,17,18]

25.5 Clinical and Diagnostic Imaging Pearls

- Smooth, well-defined cortication of the round-shaped ossicle and the superior margin of the hypoplastic odontoid favor the diagnosis of os odontoideum, orthotopic subtype.
- Flexion–extension radiographs are needed as the os odontoideum almost always has some degree of C1–C2 instability that strongly influences the surgeon's management decision.

25.6 Essential Information about the Os Odontoideum

25.6.1 Embryology of C2 and Its Odontoid Process

- C2 is embryologically unique:
  - Whereas most vertebral bodies arise from two sclerotomes, C2 and its odontoid process are derived from three sclerotomes: C0 (proatlas [PA]), C1, and C2 (▶ Fig. 25.6).
- The PA:
  - The PA normally regresses and is not found in man as a complete vertebra but rather gives rise to the occipital condyles, and the portion of the skull base surrounding the foramen magnum, including the basion; the terminal portion of the dens and the apical ligament; the superior aspect of the C1 lateral masses and the superior aspect of the posterior arch of C1.
  - The terminal tip (or apical segment) of the odontoid is derived from the PA centrum.
- PA hypochordal bow:
  - PA hypochordal bow (PA-Hb) refers to the mesenchymal tissue ventral to the notochord and is found in the region of the PA and C1 sclerotomes where it normally gives rise to the clival tubercle and the anterior arch of C1, respectively.
  - Anomalous persistent PA-Hb, whether complete, midline, or lateral, gives rise to the prebasioccipital arch, the condylus tertius, or the basilar process, respectively.
  - Hypochordal tissue derivatives are not found caudal to C1.
- The body of C2 and its odontoid process:
  - The basal segment of the odontoid process arises from the C1 sclerotome and has two bilateral primary ossification

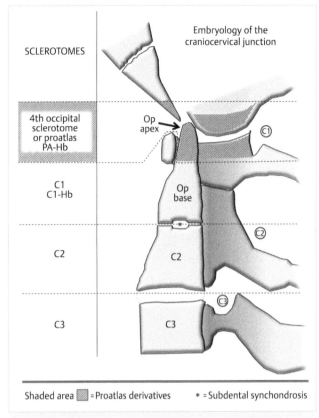

Fig. 25.6 Embryology of the craniocervical junction.[4,8,14,15,17,18,19,20,21,22,23,24] (Illustration by Dr. Susana Calle.)

centers, which normally fuse in utero prior to birth at approximately 8 months of prenatal age.
  - The odontoid process is separated from the body of C2 (the centrum) by the SDS, which is also called the lower dental synchondrosis or dentocentral synchondrosis.
  - The SDS is a remnant of the C1–C2 intervertebral disk, an epiphyseal growth plate, which is open until 5 to 7 years of age. It lies well within the body of C2 in the adult.
  - The body and neural arches of C2 arise from the C2 sclerotome.

25.6.2 Os Odontoideum: Classification Schemes

- There are two anatomic types based on the position of the ossicle[5,25,26,27]:
  - Orthotopic: The ossicle is in normally expected, anatomic, position of the dens.
  - Dystopic: The ossicle is located near the foramen magnum and may be fused to the clivus or the anterior arch of C1 or even subluxed anteriorly to the residual odontoid base. Os avis, so termed as it is a normal structure in birds, is an example of a dystopic type where the os odontoideum is fused to the clivus.[8]

25.6.3 Controversial Etiology

Is the os odontoideum a congenital abnormality or the sequelae of early trauma?

- The argument for a congenital etiology:
  - Os odontoideum frequently coexists with other congenital segmentation anomalies such as assimilation of C1 to skull base and Klippel–Feil syndrome.
  - C1 assimilation and os avis (the dystopic form of os odontoideum where the ossicle is fused to the basiocciput) have been mimicked in mice knockout experiments involving the *Hox* genes.[28,29]
  - There are multiple case reports involving identical twins as well as familial os odontoideum in multiple generations.[29,30,31,32]
  - Not all cases of delayed os odontoideum development can be explained by the "posttraumatic dislocation of the ossiculum terminale theory" as evidenced by case reports of "coexisting ossiculum terminale persistens and os odontoideum."[33,34]
- The argument for a traumatic origin:
  - There are many case reports of posttraumatic development of an os odontoideum in young children in whom a normal odontoid process had been documented on prior plain films.[16,23,35,36,37,38]
  - There are two case reports in young children of traumatic ossiculum terminale dislocation, documented by MR and CT, which subsequently gave rise to an os odontoideum.[9,10]
  - The blood supply to the odontoid process makes the basal segment vulnerable to necrosis and resorption should traumatic disruption occur. The apical segment, however, is supplied via an arcade, which can maintain separate blood flow to the ossiculum terminale and allow its growth to continue even if separated from the base.[35]

25.7 Companion Cases

25.7.1 Case 1: Type 2 Odontoid Fracture

Coronal (▶ Fig. 25.7a) and sagittal (▶ Fig. 25.7b) reformatted CT images reveal the distal fracture fragment (see *asterisk* in ▶ Fig. 25.7b) is not rounded but rather has a peglike shape with a jagged proximal margin complementing the distal aspect of the proximal dens. The anterior arch of C1 (*arrow* in ▶ Fig. 25.7b) has associated dystrophic calcification but retains its half-moon configuration and is not rounded or hypertrophied.

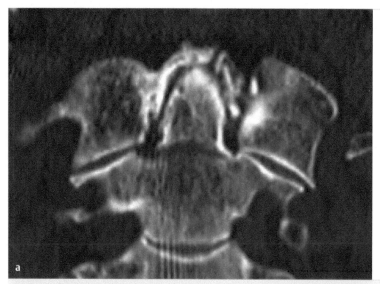
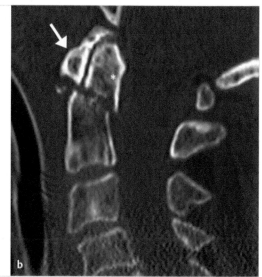

Fig. 25.7 (a, b)

25.7.2 Case 2: Chronic Odontoid Fracture with Nonunion

The ossicle (see *asterisk* in ▶ Fig. 25.8) has the shape of the distal tip of the odontoid that matches the proximal aspect of the dens and is not well rounded. There was a history of remote trauma. This appearance is most compatible with an old type 2 odontoid fracture with chronic nonunion.

25.7.3 Case 3: Os Terminale Persistens

Coronal reformation of a craniocervical junction CT scan (▶ Fig. 25.9) reveals an ossiculum terminale persistens (*arrow*) found incidentally in a 16-year-old adolescent boy. Note the sclerotic remnant of the SDS (*arrowhead*).

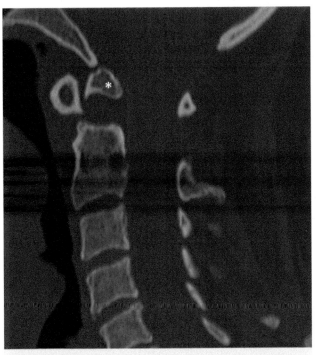

Fig. 25.8

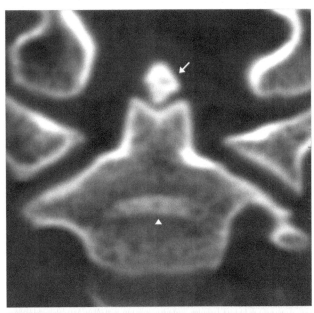

Fig. 25.9

25.7.4 Case 4: Os Odontoideum versus Large Os Terminale

The ossicle has a well-corticated rounded appearance (see *asterisk* in ▸ Fig. 25.10) and there is minimal hypoplasia of the proximal odontoid process. This appearance is most compatible with a large os terminale. However, it could be termed an os odontoideum. Practically, the next step in management would not depend on the nomenclature but rather radiographs in flexion and extension as well as the patient's physical examination and symptoms.

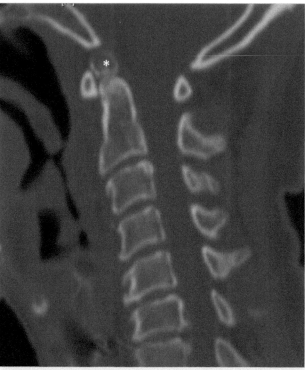

Fig. 25.10

25.7.5 Case 5: Os Odontoideum

In this case, the anterior arch of C1 is hypertrophied (*arrow* in ▸ Fig. 25.11) and has a bizarre shape that matches the ossicle (*asterisk*), compatible with the jigsaw sign previously described in os odontoideum.[39]

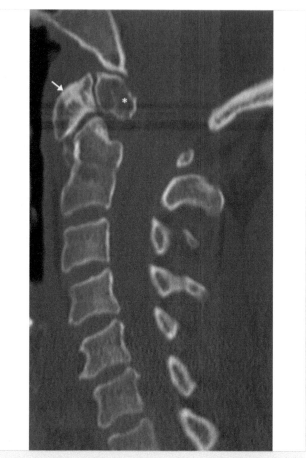

Fig. 25.11

25.7.6 Case 6: Massive "Os Odontoideum"

Sagittal CT scan reformation (▶ Fig. 25.12a) and sagittal T1-weighted MR image (▶ Fig. 25.12b). This patient presented with a long history of neck pain and subtle evidence of chronic spinal cord compression on physical examination, which was due to long-standing AAI and ventral spinal cord compression. A massive "os" (*asterisk*), which has fused with the anterior arch of C1, is present in association with hypoplasia of the proximal odontoid and clivus. Hypoplasia of the clivus raises the possibility of a PA segmentation anomaly that may also be incorporated within the "mass."

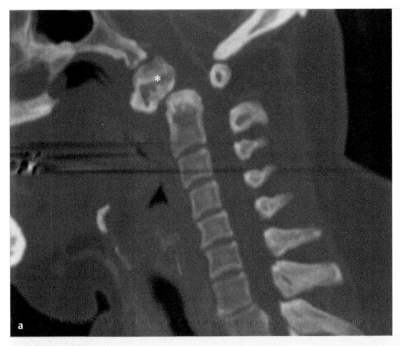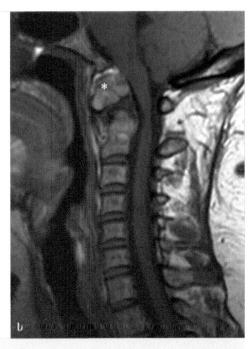

Fig. 25.12 (a, b)

25.7.7 Case 7: Basilar Process Mimicking a Condylus Tertius

On sagittal midline reformatted CT image (▶ Fig. 25.13a), there appears to be a small ossicle (*arrow*) fused to the clivus. This raised the possibility of a condylus tertius with degenerative change in the odontoid tip versus an os avis. However, the coronal reformation (▶ Fig. 25.13b) revealed that there are two asymmetric processes that have cortical continuity with the basion. The larger one (*long arrow*) articulates asymmetrically with the odontoid process like a condylus tertius, whereas the smaller process (*short arrow*) and the central cleft between them has an appearance consistent with a basilar process. Incidental note is made of assimilation of the posterior arch of C1 to the skull base, which is thought to be a segmentation anomaly of the PA.[17]

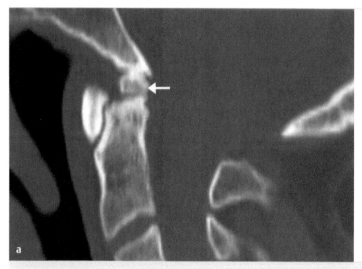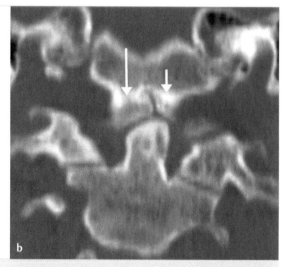

Fig. 25.13 (a, b)

25.7.8 Case 8: Dystrophic Ossification in the Region of the Dens

CT reformatted images from two different patients (▶ Fig. 25.14) reveal a well-formed odontoid process, helping distinguish the nearby dystrophic calcification from an os odontoideum. In ▶ Fig. 25.14b, the dystrophic calcification (*arrow*) has formed in the expected location of the alar ligament and may be secondary to an old avulsion injury.

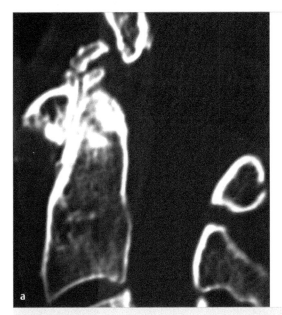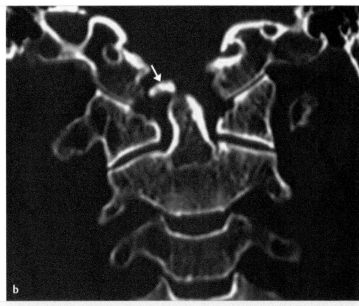

Fig. 25.14 (a, b)

25.8 Neurosurgery Questions and Answers

1. **What are the typical presentations of patients with os odontoideum?**

   Common presenting symptoms include occipitocervical neck pain, myelopathy, signs and symptoms of vertebrobasilar insufficiency and an incidental finding. Most patients who present are neurologically intact,[26] but often have AAI.[40]

2. **What additional testing, if any, is required or recommended in the workup?**

   Lateral radiographs of the cervical spine in flexion and extension are very important to determine if there is significant AAI, which would help determine the management. In the presence of paresthesias or any other neurologic findings, it is critical to identify compression of the neural elements. MRI cervical spine was obtained that showed no spinal cord compression.

   It is critical to rule out C1–C2 instability. The presence of myelopathy does not correlate with the degree of instability, but it is known that canal diameter less than 13 mm correlates with myelopathy.[41] Cervical spine coned down lateral, anteroposterior, and open mouth odontoid views are helpful to evaluate the anatomy of the dens.

   Alternatively, a noncontrast CT of the cervical spine may be used. Lateral flexion–extension views are critical to determine dynamic changes that occur at the C1–C2 junction with motion. MRI of the cervical spine may be helpful to determine the degree of spinal cord impingement or to look for evidence of spinal cord myelomalacia or spinal cord contusion.[42]

3. **What is the etiology and natural history of the condition that would assist in decision-making?**

   According to the literature, the natural history is highly variable. Factors to accurately predict deterioration in asymptomatic patients have not been identified. Some series report both symptomatic and asymptomatic patients remain without new problems for many years. Others report spinal cord injuries after minor trauma. Because of this, all patients with demonstrable AAI on flexion–extension X-rays should be considered at risk for spinal cord injury.[42]

4. **If electing to follow, what is the suggested time interval and modality? Are there any AANS (American Association of Neurological Surgeons)/CNS (Congress of Neurological Surgeons) published guidelines for the management of this condition?**

   Patients with no evidence of C1–C2 instability can be followed conservatively but should be reevaluated for development of instability.[43] Controversy exists surrounding what action should be taken for asymptomatic patients with evidence of C1–C2 instability on flexion–extension X-rays. Presently, it is a level III recommendation that patients without neurologic symptoms can be followed with clinical and radiographic surveillance even if C1–C2 instability is present. However, there is literature suggesting at least some risk of spinal cord injury.[44]

Conservative management can be considered for patients who are asymptomatic and stable on flexion–extension X-rays and have no compression of the neural elements.[42] A series of 279 patients with craniocervical instability due to os odontoideum, who underwent surgery, demonstrated high rates of fusion, low rates of complication, and improved functional scores (see ▶ Fig. 25.15).[45]

5. **Why are the indications for surgery? What are the surgical options/risks?**

   Surgery should be considered in asymptomatic patients when they are young, there is evidence of instability, and anatomy is favorable for surgery. Surgery in a young healthy patient is very safe with nearly 100% fusion rate.[1]

   If treatment is necessary, surgery is recommended. For patients with congenital or chronic nonunion fracture, it is unlikely that fusion will occur from external immobilization. If neurologic signs or symptoms of myelopathy are present secondary to C1–C2 instability, patients need C1–C2 posterior spinal fusion.[1,40]

   Surgical options have historically included posterior wiring and fusion with a halo, which was largely replaced with C1–C2 transarticular screw fixation and fusion. This technique, however, carries with it the risk of vertebral artery injury and, therefore, C1 lateral mass and C2 pedicle screw fixation has gained in popularity.[8,46] For patients with irreducible compression or associated atlantooccipital instability, occipital cervical fusion should be considered. Transoral decompression should be considered for irreducible ventral cervicomedullary decompression.[8,41,42] Odontoid screw is contraindicated as the os is well corticated similar to a sclerotic fracture fragment in a type II odontoid fracture with chronic nonunion.

6. **If conservative management and follow-up imaging is recommended, what restrictions are placed on patients with os odontoideum? Can they play sports?**

   According to small case series, all pediatric patients (symptomatic or asymptomatic) with AAI are at risk for spinal cord injury even with minor trauma. The authors of these series suggested that young patients with AAI should undergo prophylactic surgery.[44,47] This is particularly relevant to children who desire to play contact sports. If a child with os odontoideum desires to play contact sports, it would be advisable to undergo C1–C2 stabilization. For patients with os odontoideum without abnormal motion on flexion–extension films, the answer is less clear. Patients should be evaluated on a case-by-case basis and counseled about risks/benefits of surgical versus conservative management.

7. **What instructions are given to patients regarding return to neurosurgeon?**

   Patients with os odontoideum should immediately seek neurosurgical evaluation if they experience any of the following: persistent or worsening neck pain, sensory disturbances, motor weakness, gait instability, muscle spasticity, and bladder or bowel dysfunction. These may all be signs of spinal instability and neurologic injury due to spinal cord compression and warrant prompt neurosurgical evaluation.

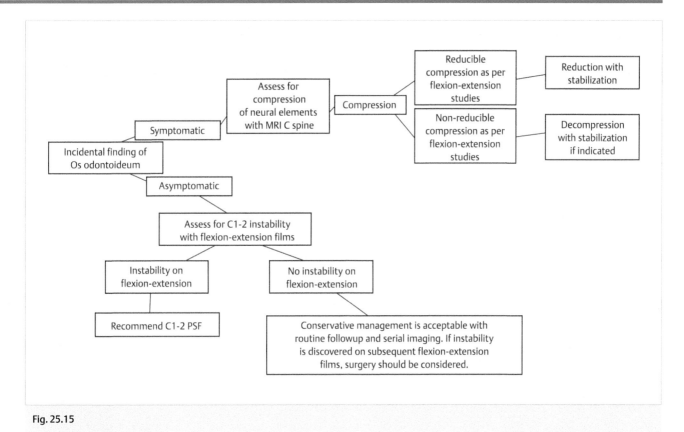

Fig. 25.15

25.9 Key Point Summary

- The os odontoideum is a smoothly corticated ossicle between the skull base and hypoplastic odontoid process.
- Assessment for possible AAI, which is often present, is the most important factor in determining management.
- If it is an incidental finding with no instability, decision-making is on a case-by-case basis as there is no high-quality class I or II evidence to determine management guidelines.

References

[1] Klimo P, Jr, Coon V, Brockmeyer D. Incidental os odontoideum: current management strategies. Neurosurg Focus. 2011; 31(6):E10

[2] Anderson LD, D'Alonzo RT. Fractures of the odontoid process of the axis. J Bone Joint Surg Am. 1974; 56(8):1663–1674

[3] Holt RG, Helms CA, Munk PL, Gillespy T, III. Hypertrophy of C-1 anterior arch: useful sign to distinguish os odontoideum from acute dens fracture. Radiology. 1989; 173(1):207–209

[4] Wollin DG. The os odontoideum: separate odontoid process. J Bone Joint Surg Am. 1963; 45(7):1459–1471

[5] Torklus D, Gehle W. The Upper Cervical Spine. Stuttgart: Thieme; 1972: 47–50

[6] Swischuk LE, John SD, Moorthy C. The os terminale-os odontoideum complex. Emerg Radiol. 1997; 4(2):72–81

[7] Cattell HS, Filtzer DL. Pseudosubluxation and other normal variations in the cervical spine in children. A study of one hundred and sixty children. J Bone Joint Surg Am. 1965; 47(7):1295–1309

[8] Kim DH, Vaccaro AR, Dickman CA, Cho D, Lee S, Kim I. Surgical Anatomy and Techniques to the Spine. 2nd ed. Philadelphia, PA: Saunders; 2013

[9] Hammerstein J, Russo S, Easton K. Atlantoaxial dislocation in a child secondary to a displaced chondrum terminale. A case report. JBJS. 2007; 89-A: 413–417

[10] Wada F, Matsuoka T, Kawai H. Os odontoideum as a consequence of a post-traumatic displaced ossiculum terminale. A case report. J Bone Joint Surg Am. 2009; 91(7):1750–1754

[11] Sherk HH, Nicholson JT. Rotatory atlanto-axial dislocation associated with ossiculum terminale and mongolism. A case report. J Bone Joint Surg Am. 1969; 51(5):957–964

[12] Zygourakis CC, Cahill KS, Proctor MR. Delayed development of os odontoideum after traumatic cervical injury: support for a vascular etiology. J Neurosurg Pediatr. 2011; 7(2):201–204

[13] Ricciardi JE, Kaufer H, Louis DS. Acquired os odontoideum following acute ligament injury. Report of a case. J Bone Joint Surg Am. 1976; 58(3):410–412

[14] Karwacki GM, Schneider JF. Normal ossification patterns of atlas and axis: a CT study. AJNR Am J Neuroradiol. 2012; 33(10):1882–1887

[15] Weinstein SL. The Pediatric Spine: Principles and Practice. 2nd ed. Philadelphia, PA: Lippincott, Williams and Wilkins; 2001:26

[16] Schippers N, Könings P, Hassler W, Sommer B. Typical and atypical fractures of the odontoid process in young children. Report of two cases and a review of the literature. Acta Neurochir (Wien). 1996; 138(5):524–530

[17] Pang D, Thompson DNP. Embryology and bony malformations of the craniovertebral junction. Childs Nerv Syst. 2011; 27(4):523–564

[18] Prescher A. The craniocervical junction in man, the osseous variations, their significance and differential diagnosis. Ann Anat. 1997; 179(1):1–19

[19] Akobo S, Rizk E, Loukas M, Chapman JR, Oskouian RJ, Tubbs RS. The odontoid process: a comprehensive review of its anatomy, embryology, and variations. Childs Nerv Syst. 2015; 31(11):2025–2034

[20] Bradford D, Hensinger R. The Pediatric Spine. New York, NY: Thieme; 1985

[21] Muhleman M, Charran O, Matusz P, Shoja MM, Tubbs RS, Loukas M. The proatlas: a comprehensive review with clinical implications. Childs Nerv Syst. 2012; 28(3):349–356

[22] Tubbs RS, Lingo PR, Mortazavi MM, Cohen-Gadol AA. Hypoplastic occipital condyle and third occipital condyle: review of their dysembryology. Clin Anat. 2013; 26(8):928–932

[23] Weinstein SL. The Pediatric Spine: Principles and Practice. 2nd ed. Philadelphia, PA: Lippincott, Williams and Wilkins; 2001:15

[24] Christ B, Wilting J. From somites to vertebral column. Ann Anat. 1992; 174(1): 23–32

[25] Hawkins RJ, Fielding JW, Thompson WJ. Os odontoideum: congenital or acquired. A case report. J Bone Joint Surg Am. 1976; 58(3):413–414

[26] Fielding JW, Hensinger RN, Hawkins RJ. Os odontoideum. J Bone Joint Surg Am. 1980; 62(3):376–383

[27] Matsui H, Imada K, Tsuji H. Radiographic classification of os odontoideum and its clinical significance. Spine. 1997; 22(15):1706–1709

[28] Condie BG, Capecchi MR. Mice homozygous for a targeted disruption of Hoxd-3 (Hox-4.1) exhibit anterior transformations of the first and second cervical vertebrae, the atlas and the axis. Development. 1993; 119(3):579–595

[29] Wang S, Wang C. Familial dystopic os odontoideum: a report of three cases. J Bone Joint Surg Am. 2011; 93(9):e44

[30] Morgan MK, Onofrio BM, Bender CE. Familial os odontoideum. Case report. J Neurosurg. 1989; 70(4):636–639

[31] Straus D, Xu S, Traynelis VC. Os odontoideum in identical twins: comparative gene expression analysis. Surg Neurol Int. 2014; 5:37

[32] Kirlew KA, Hathout GM, Reiter SD, Gold RH. Os odontoideum in identical twins: perspectives on etiology. Skeletal Radiol. 1993; 22(7):525–527

[33] Wackenheim A. Dens tripartitus. Neuroradiology. 1974; 8:181

[34] Sakaida H, Waga S, Kojima T, Kubo Y, Niwa S, Matsubara T. Os odontoideum associated with hypertrophic ossiculum terminale. Case report. J Neurosurg. 2001; 94(1) Suppl:140–144

[35] Schiff DCM, Parke WW. The arterial supply of the odontoid process. J Bone Joint Surg Am. 1973; 55(7):1450–1456

[36] Freiberger RH, Wilson PD, Jr, Nicholas JA. Acquired absence of the odontoid process: a case report. J Bone Joint Surg Am. 1965; 47:1231–1236

[37] Fielding JW. Disappearance of the central portion of the odontoid process: a case report. J Bone Joint Surg Am. 1965; 47:1228–1230

[38] Fielding JW, Griffin PP. Os odontoideum: an acquired lesion. J Bone Joint Surg Am. 1974; 56(1):187–190

[39] Fagan AB, Askin GN, Earwaker JWS. The jigsaw sign. A reliable indicator of congenital aetiology in os odontoideum. Eur Spine J. 2004; 13(4):295–300

[40] Menezes AH, Ryken TC. Craniovertebral abnormalities in Down's syndrome. Pediatr Neurosurg. 1992; 18(1):24–33

[41] Hadley MN, Walters BC, Grabb PA, et al. Section on Disorders of the Spine and Peripheral Nerve of the AANS and CNS. Os odontoideum. Neurosurgery. 2002; 50(3) Suppl:S148–S155

[42] Greenberg MS. Hand Book of Neurosurgery. 7th ed. New York, NY: Thieme; 2010:966–967

[43] Clements WDB, Mezue W, Mathew B. Os odontoideum: congenital or acquired?—that's not the question. Injury. 1995; 26(9):640–642

[44] Karmakar PS, Karmakar PS, Mitra R, Basu S, Ghosh A. Sudden onset quadriparesis after minor injury to neck in a male with os odontoideum. J Assoc Physicians India. 2013; 61(2):138–139

[45] Zhao D, Wang S, Passias PG, Wang C. Craniocervical instability in the setting of os odontoideum: assessment of cause, presentation, and surgical outcomes in a series of 279 cases. Neurosurgery. 2015; 76(5):514–521

[46] Inamasu J, Kim DH, Klugh A. Posterior instrumentation surgery for craniocervical junction instabilities: an update. Neurol Med Chir (Tokyo). 2005; 45(9):439–447

[47] Zhang Z, Wang H, Liu C. Acute traumatic cervical cord injury in pediatric patients with os odontoideum: a series of 6 patients. World Neurosurg. 2015; 83(6):1180.e1–1180.e6

26 Tarlov's Cyst

Leo Hochhauser, Kaye D. Westmark, and Karl Schmitt

26.1 Introduction

Tarlov's cysts (TCs) are one of the most common incidental findings on MRI examinations of the spine. The vast majority of these cysts do not cause symptoms and will not need treatment. We review the imaging characteristics of TCs and discuss imaging features that allow their distinction from cystic tumors and other types of meningeal cysts of the spine. In the rare case in which the TC is determined to be symptomatic, treatment options and their risks and benefits are discussed.

26.2 Case Presentation

26.2.1 History and Physical Examination

A 45-year-old woman with a history of lower back pain and bilateral lower extreme (LE) numbness and tingling. Her past medical history was significant for obesity and diabetes.

There was patchy, nondermatomal decrease in sensation in her lower extremities bilaterally in a "stocking-type" distribution.

26.2.2 Imaging Analysis

Parasagittal T1-weighted image (T1WI; ► Fig. 26.1a) and T2WI (► Fig. 26.1b) reveal a small, 1-cm cyst associated with the left S1 nerve root (*arrowhead* in ► Fig. 26.1a,b). There is a smaller cyst associated with the exiting left L3 nerve root (*arrow* in ► Fig. 26.1a,b). The cysts' signal intensity is identical to cerebrospinal fluid (CSF) on both T1 W and T2WIs.

The axial T2WI reveals the left S1 neural foramen is smoothly expanded by the cyst (*arrow* in ► Fig. 26.1c).

The Tarlov cyst, or type II perineural cyst in the Nabors classification scheme, is a common incidental finding.

26.3 Clinical Evaluation

The vast majority of TCs are incidental findings. Even if there are radicular complaints, alternative explanations for the patient's symptoms should be sought as these cysts are rarely symptomatic. In this case, the bilateral nature of the patient's complaint, which was primary stocking-type sensory loss, was felt secondary to a peripheral neuropathy due to her diabetes. No further investigation or surgical intervention was warranted.

26.4 Differential Diagnosis

- **TC (Nabors' type II spinal meningeal cyst):**
  - Intraspinal cysts that are most commonly found in the lower lumbar, sacral, and coccygeal regions.
  - Nerve fibers are present within the wall of a TC and are intimately associated with a spinal nerve.
  - They are often located off the midline and may enlarge the neural foramen.
- Juxta-articular, synovial facet joint cyst:
  - They arise from fluid-filled, hypertrophic facet joints.
  - They often have thickened walls and septations that may be dark on T2WIs due to synovial hypertrophy and/or prior hemorrhage.
- Intrasacral meningocele (Nabors' type Ib spinal meningeal cyst):
  - Intrasacral meningoceles are frequently midline. Although they may cause bony pressure remodeling, this is less commonly seen than with TCs.
- Epidermoid:
  - Unlike spinal meningeal cysts, epidermoids will not precisely mimic CSF on all pulse sequences. Importantly, they cause restricted diffusion and therefore appear high in signal on diffusion-weighted images. Similar to spinal meningeal cysts, they will not enhance with gadolinium. Epidermoids are usually midline, within the thecal sac, near the level of the conus.
- Cystic schwannoma:
  - Fluid contents do not precisely follow CSF on all sequences.
  - A solid, nodular, enhancing component is most often present.

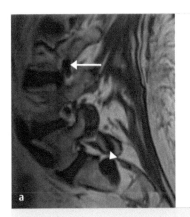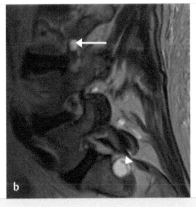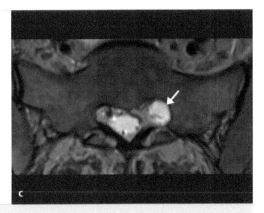

Fig. 26.1 (a–c)

26.5 Diagnostic Pearls

- Although TCs have signal intensity similar to CSF on all pulse sequences, their signal intensity on T2WIs is often slightly higher than CSF due to lack of pulsatile flow that causes some normal dephasing of CSF signal within the thecal sac.
- Original literature suggested that TCs would not fill with oil-based myelographic contrast. After water-soluble contrast media were used, they were shown to fill although often in a very delayed fashion. It is now known that both type I and II spinal meningeal cysts may fill with aqueous myelographic contrast media.
- Cysts that do not fill readily with myelographic contrast may fill slowly via a "ball-valve mechanism." These cysts may be more likely to become symptomatic and create pressure erosions of the sacrum and neural foramen.

26.6 Essential Information about Spinal Meningeal Cysts

- The Nabors classification system of spinal meningeal cysts:
  - Type I: extradural meningeal cysts without spinal nerve root fibers:
    - Ia: extradural spinal arachnoid cyst.
    - Ib: sacral meningocele.
  - Type II: extradural meningeal cyst with spinal nerve root fibers (e.g., TC).
  - Type III: spinal intradural arachnoid cysts.

26.7 Companion Case

26.7.1 History and Physical Examination

A 35-year-old woman with a history of buttock pain. The patient was neurologically normal.

26.7.2 Imaging Analysis

Initial images from a CT myelogram reveal a mass that is compressing the caudal most portion of the thecal sac, which does not fill with contrast (▶ Fig. 26.3a,b).

A midline sagittal reformation of the CT scan performed after the myelogram (▶ Fig. 26.3c) reveals that contrast did enter the sacral cyst although in a delayed fashion as is often the case.

These findings are consistent with large sacral TCs causing bony remodeling of the sacrum.

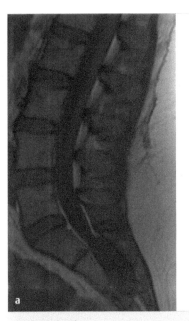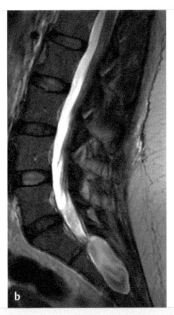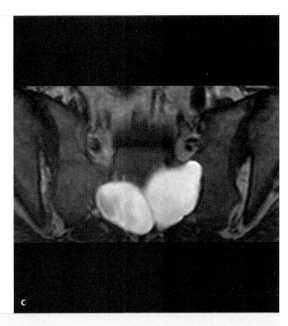

Fig. 26.2 (a–c)

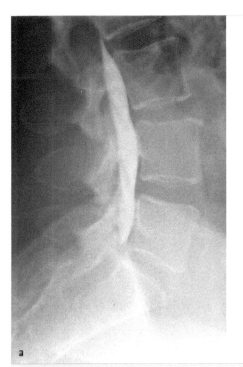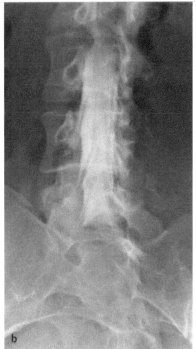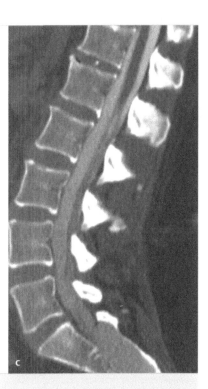

Fig. 26.3 (a–c)

26.7.3 Clinical Evaluation

TCs are commonly found in the sacral region. In this case, conservative pain management referral was made and no operative intervention was offered.

26.8 Neurosurgery Questions and Answers

1. **What is the natural history and prevalence of the TC and its supposed etiology?**

   TCs were first described by I.M. Tarlov in 1938.[1] They are common incidental findings most often involving sacral and coccygeal nerve roots in approximately 4.6 to 9% of the population.[2,3,4] The vast majority of these lesions are considered asymptomatic, incidental findings.

   Only 1% of these cysts become symptomatic, possibly secondary to cystic dilation and nerve root irritation or leakage of CSF from the cyst leading to CSF hypotension.[3,5,6] Possible presenting symptoms are nonspecific and include pelvic pain, radicular complaints, and bowel, bladder, or sexual dysfunction. Symptoms of CSF leakage have been described to include tinnitus, orthostatic headache, and, when severe, cranial nerve dysfunction.[5,6] Several studies have found that women appear to develop symptomatic TCs more often than men.[7,8]

   The etiology of TC in the original description was postulated as inflammatory or perhaps secondary to prior trauma.[1,9] Others consider a possible congenital origin as multiple TCs have been associated with other connective tissue disorders and nerve root sheath duplications.[9,10,11]

2. **Is the finding of a purely cystic lesion in the intra- or extra-dural compartments of the spine pathognomonic of a TC? How is this different from a meningeal or arachnoid cyst?**

   By definition, a TC must have the presence of spinal nerve root fibers in the wall or within the cavity of the cyst and, therefore, in the most proper sense, it is a pathological and not radiological diagnosis.[2,5,6] The cyst is located between the peri- and endoneurium of the spinal nerve root sheath at, or distal to, the junction of the nerve and its dorsal root ganglion (DRG).[1,9] Recently, Nabors et al classified spinal meningeal cysts into three categories: type I—extradural meningeal cysts without spinal nerve root fibers; type II—extradural meningeal cysts with spinal nerve root fibers (i.e., TCs); and type III—spinal intradural meningeal cysts.[12] They demonstrated that TCs and spinal nerve root diverticula are actually the same lesion and communicate with the subarachnoid space, that is, filling with water-soluble contrast on a postmyelogram CT but usually in a delayed fashion. Meningeal diverticula, however, fill rapidly with contrast and occur proximally to the DRG and have no nerve root fibers within the cyst on histopathologic examination.[1,9] Arachnoid cysts, when intradural, are Nabors type III cysts and usually occur secondary to prior infection or hemorrhage. Arachnoid cysts occurring extradurally are Nabors type I cysts. Again, lack of association with a spinal nerve distinguishes these entities from the TC.

   TCs are much more common in the lower lumbar, sacral, and coccygeal area where they may create pressure erosion and deformity of the adjacent bony structures.

3. **What findings on physical examination or elements of the history are important in determination that the TC is truly an incidental finding and asymptomatic?**

   In the vast majority of cases, the TC should be considered a common incidental finding. If a patient presents with radicular pain in the nerve root distribution of a TC, a thorough review of the patient's imaging for other pathology (disk protrusion, osteophyte, lateral recess stenosis, facet joint synovial cyst, etc.) at that level should be performed. In the vast majority of cases, we advocate treatment of the primary pathology, rather than the TC, as this is often found to be successful.[13]

   There are case reports of TCs that, after extensive evaluation, were considered the cause of radicular pain. Radiographic features that were associated with a greater likelihood of successful surgical treatment included a cyst size of ≥ 1.5 cm and solitary rather than multifocal TC formation.[7] In addition, some authors have stated that cysts that show delayed filling with contrast on CT myelography are more likely to cause symptoms.[14]

   Clinical features that suggested surgical success were younger patients with shorter duration of complaints and patients with exacerbation of symptoms with postural changes or a Valsalva maneuver, definite radicular symptoms in clear anatomic relationship to the compressive TC, and no other demonstrable pathology that could explain the patient's symptoms.[7,15,16]

4. **What treatment options have been described for TCs?**

   Intervention is neither required nor recommended for an asymptomatic, incidental TC. Surgical treatment of the symptomatic TC is also controversial and should be considered only when there is definite anatomic relationship between the cyst and the patient's complaints, no alternative pathology is demonstrated, and conservative management has failed.

   Neurosurgical techniques described include decompressive laminectomy, cyst and/or nerve root excision, and cyst fenestration and imbrication.[2,7,8,9,17] Decompressive laminectomy has been found to have a low success rate and risks dural tear or nerve injury.[2,15] In one series of 23 patients undergoing laminectomy, microsurgical exposure and/or imbrication and paraspinous muscle flap closure, there was a 22% rate of postoperative complications including infection and intracranial hypotension due to persistent CSF leakage.[17]

   In the rare case in which a surgeon elects to treat a symptomatic TC, we recommend microsurgical cyst fenestration and cyst wall resection with a fat or muscle graft reinforced closure as previously described by Acosta et al and Mummaneni et al.[2,5,6] Close follow-up for CSF leak will be necessary and prolonged CSF drainage or reoperation may be required should this occur.

   Less invasive procedures, performed for treatment, and sometimes as a diagnostic tool, include percutaneous CT aspiration, which is unfortunately associated with a very high recurrence rate.[3] Voyadzis et al reported a series of 10 patients with symptomatic TC that were treated. Of the three patients they treated with percutaneous aspiration, none improved and one experienced marked worsening felt due to hemorrhage of the cyst wall or nerve root injury.[7]

Percutaneous drainage with fibrin glue to prevent recurrence has also been reported, but in one series it was found to have a high, 75%, incidence of postprocedural aseptic meningitis.[18,19] Murphy et al reported a large series of patients treated by CT-guided fibrin glue cyst injection and found that 65% had improvement in their symptoms and therefore recommended this procedure as a first treatment option prior to consideration for open surgery.[20] Lumboperitoneal shunting, after CSF drainage test, to lower CSF pressure has also been described as a possible treatment although the risks of shunt infection must be considered.[14,21] In the Kunz et al series of 16 patients that compared surgical treatment versus conservative management, the authors did not find a significant difference in improvement between the two groups; however, they concluded that surgery may be of slight benefit for patients with a shorter duration of pain complaint and with a neurological deficit clearly associated with the cyst.[22]

5. **For an incidentally detected TC, is any follow-up needed?**
Incidentally detected TCs require no treatment and, in the asymptomatic patient, require no additional follow-up. In patients in whom there is clinical concern for CSF hypotension, however, the finding of a spinal meningeal diverticulum is exceptionally important as it may be the source of CSF leakage.[23]

References

[1] Tarlov IM. Perineurial cysts of the spinal nerve roots. Arch Neurol Psychiatry. 1938; 40:1067–1074

[2] Acosta FL, Jr, Quinones-Hinojosa A, Schmidt MH, Weinstein PR. Diagnosis and management of sacral Tarlov cysts. Case report and review of the literature. Neurosurg Focus. 2003; 15(2):E15

[3] Paulsen RD, Call GA, Murtagh FR. Prevalence and percutaneous drainage of cysts of the sacral nerve root sheath (Tarlov cysts). AJNR Am J Neuroradiol. 1994; 15(2):293–297, discussion 298–299

[4] Smith DT. Cystic formations associated with human spinal nerve roots. J Neurosurg. 1961; 18:654–660

[5] Mummaneni PV, Pitts LH, McCormack BM, Corroo JM, Weinstein PR. Microsurgical treatment of symptomatic sacral Tarlov cysts. Neurosurgery. 2000; 47(1):74–78, discussion 78–79

[6] Neulen A, Kantelhardt SR, Pilgram-Pastor SM, Metz I, Rohde V, Giese A. Microsurgical fenestration of perineural cysts to the thecal sac at the level of the distal dural sleeve. Acta Neurochir (Wien). 2011; 153(7):1427–1434, discussion 1434

[7] Voyadzis JM, Bhargava P, Henderson FC. Tarlov cysts: a study of 10 cases with review of the literature. J Neurosurg. 2001; 95(1) Suppl:25–32

[8] Nishiura I, Koyama T, Handa J. Intrasacral perineurial cyst. Surg Neurol. 1985; 23(3):265–269

[9] Tarlov IM. Spinal perineurial and meningeal cysts. J Neurol Neurosurg Psychiatry. 1970; 33(6):833–843

[10] Bergland RM. Congenital intraspinal extradural cyst. Report of three cases in one family. J Neurosurg. 1968; 28(5):495–499

[11] Nathan H, Rosner S. Multiple meningeal diverticula and cysts associated with duplications of the sheaths of spinal nerve posterior roots. J Neurosurg. 1977; 47(1):68–72

[12] Nabors MW, Pait TG, Byrd EB, et al. Updated assessment and current classification of spinal meningeal cysts. J Neurosurg. 1988; 68(3):366–377

[13] Langdown AJ, Grundy JR, Birch NC. The clinical relevance of Tarlov cysts. J Spinal Disord Tech. 2005; 18(1):29–33

[14] Lucantoni C, Than KD, Wang AC, et al. Tarlov cysts: a controversial lesion of the sacral spine. Neurosurg Focus. 2011; 31(6):E14

[15] Caspar W, Papavero L, Nabhan A, Loew C, Ahlhelm F. Microsurgical excision of symptomatic sacral perineurial cysts: a study of 15 cases. Surg Neurol. 2003; 59(2):101–105, discussion 105–106

[16] Mezzadri J, Abbati SG, Jalon P. Tarlov cysts: endoscope-assisted obliteration of the communication with the spinal subarachnoid space. J Neurol Surg A Cent Eur Neurosurg. 2014; 75(6):462–466

[17] Burke JF, Thawani JP, Berger I, et al. Microsurgical treatment of sacral perineural (Tarlov) cysts: case series and review of the literature. J Neurosurg Spine. 2016; 24(5):700–707

[18] Patel MR, Louie W, Rachlin J. Percutaneous fibrin glue therapy of meningeal cysts of the sacral spine. AJR Am J Roentgenol. 1997; 168(2):367–370

[19] Kumar K, Malik S, Schulte PA. Symptomatic spinal arachnoid cysts: report of two cases with review of the literature. Spine. 2003; 28(2):E25–E29

[20] Murphy KJ, Nussbaum DA, Schnupp S, Long D. Tarlov cysts: an overlooked clinical problem. Semin Musculoskelet Radiol. 2011; 15(2):163–167

[21] Bartels RH, van Overbeeke JJ. Lumbar cerebrospinal fluid drainage for symptomatic sacral nerve root cysts: an adjuvant diagnostic procedure and/or alternative treatment? Technical case report. Neurosurgery. 1997; 40(4):861–864, discussion 864–865

[22] Kunz U, Mauer UM, Waldbauer H. Lumbosacral extradural arachnoid cysts: diagnosis and indication for surgery. Eur Spine J. 1999; 8:218–222

[23] Schievink WI, Maya MM, Louy C, Moser FG, Tourje J. Diagnostic criteria for spontaneous spinal CSF leaks and intracranial hypotension. AJNR Am J Neuroradiol 2008; 29(5):853–856

27 Approach to the Solitary Vertebral Lesion on Magnetic Resonance Imaging

Behrang Amini, Krina Patel, Richard M. Westmark, Kaye D. Westmark, and Anneliese Gonzalez

27.1 Introduction

The detection of multiple bone lesions on MRI, in combination with clinical data, most commonly leads to the diagnosis of metastatic disease or multiple myeloma. The evaluation of a solitary bony lesion in the spine may be more challenging and will often require additional diagnostic testing if benign imaging features are not present on MRI.[1] When the vertebral lesion has no benign features, especially in the older adult patient, metastatic disease is always a significant consideration. It is important to realize that the majority of the spine and the entire nonaxial skeleton will not be visualized on a routine lumbar spine MR. Therefore, the incidentally detected, indeterminant "solitary" vertebral lesion may, in fact, be one of multiple lesions. Even in patients with a known primary malignancy, however, the diagnosis is not certain from imaging alone as it has been found that a solitary bone lesion has a 12% chance of being either benign or due to metastatic disease with a different histopathology than the known primary.[2]

This section will begin with a case presentation of the most commonly detected incidental bone tumor in the spine, the hemangioma. We will then present a more generalized approach to any solitary, incidentally detected bone lesion on MRI. With increased utilization of spine MRI, it is expected that incidental bone lesions will be frequently detected. It is therefore important to differentiate benign lesions, which need no treatment or follow-up, from those that will require additional evaluation and possibly affect patient management.

27.2 Case Presentation

27.2.1 History and Physical Examination

A 30-year-old woman presented with lower back pain at the L5–S1 level for which an LS spine MRI was performed. Her physical examination was normal. A lesion within T12 was incidentally detected.

27.2.2 Imaging Analysis

There is a focal lesion within the T12 vertebral body that is high in signal on both T1WIs and T2WIs (▶ Fig. 27.1). Linear areas of decreased signal are seen within the lesion on the T2WI. The appearance of this lesion is consistent with a typical vertebral hemangioma.

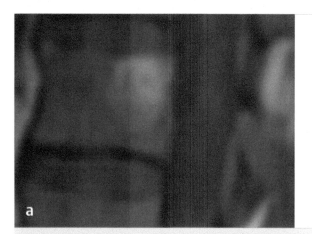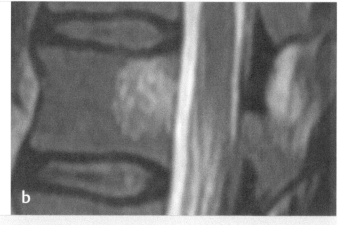

Fig. 27.1 (a, b)

27.3 Recommended Management

A focal, well-defined lesion in the vertebrae that has increased signal on both the T1W and T2WIs is considered to most likely be a benign hemangioma and no further workup or follow-up imaging is needed.

27.4 Differential Diagnosis for a Focal Vertebral Lesion on MRI That Is Hyperintense T1-Weighted Images

- Hemangioma:
  - The most common benign bone tumor consisting of both vascular and fatty elements the ratio of which determines its signal characteristics. The greater the amount of fat, the more indolent the lesion, the higher the signal on T1WI and the more complete the suppression of signal on fat-suppressed images.
  - Typical hemangiomas are asymptomatic, incidental, discrete lesions that are high in signal on both T1WIs and T2WIs that most often occur in the vertebral bodies.
  - Linear areas of decreased signal often seen on the T2WI correspond to coarsened trabeculae.
  - Most commonly, their signal does not completely suppress on fat-suppressed T2WIs due to the vascular stroma component.
  - Discrete lesion may be seen on CT with characteristic corduroy pattern.
- Focal fatty marrow:
  - It is commonly seen in adults with patchy, progressive conversion of red to yellow marrow.
  - It suppresses completely on short tau inversion recovery (STIR) and other fat-suppression sequences.
  - No discrete lesion is typically seen on CT.
- Intraosseous lipomas:
  - These are benign, rare lesions in the spine.
  - They are uniformly high in signal on both the T1WIs and fast spin echo (FSE) T2WIs.
  - Complete signal suppression is found on fat-suppressed sequences.
  - Discrete low attenuation lesion is seen on CT with no coarsened trabeculae.
- Degenerative end plate changes, Modic type II:
  - Fatty infiltration of the end plates, high in signal on both T1WI and T2WI, adjacent to a degenerative disk.
  - Signal suppresses completely on fat-suppressed sequences.
- Bone infarction:
  - Geographic area of increased signal intensity on the T1WIs with a rim of marked decreased signal.
  - The dark rim is surrounded by increased signal on the T2WIs.
  - Typically found in the watershed zone of vertebral body that has been described as predominantly in the anterior half or in multiple areas near the end plate and/or deep medullary portion of the vertebral body involving several levels.[3]

- It is often associated with steroid use. Subchondral region of the femoral heads is most often affected and may be seen on scout images of lumbar spine MRI.
- Chronic or healing infectious process:
  - Associated with disk space abnormality and edematous soft-tissue changes.
- Metastatic melanoma:
  - Melanin has increased signal on noncontrast T1WIs.
  - Hyperintense signal on T1W images from melanoma bone metastases is exceedingly rare.
  - Hemorrhagic foci appearing as areas of decreased signal on T2WI that bloom on gradient echo (GRE) and susceptibility weighted imaging (SWI) sequences are common.
  - It is an extremely rare cause of a solitary bone lesion as usually lesions are multiple and the patient, in the vast majority of cases, has a known diagnosis of metastatic melanoma.

27.5 Clinical and Diagnostic Imaging Pearls: An Approach to the Solitary Vertebral Lesion Detected Incidentally on MRI

I. Prime considerations when evaluating the MRI

Signal intensity on T1WIs:

- Hyperintense lesions on noncontrast T1WIs are virtually always benign.
  - High signal on noncontrast T1WIs is most often due to fat.
  - The most commonly encountered lesions are the typical hemangioma, focal fatty marrow, and degenerative Modic type II end plate changes.
- Hypointense lesions on T1WIs that are hyperintense on the fat-suppressed T2WIs are indeterminate on MRI and often need further evaluation. The most commonly encountered lesions are described as follows:
  - Islands of red marrow are a fairly common benign finding in younger patients but may also occur in times of hematopoietic stress and reconversion of fatty replaced marrow.
    - ○ Red marrow is lower in signal on T1WIs than surrounding fatty marrow but is typically NOT lower in signal than intervertebral disks or skeletal muscle. On fat-suppressed T2WIs, it is iso- to slightly hyperintense relative to skeletal muscle but should not be extremely bright.[4]
    - ○ The "bull's eye sign," focal internal islands of preserved high signal on T1WIs, indicates the lesion is very likely to be benign.[5]
    - ○ MR in-phase/opposed-phase imaging may be very helpful to confirm focal red marrow as a drop in signal on the out-of-phase images by more than 20% is due to the presence of both water and fat signal within the lesion, which suggests a benign lesion as most tumors, with myeloma being the exception, completely displace normal marrow fat.[6,7,8]
    - ○ Fat content (fat fraction) can also be measured by use of m-Dixon fat suppression techniques and has been shown in some studies to help differentiate focal red marrow from malignant lesions.[9,10]

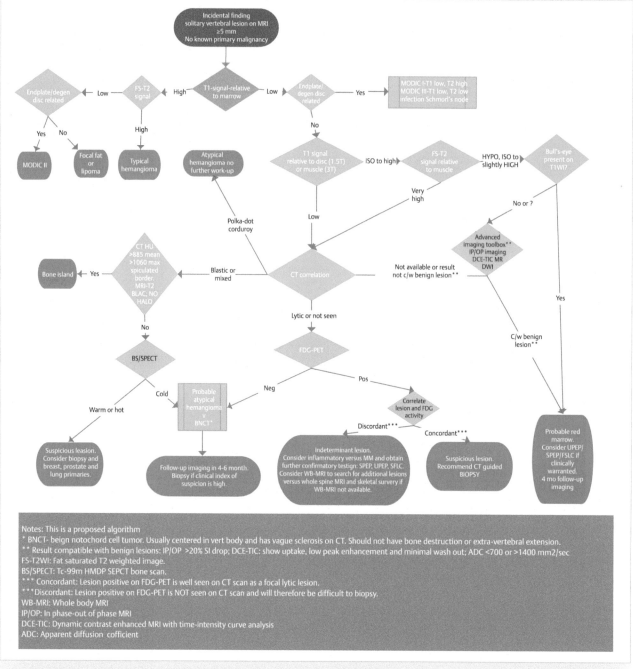

Fig. 27.2 Proposed workup algorithm for an incidental solitary bone lesion found on MRI.

○ Gadolinium contrast enhancement may also be helpful as although red marrow enhances to a greater extent than yellow marrow, marked enhancement is atypical. Normal red marrow on DCE (dynamic contrast-enhanced) MRI time intensity curves (TICs) shows a slow wash-in, low maximal peak, and either minimal or no apparent washout. Pathological marrow enhances much more quickly, reaches a higher absolute level, and shows significant contrast washout. Morales et al found that a high K-trans and, most importantly, higher plasma volume was indicative of metastatic disease rather than atypical hemangiomata as these parameters reflect the increase vascular permeability and increase in number of immature vessels in neoangiogenesis, the hallmark of neoplastic lesions.[11]

– Atypical hemangioma:
  ○ Low signal on T1WIs but high in signal on T2WIs. Confirmation with CT revealing typical, coarsened trabecula is diagnostic. If the lesion is indeterminate on MRI and CT, and there is no known primary malignancy, FDG-PET/CT is useful as atypical hemangioma do not have increased uptake.

– Hematological malignancies:
  ○ Signal intensity is often much lower than intervertebral disks and skeletal muscle on T1WIs and markedly increased on fat-suppressed T2WIs.

Table 27.1 Imaging modalities to be considered in the workup of solitary vertebral lesions[18,19]

Testing modality	Sensitivity (%)	Specificity (%)	Comments
CT	73–79	92–95	Workup of bone lesion: Lytic vs. sclerotic; evaluates matrix and best defines anatomy of bony involvement Pros: Chest, abdomen and pelvic CT scan simultaneously screens for primary cancer; superior to skeletal survey in multiple myeloma (MM); > 885 HU (mean), 1,060 HU (maximum) compatible with bone island rather than osteoblastic metastatic disease[11] Cons: Cortical destruction usually needed for detection; poor sensitivity for lesions that infiltrate bone marrow without cortical involvement
MRI	91–95	90–95	Workup of bone lesion: Fat within lesion implies benignity; low signal on T1WI and T2WI suggests sclerotic lesion; halo of high signal on T2WIs on MRI around a lesion that has been shown to be sclerotic on CT suggests osteoblastic metastatic disease as opposed to bone island[5] Pros: Best screen for metastatic disease to the spine; highest sensitivity for marrow infiltration; also defines extraosseous spread of disease. Cons: Motion sensitive; limited FOV unless WB-MRI is available
MRI + DWI			Improves sensitivity of MRI for metastatic disease but lowers specificity. Most sensitive test for prostate cancer metastasis
FDG PET/CT	90–100% for lytic lesions; 16–18% for sclerotic lesions like metastatic prostate cancer	81–97	Workup of bone lesion: Concordance (increased FDG-PET correlates with bony lesion on CT) is highly predictive (98%) of metastatic disease[20] Pros: Best screen for lung cancer, melanoma, and MM. Evaluates not only the bone lesion but also provides complete TNM staging for most solid tumors. Cons: Poor sensitivity for metastatic disease due to osteoblastic primaries like prostate cancer. Poor for non-FDG-avid primaries like myxoid GI; low-grade tumors; renal cell cancer
Bone scan	80	63	Workup of bone lesion: If sclerotic lesion is cold, probability of osteoblastic metastatic disease is low. If lesion is solitary, sclerotic, and warm, the test is not helpful, as bone islands may also have increased activity. Pro: Excellent, inexpensive screening test of whole body to determine if there are multiple lesions suggestive of metastatic disease. Cons: MM, lymphoma, and highly aggressive tumors and purely lytic metastatic disease (like renal cell cancer) are often negative on bone scan. Very nonspecific as infection, degenerative change, and trauma may cause false positives
Bone scan SPECT	90.3	86	As above but with significant increased sensitivity and specificity in comparison to planar bone scan
Bone scan SPECT/CT	90.5	90	As above but with increased specificity. Considered excellent test for metastatic prostate cancer

Abbreviations: DWI, diffusion-weighted imaging; FDG, fluorodeoxyglucose; FOV, field of view; GI, gastrointestinal; SPECT, single-photon emission computed tomography; TNM, tumor size, node involvement, and metastasis status; WB-MRI, whole body MRI.

– Metastatic disease:
  ○ Lytic metastases most often appear as well-defined, focal areas of decreased signal on the T1WIs with increased signal on T2WIs.
• Hypointense lesions on both T1WIs and fat-suppressed T2WIs are less common and further workup is sometimes required (also see ▶ Table 27.1). The most common lesions are as follows:
  – Modic type III (fibrosis) degenerative change. Linear area of decreased signal on T1 W and T2WIs associated with degenerative intervertebral disk disease.
  – Bone island (enostosis). Island of dense cortical bone within cancellous bone that is markedly dense (mean ≥ 885 HU and maximum ≥ 1,060 HU) and often oval in shape with a spiculated border.[12] A cold bone scan is helpful in distinguishing bone island from an osteoblastic metastasis, whereas increased focal uptake within the solitary lesion is not of assistance, as a bone island may have increased activity.

– Osteoblastic metastatic disease. Less dense than bone island, round shape, and halo of increased signal on T2WIs surrounding the low signal lesion is highly suggestive of metastatic disease.[5]

Patient's age:
• The vast majority of malignant lesions in the adult spine are due to metastatic disease and multiple myeloma/plasmacytoma rather than primary bone tumors, which are rare.
• In patients older than 40 years of age, the majority of metastases to vertebrae are due to breast, lung, prostate, kidney, and thyroid primary cancers, all of which are extremely rare in children.
• Breast and prostate cancers have a very high propensity to develop skeletal metastatic disease.
• In children and young adults, eosinophilic granuloma (EG), the solitary bone involvement form of Langerhans cell histiocytosis (LCH), and osteoid osteomas may present as an

incidental finding but when discovered in the spine, the majority manifest with complaints of back or neck pain and therefore would seldom be incidentally detected, asymptomatic lesions.

Location of the lesion, whether centered in the vertebral body versus the posterior elements, may provide guidance as to the most likely diagnosis:

- Vertebral body:
  - Areas of focal red marrow.
  - Intervertebral degenerative disk disease related or Schmorl's node.
  - Hemangioma.
  - Metastatic disease.
  - Plasmacytoma/multiple myeloma.
  - Bone island.
  - Intraosseous lipoma.
  - Benign notochordal cell tumor.
  - Paget's disease.
  - Chordoma.
  - Leukemia/lymphoma.
  - Giant cell tumor.
  - Osteosarcoma.
  - LCH.
  - Infection.
  - Fibrous dysplasia.
- Posterior elements: Lesions arising in the posterior elements are more likely to be primary bone tumors.
  - Osteochondroma.
  - Osteoid osteoma.
  - Osteoblastoma.
  - ABC.
  - Osteosarcoma.
  - Chondroblastoma.
  - Chondrosarcoma.
- Continuity with a severely degenerative disk and irregular vertebral end plates:
  - Degenerative end plate changes have been characterized into three types based on MRI appearance that relates to their chronicity by Modic et al[13]:
    ○ Modic type I is consistent with more acute edematous change and is T1 signal hypointense and T2 signal hyperintense. Focal enhancement is often present.
    ○ Modic type II is consistent with more chronic change and fatty infiltration and is therefore hyperintense on both T1 and FSE-T2 sequences.
    ○ Modic type III represents chronic degenerative, sclerotic reaction and is therefore hypointense on both T1 W and T2WIs.
  - Although rarely an incidental finding, infectious spondylitis should also be considered in the differential diagnosis of edematous end plates adjacent to an abnormal disk space and additional clinical correlation sought. Extensive enhancement of end plates, disk space, and especially the paravertebral soft tissues may occur in advanced degenerative change but is worrisome for infection so that clinical correlation and laboratory testing for infection, erythrocyte sedimentation rate (ESR), and C-reactive protein is indicated.

- A Schmorl node, which is a herniation of the disk through a weakened area in the vertebral end plate, often presents as an incidental finding, although it may be a cause of pain acutely. Identification of an end plate defect adjacent to the area of marrow signal abnormality is helpful in making this diagnosis. Contrast enhancement is typical.

II. Additional diagnostic testing modalities to be considered if typical benign imaging features on MRI are not present and the lesion appears to be solitary (further testing and clinical correlation will be necessary)

CT scan of the vertebral lesion is recommended to determine if the lesion is lytic or sclerotic. Practically speaking, although conventional radiographs are very helpful for assessing ribs, long bones, and the skull, they most often lack sufficient sensitivity to assist in the diagnostic workup of an indeterminate vertebral lesion detected on MRI:

- Lytic lesion. The most common tumors producing lytic lesions are as follows:
  - Multiple myeloma/plasmacytoma.
  - Non–small cell lung cancer.
  - Renal cell cancer.
  - Thyroid carcinomas (except medullary thyroid carcinoma, which is typically sclerotic or mixed).
  - Head and neck cancers.
  - Melanoma
- Sclerotic/osteoblastic lesion. The most common primary tumors producing osteoblastic lesions or mixed sclerotic/lytic lesions are the following:
  - Prostate cancer.
  - Carcinoid.
  - Transitional cell cancer.
  - Breast cancer (mixed lytic/sclerotic appearance).
  - GI primaries.
  - Medullary thyroid carcinoma.

Thorough clinical evaluation is extremely important to guide further workup as the diagnostic performance of imaging tests depends largely upon the primary malignancy:

- Metastatic lesions and multiple myeloma represent the majority of malignant tumors of the adult spine. Primary bone tumors are rare. A complete blood count, urinalysis, basic serum chemistries, as well as serum-free light chains, serum, and urine protein electrophoresis to evaluate for the possibility of multiple myeloma should be performed.[14] In women, routine gynecologist's evaluation with pelvic examination and mammography are recommended. In men, a routine clinical prostate examination and serum prostate-specific antigen (PSA) level are recommended.
- In the cases in which the lesion appears lytic with no bony reaction present, FDG-PET/CT is frequently recommended not only to identify the primary but also to provide TNM staging and hopefully identify additional lesions that may be in a location more amendable to biopsy than the spine. Two of the most common primary malignancies to result in lytic metastases are lung cancer and renal cell carcinoma. Currently, FDG-PET/CT is the staging test of choice for lung cancer. For renal cell carcinoma, however, FDG-PET/CT has decreased sensitivity due to normal uptake and excretion of the radiotracer by the kidneys.

Therefore, a chest, abdomen, and pelvis CT scan is the superior test to evaluate the kidneys and provide TNM staging. Bone scan is not recommended due to its decreased sensitivity for highly aggressive, purely lytic tumors.

- If plasmacytoma/multiple myeloma is suspected (i.e., urine protein electrophoresis [UPEP] or serum protein electrophoresis [SPEP] positive, or hypercalcemia, anemia, or renal failure in the older adult), then whole body MRI (WB-MRI) is recommended. If WB-MRI is not available, skeletal survey plus FDG-PET/CT may be utilized. MRI has the highest sensitivity for infiltration of the marrow by myeloma cells before cortical destruction occurs. The Myeloma working group recommended that patients with smoldering or asymptomatic myeloma undergo WB-MRI (or spine and pelvic MRI if WB-MRI is not available) and that the finding of more than one focal lesion of a diameter greater than 5 mm is definitional for symptomatic disease that requires therapy. In the cases of equivocal small lesions, a second MRI should be performed after 3 to 6 months, and if there is progression on MRI, the patient should be treated as having symptomatic myeloma.[15] Bone scan is not appropriate as it is very insensitive for myeloma. For many years, skeletal survey plain radiographs have been part of the standard workup in patients suspected of having multiple myeloma. Low-dose whole body CT and MRI have been proposed as alternatives to the skeletal survey as they are reported to provide higher sensitivity.[16] However, these techniques have not replaced the plain radiograph skeletal survey in many tertiary cancer centers and are more expensive and time-consuming.

For rare, primary bone tumors, analysis for presence and type of tumor matrix is very important:

- Osteoid matrix is cloudlike and may be seen in osteoid osteomas, osteoblastomas, and osteosarcomas. Osteoid osteomas and osteoblastomas occur most frequently in the posterior elements.
- Diffuse sclerosis is often seen in benign notochord cell tumors (BNCTs). Chordomas may have some internal calcification. Both chordomas and BNCTs occur in the vertebral body.
- Chondroid matrix has a classic appearance of rings and arcs of calcification and may be seen in chondrosarcoma, which has a predilection for occurring in the sacrum and posterior elements.
- Giant cell tumors lack calcified matrix, occur more frequently in the sacrum and vertebral bodies and often have a partially sclerotic border on CT. They are frequently lower in signal on T2WI than most other tumors in the differential diagnosis, (plasmacytoma, chordoma and metastatic disease) due to the presence of hemosiderin and fibrous tissue.

If the lesion is indeterminate on MR and CT/plain radiographs, there is no demonstrable primary malignancy and evidence of wider spread metastatic disease, UPEP/SPEP and serum-free light chain assay are negative, and there is no increased uptake on FDG-PET/CT (routine bone scan/SPECT if PET not available), then the indeterminate, solitary lesion may be managed conservatively with close follow-up imaging or a biospy ordered depending on the level of concern of the referring physician and patient. In these cases, the diagnosis of "atypical hemangioma" is often suggested by the radiologist. If the lesion has increased uptake on FDG-PET/CT or bone scan/SPECT, biopsy is the next step in evaluation.[14,15,17]

27.6 Essential Facts about Hemangiomas

27.6.1 Demographics

- The most common, incidentally detected, benign lesion found in 10 to 11% of the population by radiographic and autopsy series,[21,22,23,24] and as an incidental finding on 1.5% of lumbar spine MRI performed for evaluation of disk herniations.[25]
- Majority of lesions are solitary, asymptomatic lesions in the thoracic and lumbar vertebral bodies.
- Vertebral body height is usually maintained and, perhaps due to the coarsened trabecula, is rarely associated with pathologic fractures.
- Pregnancy is the only known risk factor for progression of an incidental hemangioma to become symptomatic, most often during the third trimester.[22,24,26]

27.6.2 Imaging Appearance

- CT appearance: Well-defined lesions with areas of low density, consistent with fat, interspersed among coarsened bony trabecula resulting in a "corduroy" appearance on coronal and sagittal imaging, and a "polka dot" appearance on axial images (see Companion Case 1; ▶ Fig. 27.3). CT scan may also be helpful as areas of very low attenuation (–90 to –120 HU) are diagnostic of fat. If the amount of fat in the lesion is minimal, volume averaging with adjacent tissue may raise the attenuation so that the density measurement becomes nondiagnostic.[27]
- MR appearance: Depends on the relative amount of fat and cellular components, which further classify hemangiomas into typical and atypical subtypes on imaging.
  - Typical hemangioma: It is hyperintense on T1 W and T2WIs, and is most likely to be indolent. It is well defined and confined to the vertebral body without cortical expansion or disruption.[26] For lesions incidentally detected on MR with a "T1- and T2-bright" appearance, no further evaluation is recommended. On fat-suppressed T2WIs, a typical hemangioma may have a high signal rim, which may create concern. In these cases, the high signal on the T1WIs should be reassuring (see Companion Case 6).
  - Atypical hemangioma: It is hypointense on T1WIs and hyperintense on T2WIs. It is more likely to expand beyond the cortex and create symptoms.[28] This appearance is much less specific and the differential diagnosis increases to include malignant vascular tumors, plasmacytoma, and metastatic disease. In these cases, a CT scan may be very helpful to look for typical coarsened bony trabeculae and maintained height of the vertebral body, which could confirm the lesion is a hemangioma.
  - Aggressive hemangioma: It has a variable appearance on MRI but often atypical. It is defined by the lesion breaking through the cortex and extending beyond the confines of the vertebral body, invading the spinal canal where it is most often symptomatic (see Companion Case 2).

27.7 Companion Cases

27.7.1 Companion Case 1: Typical Hemangioma

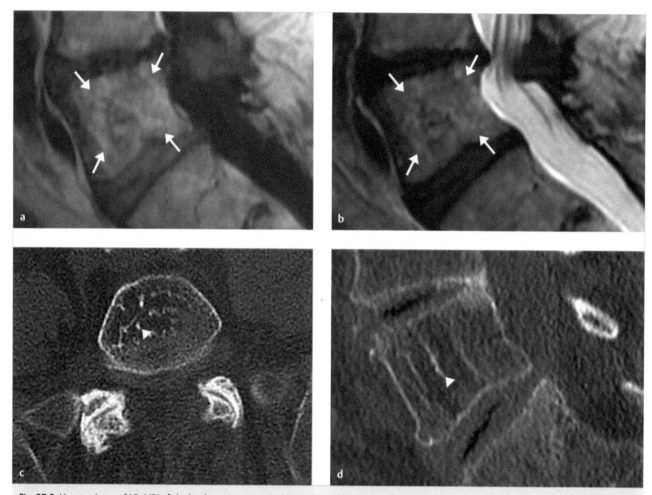

Fig. 27.3 Hemangioma of L5. MRI of the lumbar spine in sagittal T1 W **(a)** and sagittal T2 **(b)**, and noncontrast CT scan of the same patient in axial **(c)** and sagittal **(d)** planes. A T1 W/T2 W heterogeneous lesion with areas of hyperintensity on the T1WIs is seen involving the central portion of the vertebral body (*arrows* in **a** and **b**). CT images show coarse bony trabeculae inside the lesion configuring the "white polka dots" (*arrowhead* in **c**) and "corduroy" (*arrowhead* in **d**) pattern that is typical for hemangiomas.

27.7.2 Companion Case 2: Aggressive Hemangioma

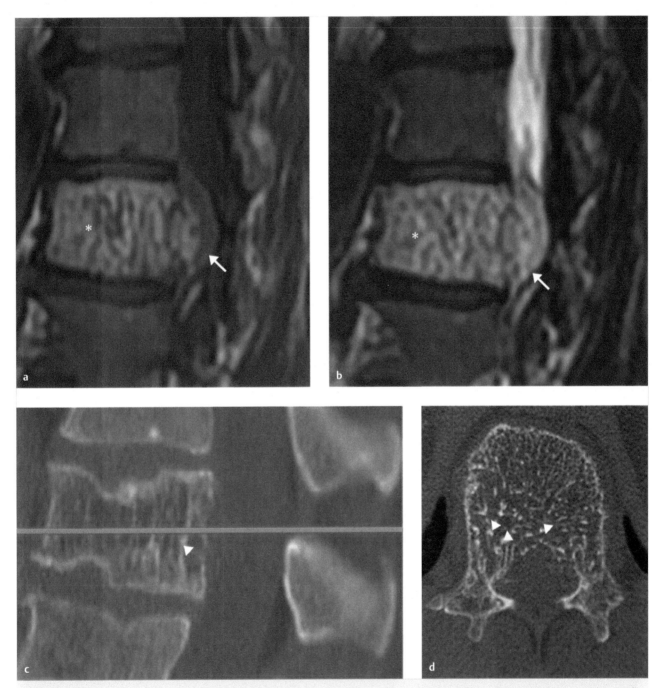

Fig. 27.4 Aggressive hemangioma of T9. MRI of the thoracic spine with sagittal T1 W **(a)** and sagittal STIR **(b)**, and noncontrast CT scan with sagittally reformatted **(c)** and axial **(d)** images. A T1 W/T2 W hyperintense lesion is seen involving the whole vertebral body (*asterisks*), disrupting the posterior cortex (*arrows*), extending into the spinal canal. CT images show the "corduroy" (*arrowhead* in **c**) and "white polka dots" (*arrowheads* in **d**) patterns, typical for hemangiomas. This case is somewhat unusual in that aggressive hemangiomas are more often low in signal on T1WIs and high in signal on T2WIs, like atypical hemangiomas. Also, identification of the classic coarsened trabeculae on CT scan is less common than with typical hemangiomas.

27.7.3 Companion Case 3: Intraosseous lipoma

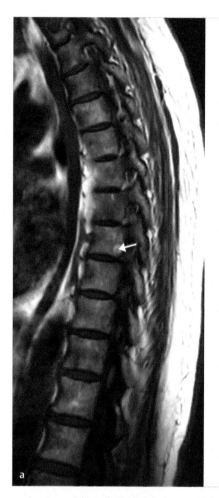
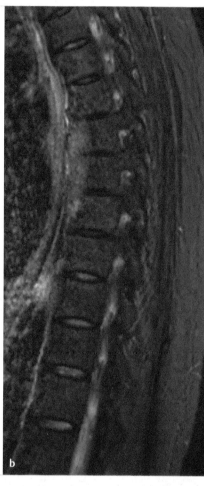

Fig. 27.5 Incidentally detected, solitary bone lesion on MRI performed for mid-thoracic back pain. Sagittal T1WI **(a)** shows a focal lesion in the posterior-inferolateral aspect of the T8 vertebral body (*arrow*), which is high in signal and completely suppresses on the STIR sequence **(b)**. It is important to realize that any tissue with a short T1 (hyperintense on T1WIs) will suppress on STIR sequences. Only a fat suppression imaging using chemical fat saturation may truly distinguish fat from other causes of T1 shortening. In any event, lesions that are hyperintense on T1WIs are almost always benign; therefore, no further workup is required. The differential diagnosis includes a small, almost entirely fatty, benign hemangioma, a focal area of fat within the marrow, and a small intraosseous lipoma.

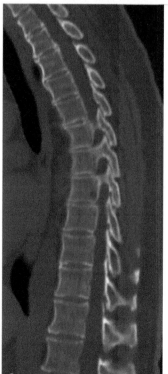
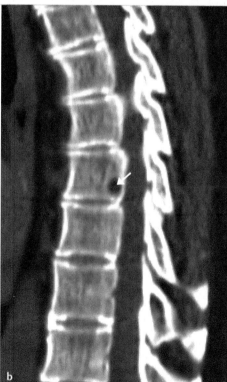

Fig. 27.6 (a, b) A CT scan had been performed in this patient shown in ▶ Fig. 27.5 for evaluation of a cough. The incidental T8 lesion can be seen in retrospect and appears well circumscribed and lytic. Narrowing the window shows that the lesion's density is similar to subcutaneous fat. An ROI measuring density found the lesion averaged −79 Hounsfield unit, which is compatible with fat. The CT confirms the lesion is therefore a focal area of fat, likely a small intraosseous lipoma. No further evaluation is necessary.

27.7.4 Companion Case 4: Atypical Hemangioma

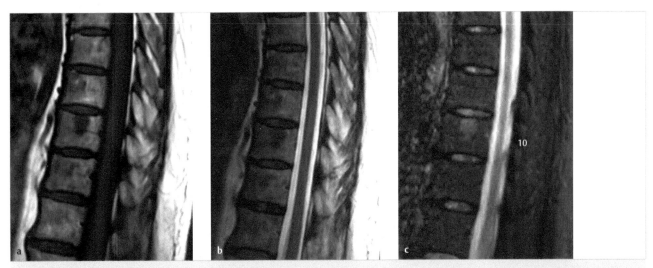

Fig. 27.7 (a–c) MRI performed for mid-thoracic back pain with no history of trauma or malignancy. Although the marrow is diffusely heterogeneous, a focal area is seen in the superior aspect of the T10 vertebral body adjacent to the end plate. The lesion is hypointense on T1WI relative to the intervertebral disk space, which, notably, is normal with no evidence of degenerative changes in the disk or end plates.

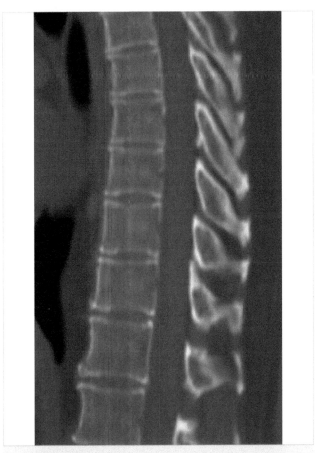

Fig. 27.8 Sagittal reconstruction from a thoracic spine CT scan reveals no evidence of a lytic or blastic lesion.

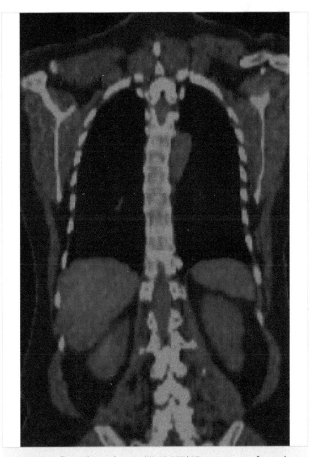

Fig. 27.9 A fluorodeoxyglucose (FDG) PET/CT scan was performed, which revealed no evidence of abnormally increased uptake in the region of the lesion in question or the remainder of the body and spine. Although the precise etiology of the lesion is uncertain, a "cold" FDG PET/CT is most compatible with an atypical hemangioma as these lesions do not have increased uptake of FDG. A follow-up MRI was recommended in 6 months.

27.7.5 Companion Case 5: Focal Red Marrow

An MRI performed in a 61-year-old woman with a remote history of colon cancer 20 years ago (▶ Fig. 27.10) revealed a sacral bone lesion. Imaging findings (shown in ▶ Figs. 27.10–27.14) are most consistent with a focal area of red marrow within the sacrum as proven by 8 years of stability. Follow-up imaging was recommended as the lesion was initially indeterminant, the patient had a remote history of prior malignancy, and it was in a difficult location to biopsy. Red marrow is lower in signal than fatty replaced marrow but typically not lower than the signal of skeletal muscle or normal intervertebral disks on T1WIs as seen in this case. Mild contrast enhancement of red marrow is typical. Although CT of focal red marrow is frequently normal, a vague area of sclerosis may be seen. Most importantly, the normal bone scan is very helpful as blastic metastatic lesions have increased uptake of the radiotracer. In this case, diffusion-weighted imaging was performed. Lack of true restriction of diffusion on the ADC image further supported a benign etiology. An alternative imaging examination to help increase confidence that the lesion is benign would be in-phase/opposed-phase imaging, which should show a decrease in signal on the out-of-phase images for red marrow.

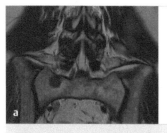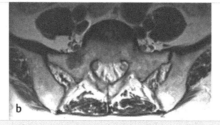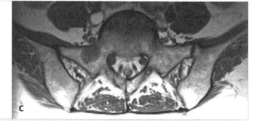

Fig. 27.10 MR images of an incidentally detected indeterminant sacral bone lesion in a 61-year-old woman with a pituitary adenoma and remote history of colon cancer 20 years prior. Coronal (a) and axial (b) non–fat suppressed T2WI and axial T1WI (c) reveal a lesion that is lower in signal than the adjacent normal bone marrow in the right sacral ala but is not lower in signal than skeletal muscle on the T1WIs. The remainder of the sacrum was normal and the lesion did not involve the sacroiliac joint or have an extraosseous component.

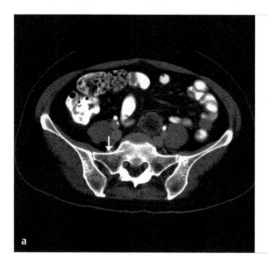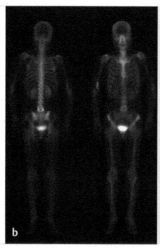

Fig. 27.11 Axial CT scan (a) and Tc-99 m hydroxydiphosphonate (HDP) bone scan (b) reveal only a vague area of possible sclerosis in the right sacral ala. The bone scan is normal without increased uptake in the sacrum.

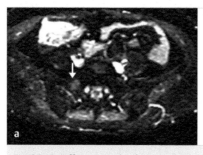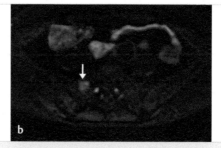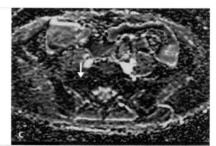

Fig. 27.12 Diffusion-weighted images, with low (a) and high (b) b-values, show increased signal on the diffusion-weighted images. However, the apparent diffusion coefficient (ADC) image reveals no evidence of restricted diffusion in comparison to the surrounding sacral bone marrow (c).

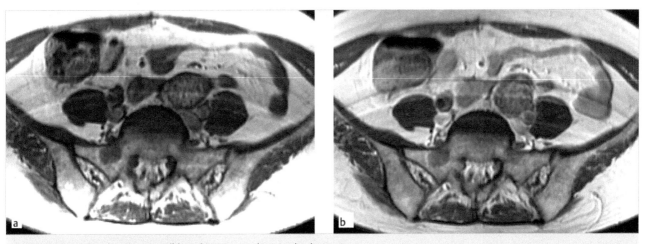

Fig. 27.13 Pre- **(a)** and postcontrast **(b)** axial T1WIs reveal minimal enhancement.

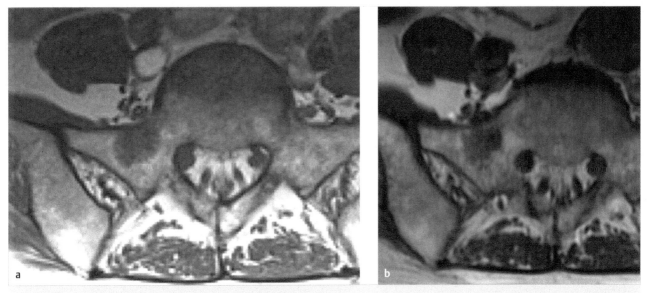

Fig. 27.14 Axial T1WIs of the lesion at presentation **(a)** and on the most recent yearly follow-up MRI performed 8 years after presentation **(b)** show that the lesion remains unchanged.

27.7.6 Companion Case 6: Appearance of a Typical Hemangioma on Fat-Suppressed T2W Images

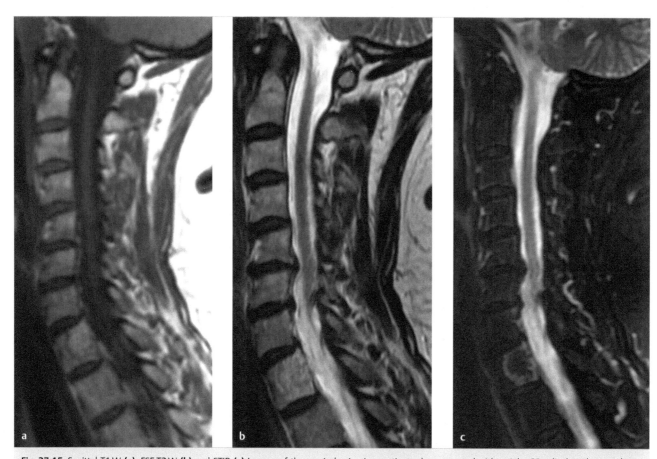

Fig. 27.15 Sagittal T1 W (**a**), FSE-T2 W (**b**) and STIR (**c**) images of the cervical spine in a patient who presented with a right C6 radiculopathy reveal an incidental lesion in the T1 vertebral body. The vast majority of the lesion is high in signal on both the T1 and non–fat suppressed T2WIs (**a, b**). There is a small rim of decreased signal on the T1WIs about the lesion. On the chemically fat-saturated T2 W sequence, fat signal within the majority of lesion is suppressed with only a bright rim surrounding the lesion. Typical hemangiomas may be recognized by their high signal on both T1 and FSE T2WIs. It is not unusual to see a bright rim surrounding these lesions on fat-suppressed T2WIs, which may create concern if one is not aware of this appearance.

References

[1] Rodallec MH, Feydy A, Larousserie F, et al. Diagnostic imaging of solitary tumors of the spine: what to do and say. Radiographics. 2008; 28(4):1019–1041

[2] Toomayan GA, Major NM. Utility of CT-guided biopsy of suspicious skeletal lesions in patients with known primary malignancies. AJR Am J Roentgenol. 2011; 196(2):416–423

[3] Yuh WT, Marsh EE, III, Wang AK, et al. MR imaging of spinal cord and vertebral body infarction. AJNR Am J Neuroradiol. 1992; 13(1):145–154

[4] Guillevin R, Vallee J-N, Lafitte F, Menuel C, Duverneuil N-M, Chiras J. Spine metastasis imaging: review of the literature. J Neuroradiol. 2007; 34(5):311–321

[5] Schweitzer ME, Levine C, Mitchell DG, Gannon FH, Gomella LG. Bull's-eyes and halos: useful MR discriminators of osseous metastases. Radiology. 1993; 188(1):249–252

[6] Hanrahan CJ, Christensen CR, Crim JR. Current concepts in the evaluation of multiple myeloma with MR imaging and FDG PET/CT. Radiographics. 2010; 30(1):127–142

[7] Seiderer M, Staebler A, Wagner H. MRI of bone marrow: opposed-phase gradient-echo sequences with long repetition time. Eur Radiol. 1999; 9(4):652–661

[8] Zajick DC, Jr, Morrison WB, Schweitzer ME, Parellada JA, Carrino JA. Benign and malignant processes: normal values and differentiation with chemical shift MR imaging in vertebral marrow. Radiology. 2005; 237(2):590–596

[9] Yoo HJ, Hong SH, Kim DH, et al. Measurement of fat content in vertebral marrow using a modified dixon sequence to differentiate benign from malignant processes. J Magn Reson Imaging. 2017; 45(5):1534–1544

[10] Kim YP, Kannengiesser S, Paek MY, et al. Differentiation between focal malignant marrow-replacing lesions and benign red marrow deposition of the spine with T2*-corrected fat-signal fraction map using a three-echo volume interpolated breath-hold gradient echo Dixon sequence. Korean J Radiol. 2014; 15(6):781–791

[11] Morales KA, Arevalo-Perez J, Peck KK, Holodny AI, Lis E, Karimi S. Differentiating atypical hemangiomas and metastatic vertebral lesions: the rold of T1-weighted dynamic contrast-enhanced MRI. AJNR Am J Neuroradiol. 2018; 39(5):968–973

[12] Ulano A, Bredella MA, Burke P, et al. Distinguishing untreated osteoblastic metastases from enostoses using CT attenuation measurements. AJR Am J Roentgenol. 2016; 207(2):362–368

[13] Modic MT, Steinberg PM, Ross JS, Masaryk TJ, Carter JR. Degenerative disk disease: assessment of changes in vertebral body marrow with MR imaging. Radiology. 1988; 166(1, Pt 1):193–199

[14] O'Sullivan GJ, Carty FL, Cronin CG. Imaging of bone metastasis: an update. World J Radiol. 2015; 7(8):202–211

[15] Bernard S, Walker E, Raghavan M. An approach to the evaluation of incidentally identified bone lesions encountered on imaging studies. AJR Am J Roentgenol. 2017; 208(5):960–970

[16] Dimopoulos MA, Hillengass J, Usmani S, et al. Role of magnetic resonance imaging in the management of patients with multiple myeloma: a consensus statement. J Clin Oncol. 2015; 33(6):657–664

[17] Regelink JC, Minnema MC, Terpos E, et al. Comparison of modern and conventional imaging techniques in establishing multiple myeloma-related bone disease: a systematic review. Br J Haematol. 2013; 162(1):50–61

[18] Yang HL, Liu T, Wang XM, Xu Y, Deng SM. Diagnosis of bone metastases: a meta-analysis comparing 18FDG PET, CT, MRI and bone scintigraphy. Eur Radiol. 2011; 21(12):2604–2617

[19] Liu T, Cheng T, Xu W, Yan WL, Liu J, Yang HL. A meta-analysis of 18FDG-PET, MRI and bone scintigraphy for diagnosis of bone metastases in patients with breast cancer. Skeletal Radiol. 2011; 40(5):523–531

[20] Taira AV, Herfkens RJ, Gambhir SS, Quon A. Detection of bone metastases: assessment of integrated FDG PET/CT imaging. Radiology. 2007; 243(1):204–211

[21] Dang L, Liu C, Yang SM, et al. Aggressive vertebral hemangioma of the thoracic spine without typical radiological appearance. Eur Spine J. 2012; 21(10):1994–1999

[22] Jain RS, Agrawal R, Srivastava T, Kumar S, Gupta PK, Kookna JC. Aggressive vertebral hemangioma in the postpartum period: an eye-opener. Oxf Med Case Rep. 2014; 2014(7):122–124

[23] Laredo JD, Reizine D, Bard M, Merland JJ. Vertebral hemangiomas: radiologic evaluation. Radiology. 1986; 161(1):183–189

[24] Chi JH, Manley GT, Chou D. Pregnancy-related vertebral hemangioma. Case report, review of the literature, and management algorithm. Neurosurg Focus. 2005; 19(3):E7

[25] Park H-J, Jeon Y-H, Rho M-H, et al. Incidental findings of the lumbar spine at MRI during herniated intervertebral disk disease evaluation. AJR Am J Roentgenol. 2011; 196(5):1151–1155

[26] Fox MW, Onofrio BM. The natural history and management of symptomatic and asymptomatic vertebral hemangiomas. J Neurosurg. 1993; 78(1):36–45

[27] Sen D, Satija L, Chatterji S, Majumder A, Singh M, Gupta A. Vertebral intraosseous lipoma. Med J Armed Forces India. 2015; 71(3):293–296

[28] Laredo JD, Assouline E, Gelbert F, Wybier M, Merland JJ, Tubiana JM. Vertebral hemangiomas: fat content as a sign of aggressiveness. Radiology. 1990; 177(2):467–472

28 Diffusely Abnormal Marrow Signal within the Vertebrae on MRI

Behrang Amini, Krina Patel, Kaye D. Westmark, and Anneliese Gonzalez

28.1 Introduction

Oncologists are frequently consulted to evaluate patients who have an MRI report stating: "The marrow signal is diffusely abnormal. Clinical correlation recommended." Although marrow signal that is diffusely HYPERINTENSE on the T1-weighted images (i.e., fatty replacement) is a normal feature of the adult spine, diffuse HYPOINTENSITY is cause for greater concern and most often warrants further investigation.[1,2]

In a retrospective study of patients whose MRI report stated that their marrow signal was "abnormal" or "heterogeneous," roughly 50% received a definitive diagnosis, of which 25% were found to have a malignancy (e.g., lung cancer, breast cancer, lymphoma, or multiple myeloma). The study concluded with the admonition that abnormal bone marrow findings on MRI should not be ignored.[3]

This chapter begins with a case presentation of "patchy, heterogeneous marrow signal" on a spine MRI that created concern for malignancy but was a normal variant. The two case presentations that follow demonstrate unquestionably abnormal bone

marrow signal changes, both of which were due to hematological malignancy.

Importantly, this chapter will describe the normal appearance of bone marrow on MRI and patterns of red to yellow marrow conversion and reconversion. Understanding normal, age-related changes will assist in recognizing diffuse marrow signal abnormalities that necessitate further evaluation.

28.2 Diffuse Abnormal Marrow: Normal Variant

28.2.1 Case Presentation

The patient is a 63-year-old, neurologically intact, woman with MRI of the lumbosacral (LS) spine performed for back pain (▶ Fig. 28.1).

The marrow signal was originally interpreted as "diffusely abnormal with concern for malignancy," which led to a referral to a cancer center for further evaluation.

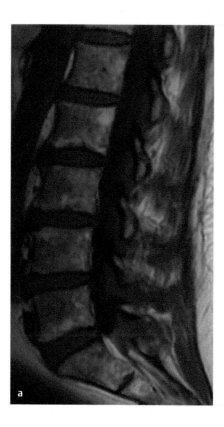
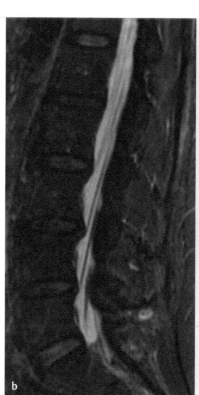

Fig. 28.1 Midline sagittal T1-weighted **(a)** and fast spin echo (FSE) T2-weighted **(b)**, fat-saturated images.

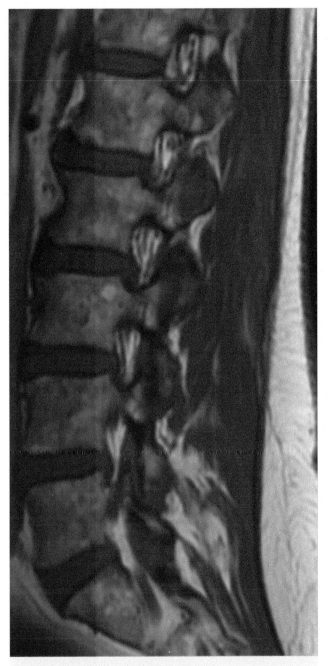

Fig. 28.2 Parasagittal T1-weighted image.

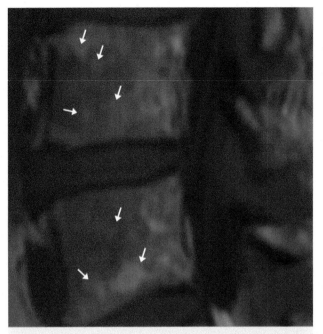

Fig. 28.3 Sagittal T1-weighted image (T1WI) shows numerous focal areas (*arrows*) of preserved hyperintensity within the heterogeneous bone marrow, the "bull's eye sign."[4]

28.2.2 Imaging Findings and Impression

The bone marrow signal is heterogeneous with large, multifocal, patchy but ill-defined, areas of slightly lower signal intensity on the T1WIs. However, these areas of heterogeneity remain higher in signal than both skeletal muscle and intervertebral disks. On the fat-suppressed T2-weighted image (▶ Fig. 28.1b; T2WI), no focal areas of increased signal are seen and the marrow remains

iso- to hypointense relative to skeletal muscle. On the T1WI, small islands of central high signal can be seen within the red marrow (*arrows*, ▶ Fig. 28.3), which has been found to be an indicator of a benign process.[4]

This heterogeneous marrow signal most likely represents patchy conversion of red to yellow marrow that is a well-described normal variant seen predominantly in older adults.[5]

It is important to understand that although patchy, heterogeneous marrow signal may be seen in the normal older population, this appearance does not exclude the possibility of metastatic disease or especially that of multiple myeloma. Multiple myeloma may present with a number of different appearances on MR including multifocal discrete lesions, diffuse decreased signal intensity, "salt-and-pepper" appearance, and finally with completely normal-appearing marrow signal.

28.2.3 Additional Testing Options

In equivocal cases, in which there is uncertainty as to whether an area of lower signal on the T1WI represents focal red marrow versus malignancy, and the "bull's eye sign" is not seen, more advanced MRI techniques may be helpful.

In-phase/opposed-phase imaging. This technique takes advantage of the lower frequency of fat-related proton spins relative to protons associated with water molecules. This difference results in fat and water signal going in and out of phase periodically.

If there is a greater than 20% signal drop on the out-of-phase images, this implies the area contains normal red marrow, whereas no signal decrease may occur in areas in which fat has been replaced by malignant infiltrating cells.[6]

m-Dixon calculation of fat fraction. This technique utilizes m-Dixon fat suppression techniques, which may be used to determine fat fraction within normal versus pathologically infiltrated bone marrow.

It has been shown to help in distinguishing normal red marrow and performed better than contrast-enhanced ratio analysis in one study.[7,8]

28.2.4 Clinical Evaluation

As the report of the MR stated there was "concern for malignancy," the patient was referred to an oncologist where a history was obtained and physical examination performed with emphasis on the presence of constitutional symptoms (fever, night sweats, weight loss, or significant fatigue), as well as symptoms or physical findings concerning the underlying malignancy. The patient was encouraged to undergo age-appropriate screening tests such as mammogram and colonoscopy. It is recommended to do a CBC (complete blood count), CMP (comprehensive metabolic panel), SPEP (serum protein electrophoresis), UPEP (urine protein electrophoresis), and serum-free light chain assay to exclude the possibility of a hematological disease, especially plasma cell disorders. If these tests are normal, no further workup is necessary.

Final Diagnosis: Patchy, heterogenous marrow is most likely due to normal, age-related conversion of red to yellow marrow.

28.2.5 Differential Diagnosis of Diffuse, Heterogeneous Marrow Signal

- Normal variant: In the adult patient, normal conversion from red to yellow marrow may be patchy in a multifocal manner. In younger patients, islands of preserved red marrow may be present. On the T1WIs, it is not lower in signal than adjacent disks or skeletal muscle. On the fat-suppressed T2WIs, it is not significantly higher in signal than skeletal muscle.
- Hematological malignancy: Especially multiple myeloma, which may present with a "salt-and-pepper" appearance.
- Red marrow reconversion (myeloid hyperplasia): This may be seen in times of hematopoietic stress. Clinical examples include severe hemolytic anemias, heart disease with chronic heart failure, heavy smoking, obesity, endurance athletics, and chemotherapy involving granulocyte colony–stimulating factors.
- Diffuse metastatic disease: Usually multifocal lesions rather than diffuse, uniform replacement.

28.2.6 Essential Information regarding Bone Marrow Signal on MRI

Normal bone marrow: red marrow distribution, appearance on MR, age-related conversion and reconversion[9,10,11,12,13]:
- In the fetus and very early neonatal period, all marrow is hypercellular red marrow. The imaging characteristics are as follows:
  - T1WI: low in signal.
  - Fat-suppressed T2WI: high in signal.

- DWI (diffusion-weighted imaging): restricted diffusion, high in signal.
  - Gradient echo (GRE) in-phase/out-of-phase imaging: no signal loss.
- **Red marrow** becomes progressively fatty infiltrated with age and is typically is 40% fat, 40% water, and 20% protein. The imaging characteristics are as follows:
  - T1WI: after the first year of life (90% of children after age 5), slightly higher in signal than intervertebral disks.
  - Fat-suppressed T2WI: isointense to slightly higher in signal than skeletal muscle
  - DWI: Typically, there is no restriction of diffusion in the bone marrow outside the neonatal period. However, at high b values, red marrow may be bright relative to fatty replaced marrow.
  - GRE in-phase/out-of-phase imaging: signal loss by greater than 20% on out-of-phase images.
- **Yellow marrow** is typically 80% fat, 15% water, and 5% protein. The imaging characteristics are as follows:
  - T1WI: very high in signal.
  - Fat-suppressed T2WI: very low in signal.
- **Red to yellow marrow conversion** occurs normally with aging and should be symmetric, beginning peripheral to central and distal to proximal: epiphysis → diaphysis → distal metaphysis →proximal metaphysis.
- **In the pelvis,** fatty marrow replacement begins around the age of 20 years in the superomedial aspect of the acetabulum.
- **The clivus and skull** should be of high signal on the T1WIs after the age of 15 years.[14,15,16]
- **In the spine,** normal fatty marrow replacement is variable, as described by Ricci et al,[5] with marrow signal remaining as low as the intervertebral disks until the age of 10 years when early fatty conversion is seen in the region of the basivertebral plexus (Ricci pattern type 1). In older adults, marrow signal becomes progressively higher in either a diffuse or a multifocal pattern. Ricci type 2 consists of bands or triangular areas of high T1 signal near the end plates, whereas Ricci type 3 consists of patchy areas of red marrow interspersed with small multifocal or large multifocal areas of higher T1 signal. Patterns 2 and 3 are seen more commonly with advancing age.
- **Adult distribution of red marrow** is reached by 25 years of age with it remaining only in the axial skeleton, flat bones, and proximal humerus and femur.
- **Marrow reconversion, from fatty to cellular red marrow**, occurs in the reverse fashion of normal maturation conversion from hematopoietic to fatty marrow. Reconversion occurs symmetrically in the central skeleton and proceeds peripherally. Within long bones, it occurs first in the proximal metaphysis, then distal metaphysis, and finally diaphysis.

28.2.7 Pearls and Pitfalls in Interpretation of Bone Marrow Signal on MRI

- The T1WIs are most important for the evaluation of bone marrow.
- Although the midline sagittal images are best for looking at marrow and disk space signal, the majority of tissue

visualized in the paraspinous compartment on the midsagittal image is ligamentous. Examine the signal intensity of paraspinous musculature in an area that is least fat infiltrated on parasagittal images, to the side of midline. Axial and coronal images can be helpful.

- Fat-suppressed T2WIs are exquisitely sensitive for detection of increased water content within the marrow from any source including malignancy, trauma, infection, and degenerative disk disease. A complete differential diagnosis should include other considerations when abnormal marrow is seen.
- The non–fat saturated FSE-T2 W sequence should not be used in the evaluation of bone marrow signal as both pathologic lesions and normal bone marrow appear high in signal. Normal fat signal must be suppressed by either inversion recovery (STIR), chemical fat saturation, or m-Dixon techniques in order for the sequence to become sensitive to pathology.
- In the normal adult, and usually after the age of 10 (90% of children older than 5 years), marrow should be higher in signal than muscle and the intervertebral disks due to the presence of fat interspersed with hematopoietic tissue on T1WIs.[17] On T1WIs at 1.5 T, hypointense marrow relative to intervertebral disk space signal was 98% accurate in predicting malignant infiltration versus normal hematopoietic marrow. Accuracy using skeletal muscle was slightly less at 94%.[18] On T1WIs at 3.0 T, highest accuracy was obtained using skeletal muscle, as the reference (89%) with a lower accuracy of 78% obtained from using intervertebral disk space signal.[19]
- The epiphyses, after the first few months of life, should be high in signal on the T1WIs. Low epiphyseal signal in an adult, indicating the presence of cellular marrow, is always suspicious for malignant infiltration unless the entirety of the marrow has already undergone reconversion.[20]
- Beyond the neonatal period, hypointense marrow signal that is lower than adjacent skeletal muscle and intervertebral disk spaces on T1WIs is almost always pathologic.[11]
- Patchy areas of red marrow, either preserved or due to reconversion of yellow marrow, may closely mimic pathologic bone marrow infiltration.

Diagnostic clues that suggest benign red marrow:
- Red marrow reconversion is symmetric and bilateral (more helpful when evaluating coronal images of the pelvis and sacrum than on a routine spine MR).

- Signal intensity of normal red marrow is only slightly greater or equal to that of skeletal muscle on fat-suppressed T2WIs. Very "bright" marrow signal on STIR is more likely to represent pathologic infiltration.
- The cortex should be intact and not expanded in red marrow reconversion.
- Bull's eye sign: Normal red marrow often has focal areas of preserved increased signal on T1WIs due to the presence of macroscopic fat. This sign has been reported to have 95% sensitivity and 99.5% specificity for benignancy.[4]
- Dynamic contrast-enhanced imaging: red marrow enhances much less than tumor on post-GBCA T1WIs and has slow wash-in, low maximal peak, and minimal to no apparent wash out.
- Diffusion-weighted imaging: normal bone marrow has low apparent diffusion coefficient (ADC), which decreases with aging. However, there is much overlap between ADC values of hypercellular, but normal, red marrow and malignancy. Infectious lesions cannot be distinguished from malignant lesions on the basis of ADC values.
- **Chemical shift imaging** is an excellent problem-solving technique and can help distinguish red marrow from pathologic infiltration. When fat and water coexist in the same voxel, their spins will be out of phase periodically due to the lower precessional frequency of fat relative to water.
  - Pearls: Red marrow, consisting of similar amounts of fat and water, shows a significant decrease in signal intensity on out-of-phase GRE images. Lack of signal intensity decrease between the in-phase and opposed-phase images suggests that normal marrow fat has been replaced completely by tumor.[6] However, it is important to recognize that completely fatty replaced marrow will also not show signal loss. Therefore, it is the combination of abnormally low signal on T1WI and lack of signal drop between the in-phase and opposed-phase GRE images that is suspicious for malignant infiltration. This technique may also help differentiate benign from malignant compression fractures based on the same principles in which a malignancy will completely replace fat with cellular tumor before causing pathologic collapse.[21]
  - Pitfalls: False negatives have been reported in multiple myeloma, sclerotic metastatic disease, and renal cell carcinoma. False positives have been reported in marrow fibrosis and hematomas.[22]

28.2.8 Companion Case: Examples of Adult Normal Bone Marrow on MRI

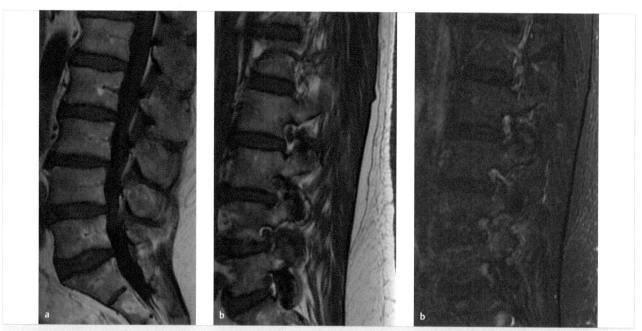

Fig. 28.4 Sagittal **(a)** and parasagittal **(b)** T1 W and parasagittal fat-suppressed T2WIs **(c)**. The marrow signal in this 65-year-old patient is uniformly of higher intensity than that of intervertebral disks and paraspinous skeletal muscle, which is better seen on the parasagittal T1WI **(b)**. The parasagittal fat-suppressed T2WI **(c)** shows that overall, the marrow signal is iso- to slightly hypointense relative to skeletal muscle. This appearance of the bone marrow is normal.

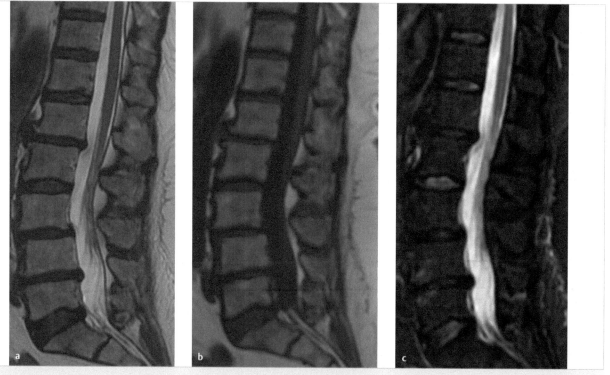

Fig. 28.5 Midline sagittal T1 W **(a)**, FSE-T2 W **(b)**, and STIR **(c)** images of the lumbar spine. The marrow signal in this 75-year-old woman is fatty replaced, which is normal. There is minimal focal bone marrow edema in the inferior aspect of the L4 and the superior aspect of the L5 vertebral bodies anteriorly (*arrows*) due to degenerative change and collapse of the L4–L5 intervertebral disk **(c)**. The marrow signal is otherwise normal as it is higher in signal than that of the intervertebral disks on the T1WIs **(a)**. Note the high sensitivity of the STIR sequence for the focal reactive bone marrow edema at L4–L5 **(c)**, which is much less apparent on the non–fat suppressed FSE-T2WI **(b)** due to the fact that both edema and adjacent normal fatty marrow signal are hyperintense unless fat saturation techniques are applied to FSE-T2 W sequences.

28.3 Diffuse Bone Marrow Signal Abnormality: Hairy Cell Leukemia

28.3.1 Case Presentation

A 65-year-old man with a 40-lb weight loss over the last 2 months had a lumbar spine MRI to evaluate his lower back pain.

28.3.2 Imaging Findings and Impression

Although the patient has typical degenerative disk disease involving L3–L4, L4–L5, and L5–S1, the more significant finding is that of diffusely abnormal bone marrow signal on the T1 and STIR images.

On the T1WIs (▶ Fig. 28.6a and ▶ Fig. 28.7a), the marrow signal in the central anterior aspect of all vertebral bodies is lower than that of the intervertebral disks and skeletal muscle, a finding that is virtually always abnormal outside of the neonatal period. There are no focal, preserved "islands" of fatty signal intensity, the so-called bull's eye sign,[23] to suggest a benign process such as red marrow reconversion. On the STIR sequence, the marrow is much higher in signal than that of skeletal muscle.

These findings are very worrisome for pathologic infiltration of the normal marrow. A hematological malignancy (myeloma, leukemia, lymphoma) or, less likely, diffuse metastatic disease should be considered and further clinical evaluation performed.

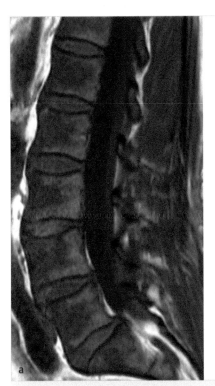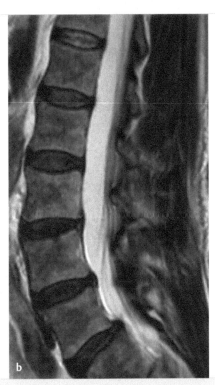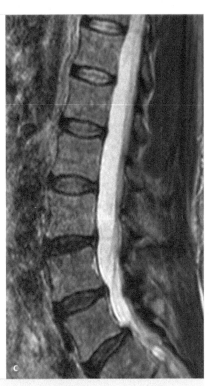

Fig. 28.6 Sagittal midline T1 W **(a)**, FSE-T2 W **(b)**, and short tau inversion recovery (STIR) **(c)** images on a 3.0-T magnet.

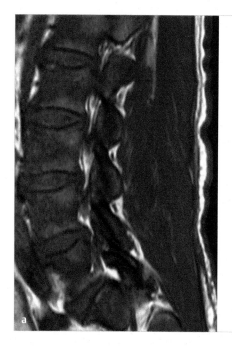
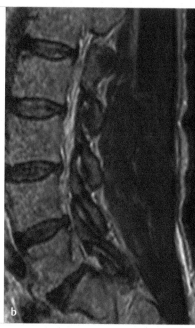

Fig. 28.7 Parasagittal T1 W **(a)** and STIR **(b)** images to allow for comparison of bone marrow signal relative to the signal of paraspinous musculature.

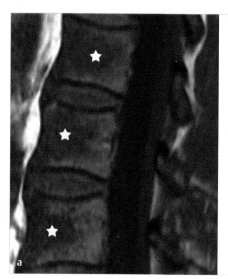
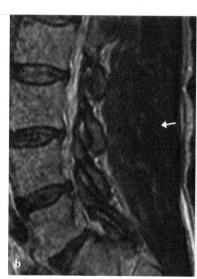

Fig. 28.8 Sagittal T1 W **(a)** and parasagittal fat-suppressed T2 W **(b)** images show confluent central areas of low signal intensity (*white stars*) within the marrow on the T1WI. On the fat-suppressed T2WI, the marrow signal is markedly hyperintense relative to skeletal muscle (*arrow*).

28.3.3 Clinical Evaluation

Hematology/Oncology Consultation

This is a 65-year-old man with diffusely abnormal marrow signal on lumbosacral (LS) spine MR performed for back pain. This finding, as well as the history of significant recent weight loss, is very worrisome for malignancy. Workup for metastatic and primary bone marrow malignancy needs to be performed, which will consist of a thorough history and physical examination, followed by laboratory testing.

Past medical history and review of systems: The patient admitted to increased fatigue and easy bruising over the last 4 to 5 months. He has no unusual occupation history or family history of malignancy.

Physical examination: Cachectic-appearing 65-year-old man with noted pallor and several ecchymotic areas present in upper and lower extremities. Splenomegaly was noted on examination, which was otherwise normal without peripheral adenopathy.

Recommended lab tests:
- Complete blood count (CBC) with differential.
- Peripheral blood smear.
- Metabolic profile.

Test results:
- CBC WBC (white blood cell): 1,700/mm³ (1,500–8,000/mL).
- RBC (red blood cell): 2.36 (4.7–6.1/mL).
- Hgb (hemoglobin): 8.2 g/dL (12–15.5 g/dL).
- Hct (hematocrit): 24.5% (38.8–50%).
- MCV (mean corpuscular volume): 104 fL/red cell (80–98 fL/red cell).
- Plt (platelet): 58K (150–450K).
- ANC (absolute neutrophil count): 200 cells/mm³ (1,500–8,000/mm³) 20% atypical lymphocytes.

Peripheral blood smear: Pancytopenia with circulating tumor cells characteristic of hairy cell leukemia (HCL).

Metabolic profile: Unremarkable with no evidence of hepatic or renal dysfunction.

Impression: A 65-year-old man with diffusely abnormal bone marrow signal on LS spine MRI and pancytopenia.

Based on the clinical presentation and lab results, a bone marrow biopsy is recommended.

Bone marrow biopsy results:
- TRAP (tartrate resistant acid phosphatase)[24] positive staining cells with extensive replacement of the marrow cavity.
- +BRAF (v-Raf murine sarcoma viral oncogene homolog B) c.1799 T > A p.V600E mutation.
- Lymphoma cells are CD20 and BCL-2 positive.

Diagnosis: Hairy cell leukemia (HCL).

Management: This patient has constitutional symptoms and pancytopenia, so he requires immediate treatment. He received one cycle of cladribine, a purine analog, cytotoxic to lymphocytes both resting and dividing cells. It induces durable complete remissions (CRs) in the majority of patients with HCL and is well tolerated.[25] Monotherapy with a purine analog is considered standard first-line treatment with the addition of rituximab in relapsed cases.[26,27] In this case, severe pancytopenia puts the patient at high risk of bleeding and infection (ANC < 1,000/μL).

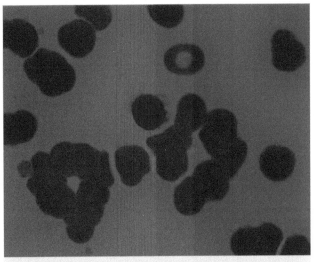

Fig. 28.9 The hairy cell leukemia (HCL) cell is usually one to two times the size of a mature lymphocyte with an eccentric nucleus. The cytoplasm is usually fairly abundant and the cytoplasmic outline is often indistinct due to the presence of varying numbers of projections, best seen on phase-contrast microscopy, giving the cell a "hairy" appearance. (This image is provided courtesy of Amer Wahed, M.D., Department of Pathology and Laboratory Medicine, University of Texas Health Science Center, Houston, TX.)

28.3.4 Differential Diagnosis of the Most Common Causes of Diffuse Abnormality of the Bone Marrow Signal (Hypointense on T1WIs)

- Hematological malignancy: leukemia, lymphoma, and multiple myeloma.
- Diffuse metastatic disease: usually multifocal lesions rather than diffuse, uniform replacement.
- Red marrow reconversion (myeloid hyperplasia) may be seen in times of hematopoietic stress. Clinical examples include severe hemolytic anemias, heart disease with chronic heart failure, heavy smoking, obesity, endurance athletics, and chemotherapy involving granulocyte colony–stimulating factors.
- Normal variant: most commonly seen in some young patients who have an increased amount of red marrow.
- Chronic illness: HIV and end-stage renal disease.
- Hemosiderosis: Secondary hemochromatosis and reticuloendothelial system (RES) iron overload. Iron accumulation occurs primarily in the RES. Therefore, decreased signal intensity on T2*WIs is seen in the liver, spleen, and bone marrow but not in the pancreas or kidneys. It is most often due to multiple transfusions and/or hemolytic anemias.[28]
- Gaucher's disease: It is the most common lysosomal storage disorder. Type I (most common form) can present in late childhood/early adult with massive splenomegaly, hepatomegaly, and bone pain due to diffuse marrow involvement and osteonecrosis. Diffuse decrease in marrow signal is seen on both T1 W and T2WIs. Vertebral bodies may be "**h**-shaped" due to microvascular infarction of the end plates (more classically seen in sickle cell anemia based on the same pathophysiology).[29,30]

- Myelodysplasia: Diffuse abnormality of the bone marrow that presents with severe anemias and is considered a preleukemia state. It presents with diffuse hypointensity on T1WIs and heterogeneous, but usually hyperintensity on T2WI early on. In later stages, the marrow may be hypointense on T2WIs. Diffuse sclerosis is seen on CT. Signal on T2*-weighted images can be low if the patient has received multiple transfusions.

28.3.5 Essential Information regarding Hairy Cell Leukemia

- This is an uncommon lymphoproliferative disorder characterized by the microscopic appearance of villous, "hairy" projections of cytoplasm from the surface of the mature B cells.
- HCL is a subtype of chronic lymphocytic leukemia (CLL) and represents approximately 2% of all leukemias.[31]
- The classic form of HCL is more common in elderly males, the majority of whom present with splenomegaly, weight loss, easy bruising, and abnormal CBC. HCL remains an incurable disease characterized by long periods of remission with eventual relapse and need for retreatment in many patients. Cladribine and pentostatin are the first-line regimens, with overall response rates (ORR) of 90 to 100% and complete responses (CR) of 80 to 95% defined as the normalization of blood counts and absence of morphologic evidence of HCL in peripheral blood and bone marrow. Remission is durable with a median progression-free survival (PFS) of approximately 9 to 11 years.[32]
- Hairy cells produce TNF-alpha (tumor necrosis factor-alpha), a cytokine, which suppresses the production of normal cells in the bone marrow and secrete IL-2 R (interleukin-2 receptor) into the serum, which can be tested for to monitor treatment.[33] The hairy cells have the oncogenic BRAF V600E mutation, which is likely responsible for their uncontrolled proliferation.[25] This has led to the application of inhibitors targeting BRAF for patients with refractory or relapsed disease.[26]

28.4 Multiple Myeloma

28.4.1 Case Presentation

A 72-year-old man with several months of diffuse back pain and fatigue presents to his primary care doctor and undergoes a lumbosacral spine MRI.

28.4.2 Imaging Findings

T1WIs (▶ Fig. 28.10 a,b) reveal a very heterogeneous appearance of the marrow signal, which remains, however, hyperintense relative to adjacent intervertebral disks and paraspinous musculature. The sagittal and parasagittal fat-suppressed T2WIs (▶ Fig. 28.11a,b) are markedly abnormal and reveal multifocal lesions that are much higher in signal than skeletal muscle. In addition, a large, focal lesion in the posterior elements of T12 is much more apparent on the fat-saturated T2WI (*arrow* in ▶ Fig. 28.11b).

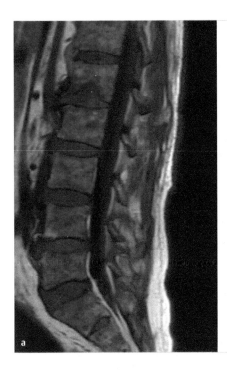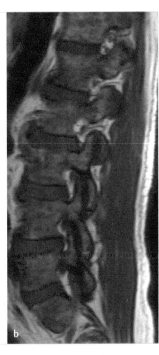

Fig. 28.10 Midline **(a)** and parasagittal **(b)** T1WIs of the lumbar spine.

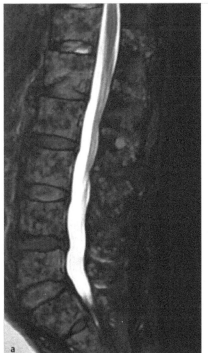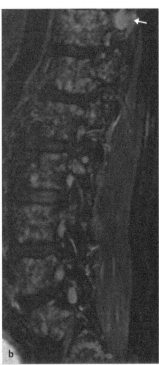

Fig. 28.11 Sagittal **(a)** and parasagittal **(b)** STIR images of the lumbar spine.

Impression

The heterogenous appearance of the marrow on T1WIs (▶ Fig. 28.10 a,b) is very subtle and could be mistaken for a normal variant as red marrow may become more fatty with advancing age, often in a multifocal manner, as described by Ricci et al,[34] patterns 3a or 3b.

The fat-suppressed T2WIs are very helpful in this case because they are markedly abnormal and make apparent the fact that multifocal pathologic lesions are responsible for the marrow heterogeneity.

Multifocal lesions on MRI that are low in signal on T1WI and very high in signal on fat-suppressed T2WIs are most likely due to multiple myeloma (MM) or diffuse metastatic disease.

Further evaluation by hematology/oncology is recommended.

28.4.3 Clinical Evaluation

Hematology/Oncology Consultation

This is a 72-year-old man with no significant past medical history (PMH) who presents with lower back pain and a lumbar spine MRI showing multifocal lesions.

Past medical history and review of systems: PMH was unremarkable. The patient did admit to mildly decreased appetite, a 5-lb weight loss over the last 2 months as well as mild shortness of breath with activities. He denies tobacco product usage.

Physical examination: The patient appeared pale on examination and complained of mild tenderness to percussion of thoracic and lumbar spine region. Cardiac examination revealed a grade 2/6 systolic murmur. There was no palpable hepatosplenomegaly or adenopathy. Note was made of mild pedal edema. Neurological examination was normal.

Impression: The patient is an older adult man with diffuse marrow abnormality and multifocal discrete lesions. The most common etiologies are MM and metastatic disease.

Additional recommended testing and results: Laboratory testing should include CBC and differential, platelet count, and examination of the peripheral blood smear. A complete metabolic profile, including calcium and albumin levels as well as lactate dehydrogenase (LDH) and beta-2 microglobulin levels should be obtained. Serum protein electrophoresis (SPEP) and serum immunofixation electrophoresis (SIFE) and serum-free light chain (SFLC) assay as well as 24-hour urine for total protein and urine protein electrophoresis (UPEP), and urine immunofixation electrophoresis (UIFE) should be obtained.

A screening chest X-ray had been performed recently and was unremarkable. Skeletal survey should be completed for further myeloma workup, while PET/CT versus whole spine MRI should be obtained if extramedullary disease is a possibility.[35] Prostate-specific antigen (PSA), colonoscopy, and whole-body PET/CT would be recommended if additional testing for MM is negative.

Testing results:
- CBC ANC: 4,700 cells/mm^3 (1,500–8,000/mm^3).
- Hgb: 8.3 g/dL (12–15.5 g/dL).
- Platelets: 100K (150–450K).
- Metabolic profile BUN (blood urea nitrogen): 60 mg/dL (7–20 mg/dL).
- Creatinine: 2.5 mg/dL (0.6–1.2 mg/dL).

- Potassium: 5.4 mEq/L (3.5–5 mEq/L).
- Calcium: 12.0 mg/dL (8.5–10.2 mg/dL).
- Phosphate: 5.6 mg/dL (2.5–4.5 mg/dL).
- Albumin: 3.2 g/dL (3.5–5.5 g/dL).
- Total protein: 9.0 g/dL (6–8.3 g/dL).
- LDH: 450 U/L (100–190 U/L in adults).
- Beta-2 microglobulin: 6.1 mg/L (0.8–2.3 mg/L).
- Uric acid: 8.2 mg/dL (2.6–7.1 mg/dL).
- SPEP M-spike was present at 3.1 g/dL.
- SIFE A band was identified as IgG (immunoglobulin G) kappa.
- SFLC kappa: 1,145 mg/L (3.3–19.4 mg/L).
- SFLC lambda: 5 mg/L (5.71–26.3 mg/L).
- SFLC kappa/SFLC lamba ratio: 229 (0.26–1.65).
- Twenty-four hour urine total volume: 1.575 mL
  - 157 mg/dL proteinuria.
  - 2,473 mg total proteinuria.
- UPEP: 1,353-mg Bence Jones protein.
- UIFE kappa.

On the basis of the above testing, bone marrow biopsy was performed. The bone marrow biopsy revealed 70% kappa-restricted clonal plasma cells.

Subsequently, metaphase cytogenetics and plasma cell fluorescence in situ hybridization (FISH) were performed, which revealed standard risk disease. Cytogenetics were normal diploid and FISH studies were negative for deletion 17p, t,4;14 t (14;16), t(14;20), amplification 1q/deletion 1p, monosomy 13, or t(11;14).

Diagnosis: The patient fulfills the criteria for active (symptomatic) MM.

Bone marrow biopsy reveals greater than 10% plasma cells and numerous MM-defining events are present, including renal insufficiency (creatinine > 2.0 mg/dL); serum calcium > 11.5 mg/dL; anemia with hemoglobin < 10 mg/dL; and multiple bone lesions that are greater than 5 mm in size on MRI.[35]

Revised International Staging System: Stage II (Beta-2 microglobulin > 5.5 mg/L, high serum LDH, albumin < 3.5, standard risk FISH).[36]

Treatment recommendations: Upfront treatment for this patient would include a triplet regimen including a proteasome inhibitor (PI) such as bortezomib or carfilzomib, an immunomodulatory drug (IMID) such as lenalidomide (renally dosed) and dexamethasone. After achieving at least a partial response (ideally a very good response or better), this patient would undergo consolidation with an autologous stem cell transplant, which consists of high-dose melphalan, followed by stem cell rescue if deemed a transplant candidate. Once they achieve optimal response with or without autologous stem cell transplant, they would continue onto maintenance therapy.

Supportive care is of great importance in this patient given his bone marrow suppression, hypercalcemia, and renal injury. Due to their hypercalcemia and possible tumor lysis syndrome, they would receive allopurinol, fluids, and renally adjusted zoledronic acid. Once their renal function improves, denosumab may be considered instead. Antiviral prophylaxis, thromboprophylaxis, and a proton pump inhibitor are indicated for prevention of shingles from the PI, deep vein thrombosis from the IMID, and steroid combination and reflux or gastritis from steroids, respectively. Vitamin D supplementation is indicated for low lab levels.

MRI of the remainder of the spine was performed to assess for additional lesions and extraosseous extension that would be concerning for imminent spinal cord compression. Cord compression is considered an oncologic emergency and would require a STAT consult to neurosurgery for possible decortication and radiation oncology. Steroids should be initiated for these patients as soon as possible as well to decrease cord edema.

28.4.4 Differential Diagnosis of Multifocal Vertebral Lesions

Common Causes

- Multiple myeloma.
- Metastatic disease (most commonly lung cancer in male and breast cancer in female patients):
  – Prostate cancer.
  – Renal cell carcinoma.
  – Gastrointestinal/genitourinary malignancies.
  – Thyroid cancer.
  – Melanoma.
  – Leukemia/lymphoma.

Uncommon Causes

- Sarcoidosis.
- Mastocytosis.

28.4.5 Pearls and Pitfalls of Imaging Interpretation in Multiple Myeloma

- Plain radiographs traditionally used for screening for lytic lesions in patients with suspected MM have a high false-negative rate, as greater than 50% of bone must be destroyed before a lesion is detectable on lateral radiographs of the spine. However, plain radiographs of the skull and ribs are still utilized as MRI and FDG-PET/CT's sensitivity for lesions in these areas is reduced.[37]
- Bone scans are typically negative in patients with MM even with widespread lytic lesions.
- Numerous lytic bone lesions in an older patient with a negative bone scan are highly suggestive of MM.
- FDG-PET/CT and WB-MRI are considered the most sensitive imaging modalities to evaluate for the presence of skeletal involvement. CT is able to detect lesions with cortical involvement and helps assess the risk of pathologic fractures. MRI has high sensitivity for the presence of bone marrow involvement and is the best imaging test for the spine as it also detects extraosseous involvement and involvement of the spinal canal.
- Preserved red marrow, often seen in younger patients or in patients receiving marrow-stimulating factors after complete remission (CR), may have an appearance on MRI identical to marrow diffusely infiltrated with myeloma cells. The differentiation can often be made clinically, however.
- Completely normal marrow signal on MRI is present in approximately 28% of MM patients and therefore does not exclude the diagnosis.[38]

28.4.6 Essential Clinical and Imaging Information Regarding Multiple Myeloma

Basic Facts

- MM is a malignancy of the plasma cells that accumulate within the bone marrow.
- The majority of MM involves clonal overproduction of heavy chain proteins that may be recognized by elevated total serum protein as well as a monoclonal spike (M-spike) on SPEP.
- A minority of patients may have light chain disease, in which only the kappa or lambda chain of the Ig are overproduced. As these proteins are small, they are excreted in the urine; therefore, the total serum protein and SPEP may be normal. The proteins within the urine (Bence Jones proteins) are associated with renal damage and may be detected by UPEP.
- MM occurs most frequently in the 65- to 74-year-old age group.

Definition of Disease and Classification Schemes[35,36]

- The International Myeloma Working Group updated the criteria for the diagnosis of active MM:
  – Greater than 10% clonal plasma cells in the bone marrow OR a biopsy-proven bony or extramedullary plasmacytoma.
  – One or more myeloma-defining events (CRAB OR biomarkers of malignancy, SLiM).
- SLiM ≥ 60% clonal plasma cells in bone marrow; SFLC ratio of ≥ 100 provided involved light chain is at least 100 mg/L; greater than one focal lesion on MRI that is ≥ 5 mm in size.
- CRAB features are evidence of end organ damage from MM and include hypercalcemia, renal insufficiency, anemia, and bone lesions (≥ 1 osteolytic lesion on skeletal radiographs, CT, or PET/CT).
- New updated diagnostic criteria no longer require evidence of end organ damage (CRAB features) to make the diagnosis of active MM; therefore, more than one 5-mm lesion on MRI may define active MM.
- More than one bone lesion distinguishes solitary plasmacytoma from MM when bone marrow has less than 10% clonal plasma cells.
- The Durie–Salmon PLUS staging system has incorporated the use of MRI and FDG-PET/CT, especially when WB-MRI is not available. Serum creatine is the only laboratory parameter. The presence of more than one focal lesion on MRI that is greater than 5 mm in size is now considered an "MM-defining event."[35]
- The R-ISS (revised international staging system) uses measurement of the serum beta-2 microglobulin, albumin LDH levels, and FISH studies of the bone marrow aspirate, which reflect the tumor cell burden and proliferative ability to determine prognosis, rather than imaging information.[36]

Imaging of Multiple Myeloma

- MRI appearances of MM are variable and include the following[39]:
  – Multiple focal lesions.
  – Diffusely low signal marrow on T1WI.

– Focal lesions and diffuse homogenous decrease in signal on T1WI (mixed pattern seen in 11% of MM patients).
– Stippled, salt-and-pepper appearance (3% of MM patients).
– Completely normal appearance of the marrow on MRI (28% of MM patients).

- MM diffusely infiltrated marrow will have a time intensity of enhancement curve that differs from normal marrow. Lesions are usually low in signal on T1WI and high in signal on fat-suppressed T2WIs. Lesions enhance with early wash-in and early washout of GBCAs.[38,39]

- FDG-PET/CT is considered a very useful test especially when WB-MRI is not available and is usually positive either focally or diffusely in active MM, whereas in MGUS (monoclonal gammopathy of uncertain significance) and smoldering myeloma, it is typically negative. FDG-PET is also used to monitor response to therapy. False-positive results on FDG-PET/CT are not uncommon and may occur due to infection, recent chemotherapy, or radiation therapy.[40]

References

[1] Moulopoulos LA, Koutoulidis V. Bone Marrow MRI. A Pattern-Based Approach. Milan, Italy: Springer-Verlag; 2015

[2] Siegel MJ. MR imaging of pediatric hematologic bone marrow disease. J Hong Kong Coll Radiol. 2000; 3:38–50

[3] Shah GL, Rosenberg AS, Jarboe J, Klein A, Cossor F. Incidence and evaluation of incidental abnormal bone marrow signal on magnetic resonance imaging. ScientificWorldJournal. 2014; 2014:380814

[4] Schweitzer ME, Levine C, Mitchell DG, Gannon FH, Gomella LG. Bull's-eyes and halos: useful MR discriminators of osseous metastases. Radiology. 1993; 188(1):249–252

[5] Ricci C, Cova M, Kang YS, et al. Normal age-related patterns of cellular and fatty bone marrow distribution in the axial skeleton: MR imaging study. Radiology. 1990; 177(1):83–88

[6] Disler DG, McCauley TR, Ratner LM, Kesack CD, Cooper JA. In-phase and out-of-phase MR imaging of bone marrow: prediction of neoplasia based on the detection of coexistent fat and water. AJR Am J Roentgenol. 1997; 169(5): 1439–1447

[7] Yoo HJ, Hong SH, Kim DH, et al. Measurement of fat content in vertebral marrow using a modified dixon sequence to differentiate benign from malignant processes. J Magn Reson Imaging. 2017; 45(5):1534–1544

[8] Kim YP, Kannengiesser S, Paek MY, et al. Differentiation between focal malignant marrow-replacing lesions and benign red marrow deposition of the spine with T2*-corrected fat-signal fraction map using a three-echo volume interpolated breath-hold gradient echo Dixon sequence. Korean J Radiol. 2014; 15(6):781–791

[9] Shah LM, Hanrahan CJ. MRI of spinal bone marrow: part I, techniques and normal age-related appearances. AJR Am J Roentgenol. 2011; 197(6): 1298–1308

[10] Hanrahan CJ, Shah LM. MRI of spinal bone marrow: part 2, T1-weighted imaging-based differential diagnosis. AJR Am J Roentgenol. 2011; 197(6): 1309–1321

[11] Siegel MJ. MR imaging of pediatric hematologic bone marrow disease. J Hong Kong Coll Radiol. 2000; 3:38–50

[12] Vande Berg BC, Malghem J, Lecouvet FE, Maldague B. Magnetic resonance imaging of the normal bone marrow. Skeletal Radiol. 1998; 27(9):471–483

[13] Steiner RM, Mitchell DG, Rao VM, Schweitzer ME. Magnetic resonance imaging of diffuse bone marrow disease. Radiol Clin North Am. 1993; 31(2): 383–409

[14] Foster K, Chapman S, Johnson K. MRI of the marrow in the paediatric skeleton. Clin Radiol. 2004; 59(8):651–673

[15] Schick RM. Normal age-related changes in bone marrow in the axial skeleton at MR imaging. Radiology. 1991; 179(3):877

[16] Okada Y, Aoki S, Barkovich AJ, et al. Cranial bone marrow in children: assessment of normal development with MR imaging. Radiology. 1989; 171(1): 161–164

[17] Sebag GH, Dubois J, Tabet M, Bonato A, Lallemand D. Pediatric spinal bone marrow: assessment of normal age-related changes in the MRI appearance. Pediatr Radiol. 1993; 23(7):515–518

[18] Carroll KW, Feller JF, Tirman PFJ. Useful internal standards for distinguishing infiltrative marrow pathology from hematopoietic marrow at MRI. J Magn Reson Imaging. 1997; 7(2):394–398

[19] Zhao J, Krug R, Xu D, Lu Y, Link TM. MRI of the spine: image quality and normal-neoplastic bone marrow contrast at 3 T versus 1.5 T. AJR Am J Roentgenol. 2009; 192(4):873–880

[20] Daldrup-Link HE, Henning T, Link TM. MR imaging of therapy-induced changes of bone marrow. Eur Radiol. 2007; 17(3):743–761

[21] Erly WK, Oh ES, Outwater EK. The utility of in-phase/opposed-phase imaging in differentiating malignancy from acute benign compression fractures of the spine. AJNR Am J Neuroradiol. 2006; 27(6):1183–1188

[22] Swartz PG, Roberts CC. Radiological reasoning: bone marrow changes on MRI. AJR Am J Roentgenol. 2009; 193(3) Suppl:S1–S4, Quiz S5–S9

[23] Schweitzer ME, Levine C, Mitchell DG, Gannon FH, Gomella LG. Bull's-eyes and halos: useful MR discriminators of osseous metastases. Radiology. 1993; 188(1):249–252

[24] Akkaya H, Dogan O, Agan M, Dincol G. The value of tartrate resistant acid phosphatase (TRAP) immunoreactivity in diagnosis of hairy cell leukemia. APMIS. 2005; 113(3):162–166

[25] Tiacci E, Trifonov V, Schiavoni G, et al. BRAF mutations in hairy-cell leukemia. N Engl J Med. 2011; 364(24):2305–2315

[26] Tiacci E, Park JH, De Carolis L, et al. Targeting mutant BRAF in relapsed or refractory hairy-cell leukemia. N Engl J Med. 2015; 373(18):1733–1747

[27] Else M, Ruchlemer R, Osuji N, et al. Long remissions in hairy cell leukemia with purine analogs: a report of 219 patients with a median follow-up of 12.5 years. Cancer. 2005; 104(11):2442–2448

[28] Queiroz-Andrade M, Blasbalg R, Ortega CD, et al. MR imaging findings of iron overload. Radiographics. 2009; 29(6):1575–1589

[29] Simpson WL, Hermann G, Balwani M. Imaging of Gaucher disease. World J Radiol. 2014; 6(9):657–668

[30] Terk MR, Esplin J, Lee K, Magre G, Colletti PM. MR imaging of patients with type 1 Gaucher's disease: relationship between bone and visceral changes. AJR Am J Roentgenol. 1995; 165(3):599–604

[31] Fanta PT, Saven A. Hairy cell leukemia. In: Ansell SM, eds. Rare Hematological Malignancies. Boston, MA: Springer; 2008:193–209

[32] Goodman GR, Burian C, Koziol JA, Saven A. Extended follow-up of patients with hairy cell leukemia after treatment with cladribine. J Clin Oncol. 2003; 21(5):891–896

[33] Wintrobe MM. Wintrobe's Clinical Hematology. In: Greer JG, Foerster J, Lukens JN, Rodgers GM, Paraskevas F, eds. 11th ed. Hagerstown, MD: Lippincott Williams & Wilkins; 2004:2465–2466

[34] Ricci C, Cova M, Kang YS, et al. Normal age-related patterns of cellular and fatty bone marrow distribution in the axial skeleton: MR imaging study. Radiology. 1990; 177(1):83–88

[35] Rajkumar SV, Dimopoulos MA, Palumbo A, et al. International Myeloma Working Group updated criteria for the diagnosis of multiple myeloma. Lancet Oncol. 2014; 15(12):e538–e548

[36] Palumbo A, Avet-Loiseau H, Oliva S, et al. Revised International Staging System for Multiple Myeloma: a report from International Myeloma Working Group. J Clin Oncol. 2015; 33(26):2863–2869

[37] Regelink JC, Minnema MC, Terpos E, et al. Comparison of modern and conventional imaging techniques in establishing multiple myeloma-related bone disease: a systematic review. Br J Haematol. 2013; 162(1):50–61

[38] Baur-Melnyk A, Buhmann S, Dürr HR, Reiser M. Role of MRI for the diagnosis and prognosis of multiple myeloma. Eur J Radiol. 2005; 55(1):56–63

[39] Dutoit JC, Verstraete KL. MRI in multiple myeloma: a pictorial review of diagnostic and post-treatment findings. Insights Imaging. 2016; 7(4):553–569

[40] Cavo M, Terpos E, Nanni C, et al. Role of 18F-FDG PET/CT in the diagnosis and management of multiple myeloma and other plasma cell disorders: a consensus statement by the International Myeloma Working Group. Lancet Oncol. 2017; 18(4):e206–e217

29 Filum Terminale Lipoma

Cole T. Lewis, Octavio Arevalo, Rajan P. Patel, and David I. Sandberg

29.1 Case Presentation

29.1.1 History

A 9-year-old male patient presents with a history of nonspecific back pain.

29.2 Imaging Analysis

Lumbosacral spine MRI from a 9-year-old male patient with nonspecific back pain was performed. Sagittal T1-weighted (T1w; ▶ Fig. 29.1a), sagittal short tau inversion recovery (STIR; ▶ Fig. 29.1b), axial T1w (▶ Fig. 29.1c), and axial T2-weighted (T2w) with fat suppression (▶ Fig. 29.1d) images. An intrathecal linear hyperintensity is seen in T1w sagittal and axial images (*arrows* in ▶ Fig. 29.1a,c), in close relationship with the filum terminale; its high T1w signal intensity is suppressed in the series with fat saturation (*arrows* in ▶ Fig. 29.1b,d). Note the normal morphology and position of conus medullaris (*asterisk* in ▶ Fig. 29.1b) with tip located at the superior end plate of L2 level (*arrowhead* in ▶ Fig. 29.1b).

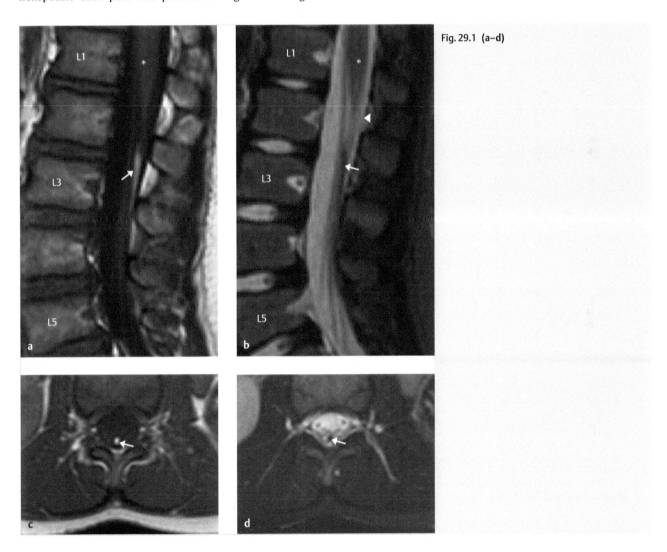

Fig. 29.1 (a–d)

29.3 Differential Diagnosis

- Filum terminale lipoma:
  - It is seen as a linear hyperintensity within the filum terminale on T1w images, 1- to 5-mm wide and of variable length, and follows fat signal intensity in all MRI sequences.[1,2,3]
- Tethered cord with terminal lipoma:
  - The cord extends abnormally inferiorly than the normal level of mid-L2, and there is a thick lipoma at its caudal termination.
  - Indistinct cord termination with a smooth transition between conus and filum.[4,5]

29.4 Diagnostic Pearls

- **Filum terminale lipoma:**
  - Small amounts of fat within the filum may be an incidental, asymptomatic finding, especially if the conus terminates normally.
  - Patients may be or may become symptomatic with tethered cord symptoms at any age and, therefore, clinical correlation is necessary to determine the significance of the finding.

29.5 Essential Information about Filum Terminale Lipoma

Etiology:

- It is believed that entity is secondary to an alteration of normal apoptosis and of the elongation process of the filum during fetal development.

Follow-up:

- If asymptomatic, and the conus ends at a normal level, no imaging follow-up is needed. Neurosurgical consultation is recommended to determine whether the lesion is symptomatic, especially if it is associated with a low-lying conus.

29.6 Neurosurgery Questions and Answers

1. **What is the etiology and natural history of the condition that would assist in decision-making?**
   Filum terminale lipomas are a type of spinal dysraphism that is thought to be a result of a disorder of secondary neurulation.[6] Fatty tissue within the filum can affect the natural flexibility of the filum and may result in tethered cord syndrome.[6] Filum terminale lipomas typically exhibit benign clinical courses.[7] However, urinary and motor dysfunction as well as scoliosis and foot deformities may be present.

2. **Given the presentation and imaging findings, what specific findings on physical examination and/or elements of the history are important in your determination of the diagnosis and, more importantly, in the determination as to if this probable incidental finding is truly asymptomatic?**
   Filum terminale lipomas with a normal conus level are likely to be completely incidental findings.[7] However, they should undergo thorough neurological evaluation and assessment of any symptoms that may be related to the tethered cord syndrome.

3. **What additional testing, if any, is required or recommended in the workup?**
   In patients with low-lying conus, MRI of the total neuroaxis should be performed to evaluate for the presence of syringohydromyelia or other associated CNS abnormalities. Patients should also undergo urodynamic testing for further evaluation.[8]

4. **If electing to follow, what is the suggested time interval and modality?**
   Pediatric patients with a fatty filum terminale and conus medullaris at the normal level, the L1–L2 interspace, do not need routine follow-up but should be instructed to see a neurosurgeon for back pain, weakness, or bowel/bladder dysfunction. If the conus medullaris is lower than the pedicle of L2 in the presence of a fatty filum terminale, elective surgical intervention should be considered.

5. **If electing surgical (or medical) management, then why and what are the surgical options and risks?**
   In patients presenting with symptoms consistent with the tethered cord syndrome, spinal cord untethering has been shown to be beneficial and safe. Surgical intervention in patients with asymptomatic filum terminale lipomas remains controversial, but most neurosurgeons will consider surgery if the conus is low lying.[6] Surgical intervention is accompanied by standard risks such as infection, bleeding, and anesthetic risk; however, additional risks include damage to the adjacent nervous tissue, which could result in bladder/bowel dysfunction, cerebrospinal fluid leaks, and motor/sensory deficits. The risk of spinal cord retethering, which is common in more complex conditions of spinal dysraphism, is very rare for a simple fatty filum terminale.

6. **Are there any special circumstances that would lead a surgeon to consider being more proactive?**
   Neurosurgical intervention is indicated in patients presenting with symptoms consistent with the tethered cord syndrome or progressive neurological impairments and is typically offered prophylactically in patients with a low-lying conus medullaris.

References

[1] Barkovich J. Filum terminale fibrolipoma. In: Barkovich J, ed. Diagnostic Imaging Pediatric Neuroradiology. Salt Lake City, UT: Amirsys; 2007:III-4–III-6

[2] Cools MJ, Al-Holou WN, Stetler WR, Jr, et al. Filum terminale lipomas: imaging prevalence, natural history, and conus position. J Neurosurg Pediatr. 2014; 13(5):559–567

[3] Meyers AB, Chandra T, Epelman M. Sonographic spinal imaging of normal anatomy, pathology and magnetic growing rods in children. Pediatr Radiol. 2017; 47(9):1046–1057

[4] Raghavan N, Barkovich AJ, Edwards M, Norman D. MR imaging in the tethered spinal cord syndrome. AJR Am J Roentgenol. 1989; 152(4):843–852

[5] Rufener SL, Ibrahim M, Raybaud CA, Parmar HA. Congenital spine and spinal cord malformations: pictorial review. AJR Am J Roentgenol. 2010; 194(3) Suppl:S26–S37

[6] Usami K, Lallemant P, Roujeau T, et al. Spinal lipoma of the filum terminale: review of 174 consecutive patients. Childs Nerv Syst. 2016; 32(7):1265–1272

[7] Cools MJ, Al-Holou WN, Stetler WR, Jr, et al. Filum terminale lipomas: imaging prevalence, natural history, and conus position. J Neurosurg Pediatr. 2014; 13(5):559–567

[8] Vernet O, Farmer JP, Houle AM, Montes JL. Impact of urodynamic studies on the surgical management of spinal cord tethering. J Neurosurg. 1996; 85(4):555–559

30 Ventriculus Terminalis

Cole T. Lewis, Octavio Arevalo, Rajan P. Patel, and David I. Sandberg

30.1 Case Presentation

An 18-month-old female patient presents with small shallow sacral dimple.

30.2 Imaging Analysis

MRI of an 18-month-old female patient with sagittal T1-weighted (T1w; ▸ Fig. 30.1a), sagittal short tau inversion recovery (STIR; ▸ Fig. 30.1b), axial T1w (▸ Fig. 30.1c), and axial T2-weighted (T2w; ▸ Fig. 30.1d) images. This image shows a linear-shaped cystic structure within the central portion of the conus medullaris that has similar signal intensity to cerebrospinal fluid (CSF) on T1w and T2w images (*arrowheads*). This structure corresponds to an expanded central canal without any spinal cord signal abnormality. It is important to note that conus medullaris is in normal position and the filum terminale is normal in appearance (*arrows*).

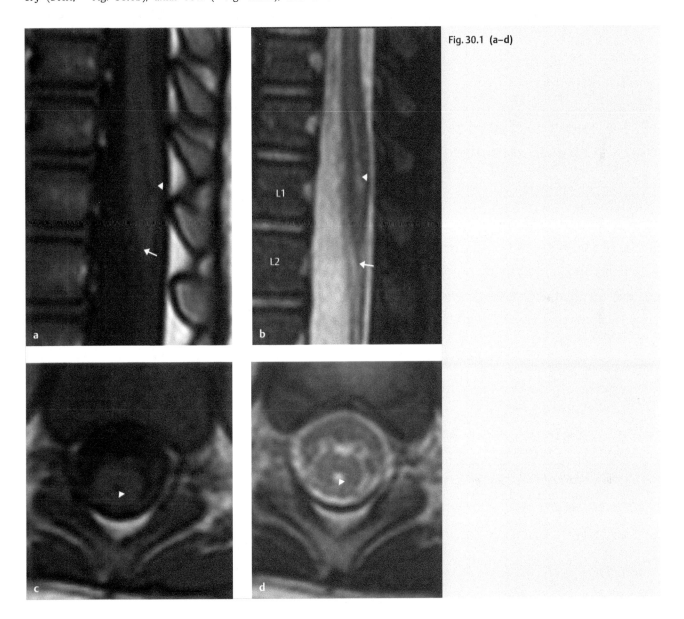

Fig. 30.1 (a–d)

30.3 Differential Diagnosis

- **Ventriculus terminalis:**
  - Normal variant representing a focal dilatation of the central canal in the conus.
- Transient dilatation of the central canal:
  - Normal variant in which there is a slight transient dilatation of the central canal during the first week of life.[1,2]
- Cystic spinal cord neoplasm:
  - The imaging landmark is cord signal abnormality, mass effect, neurologic symptoms, and contrast enhancement in solid portions.
- Syringohydromyelia:
  - Cystic dilatation of the central canal that could be isolated or associated with congenital anomalies in up to 30% of cases.[3]
- Myelomalacia:
  - Cord atrophy secondary to previous vascular, traumatic, or other injury.

30.4 Diagnostic Pearls

- This refers to an expanded central canal filled with CSF at the conus without any spinal cord signal abnormality or enhancement.
- It can be up to 2- to 3-mm wide and less than 2-cm long and has smooth, regular margins without any mass effect.
- It is important to note that the location of the conus is at T12–L2.[4,5,6]

30.5 Essential Information about Ventriculus Terminalis

30.5.1 Etiology

- The ventriculus terminalis develops around the ninth embryonic week and represents the junction between the central canal portion formed by neurulation and the portion formed by caudal cell mass canalization.

30.5.2 Imaging Pitfalls

- Gibbs' truncation artifact: Parallel lines that appear when the interface between high and low signal intensities occurs in the same plane, that is, the cord surface–CSF interface mimicking a central canal dilatation.
- If associated with filum terminalis lipoma, rule out a tethered cord by establishing a normally positioned conus.

30.5.3 Follow-up

- If asymptomatic, no imaging follow-up is needed.

30.6 Neurosurgery Questions and Answers

1. **What is the etiology and natural history of the condition that would assist in decision-making?**

   The ventriculus terminalis is an ependymal lined cystic cavity that is a normal part of the embryological development.[7] Persistent ventriculus terminalis may be present and may be a normal finding in children younger than 5 years.[8] Progressive enlargement is very rare and may be associated with either nonspecific symptoms or focal neurological deficits.

2. **Are there any special circumstances that would lead the surgeon to consider being more proactive?**

   If neurological deficits are present and/or progressive enlargement occurs, neurosurgical evaluation is necessary.

3. **What additional testing, if any, is required or recommended in the workup?**

   MRI of the lumbosacral spine with and without contrast is recommended to fully define the pathology. If urological symptoms are present, the patient should be evaluated by urology for possible neurogenic bladder by means of electrophysiological and urodynamic investigations.[8]

References

[1] Unsinn KM, Geley T, Freund MC, Gassner I. US of the spinal cord in newborns: spectrum of normal findings, variants, congenital anomalies, and acquired diseases. Radiographics. 2000; 20(4):923–938

[2] Blondiaux E, Katorza E, Rosenblatt J, et al. Prenatal US evaluation of the spinal cord using high-frequency linear transducers. Pediatr Radiol. 2011; 41(3):374–383

[3] Petit-Lacour MC, Lasjaunias P, Iffenecker C, et al. Visibility of the central canal on MRI. Neuroradiology. 2000; 42(10):756–761

[4] Moore K. Ventriculus terminalis. In: Barkovich J, ed. Diagnostic Imaging Pediatric Neuroradiology. Salt Lake City, UT: Amirsys; 2007:III-5–III-2

[5] Coleman LT, Zimmerman RA, Rorke LB. Ventriculus terminalis of the conus medullaris: MR findings in children. AJNR Am J Neuroradiol. 1995; 16(7):1421–1426

[6] Demiryurek D, Bayramoglu A, Aydingoz U, Erbil KM, Bayraktar B. Magnetic resonance imaging determination of the ventriculus terminalis. Neurosciences (Riyadh). 2003; 8(4):241–243

[7] Lotfinia I, Mahdkhah A. The cystic dilation of ventriculus terminalis with neurological symptoms: three case reports and a literature review. J Spinal Cord Med. 2018; 41(6):741–747

[8] Zeinali M, et al. Cystic dilation of a ventriculus terminalis. Case report and review of the literature. Br J Neurosurg. 2017:1–5

31 Prominent Central Canal

Cole T. Lewis, Octavio Arevalo, Rajan P. Patel, and David I. Sandberg

31.1 Case Presentation

A 16-year-old female patient with history of a motor vehicular collision presents with complaint of neck pain and thoracic region back pain.

31.2 Imaging Analysis

Spine MRI from a 16-year-old female patient with sagittal T2-wighted (T2w; ▶ Fig. 31.1a), sagittal T1-weighted (T1w; ▶ Fig. 31.1b), and axial T2w (▶ Fig. 31.1c) images. A slightly enlarged central canal is noticed (*arrows*); however, there are no additional abnormalities of the spinal cord in course, overall diameter, or surrounding parenchymal signal intensity.

31.3 Differential Diagnosis

- **Prominent central canal:**
  - This refers to a slightly expanded central canal filled with cerebrospinal fluid (CSF) without any spinal cord signal abnormality or enhancement.
- Cystic spinal cord neoplasm:
  - The imaging hallmarks are cord signal abnormality, mass effect, contrast enhancement, and associated with neurological symptoms.[1]
- Syringohydromyelia:
  - Cystic dilatation of the central canal that could be isolated or associated with congenital anomalies in up to 30% of cases.[1]
  - The entire spine MRI should be performed to rule out low-lying cerebellar tonsils (Chiari I malformation) as well as low-lying conus with or without fatty filum (tethered cord).
- Myelomalacia:
  - Cord atrophy secondary to previous vascular, traumatic, or other injury.

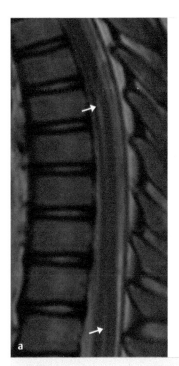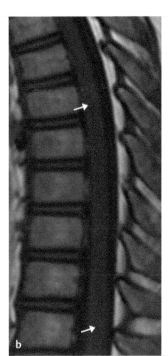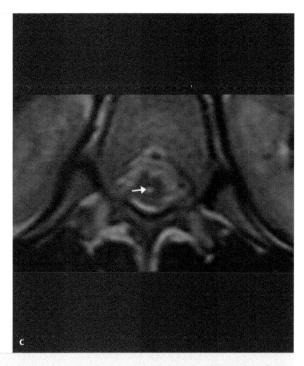

Fig. 31.1 (a–c)

31.4 Diagnostic Pearls

- Prominent central canal:
  - The diameter should be less than 1 to 2 mm, the structure perfectly round on axial images, and located between the ventral one-third and dorsal two-thirds of the spinal cord.
  - The spinal cord should not be expanded.
  - The patient should be asymptomatic without a Chiari malformation or a tethered spinal cord (i.e., low-lying conus with thickened filum).

31.5 Essential Information about Prominent Central Canal

31.5.1 Etiology

- Normal spinal cord development.

31.5.2 Imaging Pitfalls

- Gibbs' truncation artifact: Parallel lines that appear when the interface between high and low signal intensities occurs in the same plane, that is, cord surface–CSF interface mimicking a central canal dilatation.

31.5.3 Follow-up

- If asymptomatic, no imaging follow-up is needed.
- If the patient becomes symptomatic, close inspection of the craniocervical junction and the conus should be performed to exclude Chiari 1 malformation and a tethered spinal cord, respectively.
- If the patient is asymptomatic, the cord is not expanded, is normal in signal, and the fluid-filled canal is perfectly round, measuring less than 2 mm, and located between the ventral one-third and dorsal two-thirds of the spinal cord; no contrast enhancement is necessary.

31.6 Neurosurgery Questions and Answers

1. **Given the presentation and imaging findings, what specific findings on physical examination and/or elements of the history are important in your determination of the diagnosis and, more importantly, in determining whether this probable incidental finding is truly asymptomatic?**
   If the patient is symptomatic and the central canal is noted to be 1 to 2 mm, then this likely represents an incidental finding that does not require further evaluation.[2]

2. **What additional testing, if any, is required or recommended in the workup?**
   Should the patient become symptomatic, they should be evaluated for other known causes of syrinx formation. As part of such a workup, MRI of the entire neuroaxis should be performed and contrast would be necessary.[3]

3. **What is the etiology and natural history of the condition that would assist in decision-making?**
   The central canal is a space that typically decreases in patency with age.[4] A prominent central canal is often incidentally found and is asymptomatic.[4]

4. **If electing to follow, what is the suggested time interval and modality?**
   If the central canal is noted to be 3 mm or larger, then follow-up is appropriate.[2] The patient should be reevaluated at 12 months with repeat MRI to assess for central canal stability. If stability is confirmed and the patient is asymptomatic, then continued follow-up is likely not necessary.[2]

References

[1] Moore K. Ventriculus terminalis. In: Barkovich J, ed. Diagnostic Imaging Pediatric Neuroradiology. Salt Lake City, UT: Amirsys; 2007:III-5–III-2

[2] Jones BV. Cord cystic cavities: syringomyelia and prominent central canal. Semin Ultrasound CT MR. 2017; 38(2):98–104

[3] Timpone VM, Patel SH. MRI of a syrinx: is contrast material always necessary? AJR Am J Roentgenol. 2015; 204(5):1082–1085

[4] Petit-Lacour MC, Lasjaunias P, Iffenecker C, et al. Visibility of the central canal on MRI. Neuroradiology. 2000; 42(10):756–761

32 Low-Lying Conus

Cole T. Lewis, Octavio Arevalo, Rajan P. Patel, and David I. Sandberg

32.1 Case Presentation

A 9-month-old, former 30-week premature male patient, presents with a history of mosaic tetrasomy 22q (cat eye syndrome). No spine-related symptoms or signs were found at physical examination (PE).

32.2 Imaging Analysis

Sagittal short tau inversion recovery (STIR) image of the lumbar spine from a 9-month-old infant (▶ Fig. 32.1). The conus medullaris tip is located at mid L3 level (*arrow*), without any other associated cord, thecal sac, bone, or filum abnormality.

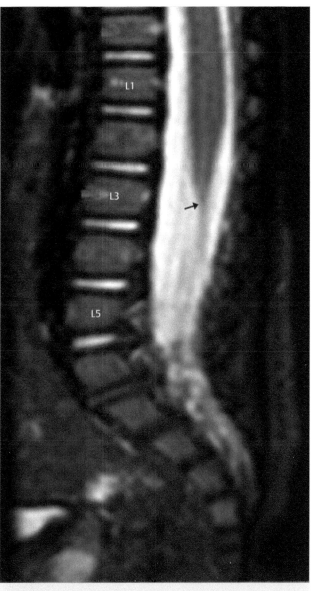

Fig. 32.1

32.3 Differential Diagnosis

- Low-lying conus medullaris:
  - It refers to a low position of a normal-appearing conus medullaris with respect to the vertebral level.
  - It is usually located between the T12–L1 and L1–L2 disk level; however, in 6.4% of population it can be found between the upper and middle third of L2.[1]
- Tethered spinal cord:
  - A low-lying conus medullaris pulled down by a thick filum terminale.
  - The conus medullaris is located at or below the inferior end plate of L2 and is attached to a thickened filum or filum lipoma.
  - In 25% of cases, there is central canal dilatation.[2]
- Open or closed spinal dysraphism:
  - This is a wide spectrum of malformations including spinal lipoma, myelomeningocele, meningocele, dermoid, and dermal sinus tract.

32.4 Imaging Pearls

- Low-lying conus medullaris:
  - The normal conus medullaris does not end below the middle third of the L2 body.[3]
  - There is no abnormality in the thecal sac, roots, or filum terminale.[3,4,5]

32.5 Essential Information about Low-Lying Conus

32.5.1 Etiology

- Failure of the ascent of the conus medullaris with respect to the adjacent vertebral column during fetal and postnatal development.

32.5.2 Imaging Pitfalls

- The termination level of the conus medullaris can be higher or lower in patients with sacralization of the fifth lumbar vertebrae or lumbarization of the sacrum, respectively.[5]

32.5.3 Follow-up

- There is still controversy surrounding the management and surveillance of patients with this finding. Some specialists prefer a conservative follow-up involving neurosurgery, neurology, and urology teams; nevertheless, when associated with lipoma or thickening of the filum, prophylactic filum sectioning might be indicated.

32.6 Neurosurgery Questions and Answers

1. **Given the presentation and imaging findings, what specific findings on PE and/or elements of the history are important in your determination of the diagnosis and, more importantly, in determining whether this probable incidental finding is truly asymptomatic?**

   A low-lying conus medullaris may be an incidental finding. If the patient is asymptomatic and neurologically intact, they may be observed if there is no evidence of a fatty filum terminale.

2. **What additional testing, if any, is required or recommended in the workup?**

   If the patient exhibits any signs of tethered cord syndrome, MRI of the total neuroaxis should be performed to evaluate for the presence of syringohydromyelia or other associated CNS abnormalities. Also, patients should also undergo urodynamic testing for further evaluation.[6]

3. **If electing surgical (or medical) management, then why … and what are the surgical options and risks?**

   If the patient has signs of neurological dysfunction with a fatty filum terminale, then the patient may benefit from surgical sectioning of the fatty filum.[7,8] Surgical intervention is accompanied by standard risks such as infection, bleeding, and anesthetic risk; however, additional risks include damage to the conus medullaris, which could result in bladder/bowel dysfunction, cerebrospinal fluid leaks, and motor/sensory deficits.

References

[1] Demiryürek D, Aydingöz U, Akşit MD, Yener N, Geyik PO. MR imaging determination of the normal level of conus medullaris. Clin Imaging. 2002; 26(6): 375–377

[2] Moore KR. Tethered spinal cord. In: Barkovich J, ed. Diagnostic Imaging Pediatric Neuroradiology. Salt Lake City, UT: Amirsys; 2007:III-6–III-24

[3] Kesler H, Dias MS, Kalapos P. Termination of the normal conus medullaris in children: a whole-spine magnetic resonance imaging study. Neurosurg Focus. 2007; 23(2):E7

[4] DiPietro MA. The conus medullaris: normal US findings throughout childhood. Radiology. 1993; 188(1):149–153

[5] Kershenovich A, Macias OM, Syed F, Davenport C, Moore GJ, Lock JH. Conus medullaris level in vertebral columns with lumbosacral transitional vertebra. Neurosurgery. 2016; 78(1):62–70

[6] Vernet O, Farmer JP, Houle AM, Montes JL. Impact of urodynamic studies on the surgical management of spinal cord tethering. J Neurosurg. 1996; 85(4): 555–559

[7] Usami K, Lallemant P, Roujeau T, et al. Spinal lipoma of the filum terminale: review of 174 consecutive patients. Childs Nerv Syst. 2016; 32(7):1265–1272

[8] Cools MJ, Al-Holou WN, Stetler WR, Jr, et al. Filum terminale lipomas: imaging prevalence, natural history, and conus position. J Neurosurg Pediatr. 2014; 13(5):559–567

33 Incidental Solitary Sclerotic Bone Lesion

Behrang Amini, Susana Calle, Octavio Arevalo, Richard M. Westmark, and Kaye D. Westmark

33.1 Introduction

Detection of a solitary sclerotic bone lesion on CT or plain radiograph often creates a diagnostic dilemma. In this chapter, we will discuss key imaging features that strongly indicate the lesion is benign and those that warn further evaluation is warranted. The differential diagnosis of bone lesions that result in bony sclerosis will be given. Finally, we conclude with a case of an incidentally presenting sclerotic vertebral body lesion.

33.2 Case Presentation

A 30-year-old woman underwent a CT of the pelvis for endometriosis and an incidental lesion was found in the sacrum. Therefore, MRI and bone scan were performed. Physical examination and past medical history were normal and noncontributory respectively.

33.3 Imaging Analysis

MRI of the sacrum: axial T1-weighted (T1w; ▸ Fig. 33.1a) and sagittal short tau inversion recovery (STIR; ▸ Fig. 33.1b), CT scan axial images (c), and bone scintigraphy (d). A T1w/T2-weighted (T2w) hypointense nonexpansile lesion is seen involving the sacrum (*asterisk*). Density measurements on CT scan revealed greater than 1,000 HU throughout the lesion. The lesion shows increased uptake of the tracer in the bone scan (*arrow* in ▸ Fig. 33.1d). This solitary, uniformly high-density lesion with neither edema in the surrounding bone marrow nor extension into the surrounding soft tissue most likely represents a giant bone island. Increased uptake on bone scan has been reported in bone islands, especially giant ones, but warrants imaging follow-up.

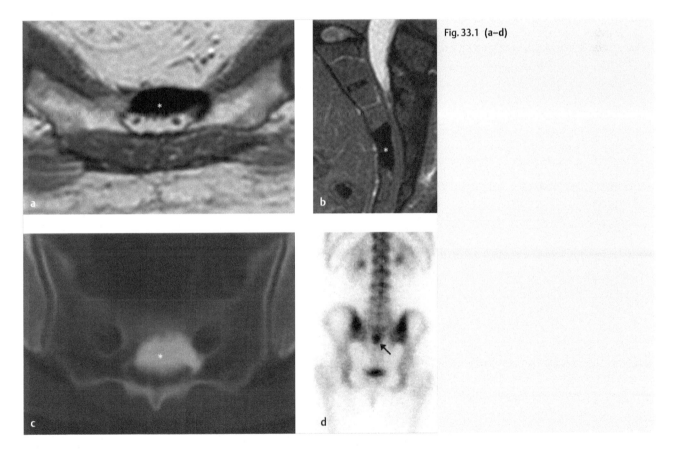

Fig. 33.1 (a–d)

33.4 Clinical Evaluation and Management

In this case, because of the increased uptake on bone scintigraphy, a follow-up MRI was recommended at 6 and 12 months. Even though plain X-ray and CT would typically be used to follow a suspected bone island, MRI was chosen as the follow-up modality because the sacrum is an area not well seen on plain films due to overlying bowel gas and concern regarding radiation dose from multiple CT scans to the pelvis of a 30-year-old woman.

At the 1-year follow-up, the lesion was completely stable and no additional follow-up was recommended in the absence of symptoms.

33.5 Imaging Differential Diagnosis

- **Bone island:**
  - Incidentally discovered, benign lesions also called enostoses, which are islands of cortical bone located in the cancellous bone.
  - Hyperdense oval-shaped lesions with spiculated or "paintbrush" margins, without distortion of the adjacent bony trabeculae.
  - A "cold" bone scan is helpful in distinguishing the bone island from a sclerotic metastasis, whereas a warm bone scan is nondiagnostic. (see diagnostic imaging pearls)
- Osteoblastic metastatic disease (see ▶ Table 33.1):
  - More often multiple with increased uptake on bone scan.
  - Halo of increased signal on T2 W images about the low signal central lesion is suggestive of metastatic disease.
  - Less dense on CT and more heterogeneous than bone islands.
- Sclerosing variant of osteosarcoma:
  - More heterogenous and irregular with bony trabecular destruction and possible extension beyond the confines of the cortex.
  - Edema often present in the surrounding bone marrow.
- Osteoid osteoma:
  - Lucent nidus is present.
  - It favors posterior elements.

Table 33.1 Primary malignancies most likely to have osteoblastic metastases

Prostate cancer (most common)
Breast cancer (usually mixed lytic/sclerotic)
Transitional cell carcinoma
Carcinoid
Medulloblastoma
Neuroblastoma
Colon, gastric cancer
Lymphoma
Treated lytic lesions

- It classically presents with nocturnal pain in young patients, painful scoliosis, and marked relief from NSAIDs (nonsteroidal anti-inflammatory drugs).
- Fibrous dysplasia:
  - Less dense than a bone island.
  - Classic ground glass appearance of the bone.

33.6 Distinguishing a Bone Island from a Solitary Sclerotic Metastasis: Diagnostic Imaging Pearls

- Bone islands do not have edema in the adjacent bone marrow or extension into surrounding soft tissue or adjacent bony destruction.[1]
- The classic bone island has a spiculated or paintbrush border and is much denser on CT than a osteoblastic metastasis. One study, using a mean attenuation of 885 HU and a maximum attenuation of 1,060 HU as cut-off values, distinguished the higher density bone islands from lower density osteoblastic metastases with 95% sensitivity and 96% specificity.[2]
- The primary utility of the bone scan is that if there is no increased uptake, sclerotic metastatic disease is highly unlikely; therefore, the lesion can be considered most likely a bone island and follow-up radiographic imaging obtained.[3]
- Increased uptake on bone scan associated with a solitary sclerotic lesion is atypical and therefore more worrisome, but largely unhelpful as there are many reports of bone islands having increased Tc-99 m hydroxydiphosphonate (HDP) uptake.[4,5,6]
- The bone scan is also helpful to look for additional sites of increased uptake that may not have been imaged, such as multiple nontraumatic rib, calvarial, or long bone lesions, which would strongly suggest the diagnosis of metastatic disease.
- In the cases in which the solitary sclerotic lesion has increased, uptake on bone scan, follow-up CT, or plain film imaging is recommended at 3-, 6-, and 12-month intervals.[5] Biopsy should be considered in atypical cases or in high-risk patients with primary malignancies associated with osteoblastic metastatic disease.[5]
- In the cases with no known primary malignancy that are being followed with serial imaging, if the lesion increases in diameter by greater than 25% at 6 months or less, or greater than 50% at 12 months, open biopsy has been recommended by Brien et al.[4]
- Although usually stable in size, bone islands may increase or decrease in size or disappear. Growth has been demonstrated well after skeletal maturity.[7]

33.7 Clinical Pearls

- Prostate cancer is the most common malignancy to present with purely sclerotic metastases to the axial skeleton.
- In patients with known prostate cancer, a prostate-specific antigen (PSA) less than 10 ng/mL has been reported to have a 99% negative predictive value for positive bone scan.[8]
- American College of Radiology (ACR) advisory committee recommends a bone scan for patients whose PSA is ≥ 20 ng/mL or with a poorly differentiated primary tumor that may not have an elevation in PSA (ACR appropriateness Criteria, 2012).

33.8 Essential Information about Bone Islands

- Bone islands are seen in around 1% of spinal x-rays and 14% of cadaveric examinations.[9,10]
- CT/X-ray appearance: Hyperdense oval-shaped lesions with spiculated or "paintbrush" margins, without distortion of the adjacent bony trabeculae, are considered characteristic.
- MR appearance: Low signal intensity on all sequences, without enhancement or bone marrow edema.
- Giant bone island: The term originally used by Smith in 1973 that was later defined as equal to or greater than 2 cm in diameter, excluding peripheral spiculation.[4,11,12]
- Osteopoikilosis is an inherited condition in which multiple bone islands are present. Lesions should be cold on bone scan and appear typical of bone islands with parallel orientation to the long axis of the bone, show symmetric size and periarticular clustering, and largely spare the axial skeleton. This is in contrast to sclerotic metastatic disease that often involves the axial skeleton and seldom affects the epiphyses.

33.9 Companion Cases

33.9.1 Case 1: Typical Bone Island on CT and MRI

Imaging Findings

There is a spiculated hyperdense lesion (*arrow* in ▶ Fig. 33.2a) in the upper anterior corner of the L4 vertebral body whose average density is 1,058 HU. This lesion is hypointense on all MRI sequences (*arrows* in ▶ Fig. 33.2b-d). This lesion has the classic appearance of a bone island.

Given the classic appearance on CT and confirmatory high density, as well as the benign appearance on MRI with no evidence of a "halo" on T2W image, the diagnosis of bone island was made and no imaging follow-up was performed.

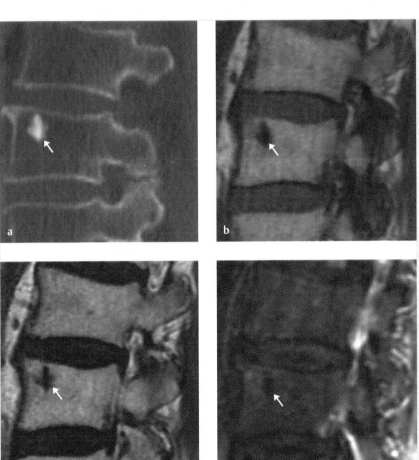

Fig. 33.2 CT sagittal reformation **(a)** and MR images of the lumbar spine, T1-weighted (T1W; **b**), T2-weighted (T2W; **c**), and short tau inversion recovery (STIR; **d**) were performed for back pain.

33.9.2 Case 2: Solitary Prostate Cancer Metastasis

Imaging Findings

A focal area of hypointensity is seen within the superior end plate of T11 (*arrow*). The lesion can be faintly seen on the fat saturated T2-weighted image sequence. An enlarged image confirms the lesion has central hypointensity with a peripheral "halo" of hyperintensity.

Fluorodeoxyglucose (FDG) PET/CT was ordered by the primary care physician.

The lesion within T11 is sclerotic and there is increase uptake of FDG (3.3 standardized uptake value; see *arrow* in ▸ Fig. 33.4a,c). In addition, a focus of abnormal, increased uptake is also seen in the right side of the prostate gland (*arrow* in ▸ Fig. 33.4b). While FDG-PET/CT does offer the advantage of TNM (tumor size, node involvement, and metastasis status) screening at the same time as evaluating unknown bone lesions, it is not typically recommended for sclerotic lesions as its sensitivity is reduced in companion with typical Tc-99 m HDP skeletal scintigraphy.

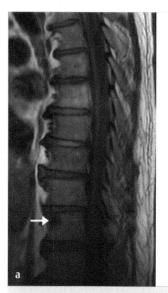 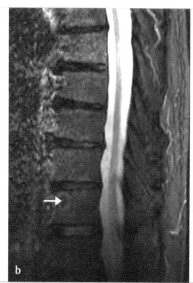 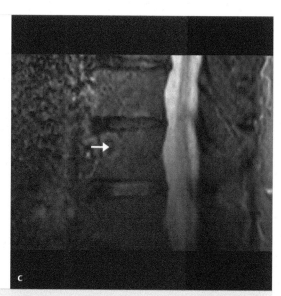

Fig. 33.3 Thoracic spine MRI was performed for mid-back pain. Sagittal T1 W **(a)**, FSE (fast spin echo) T2 W **(b)**, and T2 W images enlarged to show the area of interest at T11 **(c)** are shown.

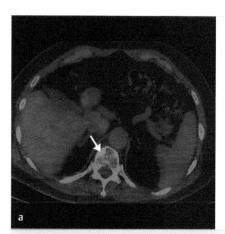 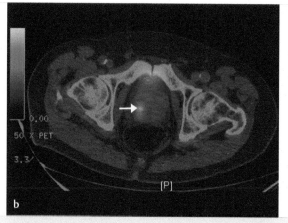 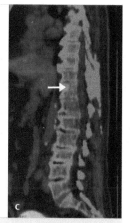

Fig. 33.4 FDG-PET/CT fused axial images at the level of T11 **(a)** and at the level of the prostate **(b)** are shown. A sagittal reformation of the CT fused with PET is also shown **(c)**.

33.9.3 Case 3: Benign Notochordal Cell Tumor

Imaging Findings

A sclerotic lesion is identified within the center of L4. The sclerosis is distinctly different from the coarsened trabecula seen in hemangioma. Even though the possibility of osteoblastic metastatic disease or osteosarcoma was considered, the central location of the lesion and diffuse sclerosis raised the possibility of a chordoma. MRI was performed for further evaluation, which is shown in ▶ Fig. 33.6.

MRI of the lumbar spine, sagittal T1 W (▶ Fig. 33.6a), T2 W (▶ Fig. 33.6b), and T1 W with gadolinium (▶ Fig. 33.6c) reveals a T1 W hypointense, T2 W hyperintense, well-defined, nonenhancing lesion in the posterior and medial aspects of the vertebral body of L4 with no extension into the paravertebral soft tissues. The low signal on the T1 W image is not compatible with a typical hemangioma, intraosseous lipoma, or other benign lesion. The very high signal intensity on T2 W image was unexpected and not compatible with a blastic metastasis or with osteoid-forming primary bone tumor. Primary bone tumors with very high signal on T2 W image are usually of chondroid origin or are typical chordomas. The matrix, diffuse sclerosis rather than rings and arcs, is typical of a chordoma rather than a chondrosarcoma. However, the complete lack of enhancement and no evidence of bony destruction are very atypical of chordoma or other primary bone tumors.

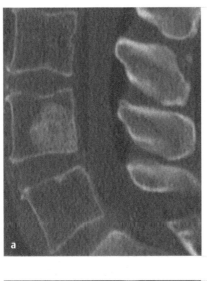
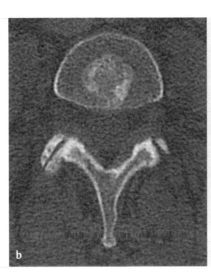

Fig. 33.5 (a, b) CT of lumbar spine without contrast was performed for minor trauma.

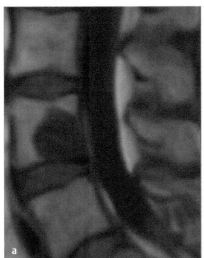
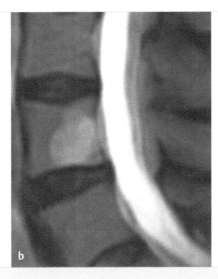
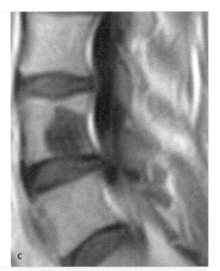

Fig. 33.6 (a–c)

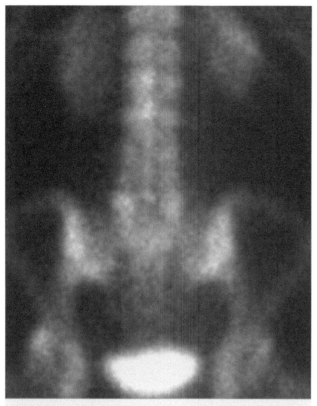

Fig. 33.7

A bone scan was obtained for further evaluation, which is shown in ▶ Fig. 33.7.

The bone scan image shows no increased uptake in the region of the tumor.

Impression

These findings are typical of a benign notochordal cell tumor (BNCT).

Differential Diagnosis

- **Benign notochordal cell tumor:**
  - The relationship between BNCT and chordoma is uncertain although both tumors have been found in the same pathologic specimen.
  - It will have positive immunohistochemistry stain for brachyura, which stains positively for any tumor that is of notochordal cell lineage.
  - It has a well-defined, central location in the vertebral body.
  - It has low signal on T1 W images and high signal on T2 W images.
  - There is no enhancement.
  - There is no increased uptake on bone scan.
  - There is no cortical disruption or extension beyond the confines of the vertebral body.
- Primary malignant bone tumor: chordoma, giant cell tumor, or chondroid malignancy:
  - Enhancement is common.
  - There is cortical and trabecular disruption.

- It commonly extends beyond the confines of the vertebral body (collar-button appearance of chordoma).
  - Chondroid malignancies are also very high in signal on T2 W images, but CT should show rings and arcs of calcification consistent with chondroid matrix rather than diffuse sclerosis.
- Atypical hemangioma:
  - It shows a well-defined, low signal on T1 W images and high signal on T2 W images, but typically enhances and has coarsened trabecula on CT scan although these findings on CT may be more difficult to detect in atypical hemangioma in comparison to typical ones.
- Lymphoma:
  - It is rarely sclerotic and usually has significant enhancement.
- Metastatic disease:
  - Sclerotic metastatic disease could appear similar on CT; however, it should have increased uptake on bone scan.
  - Sclerotic metastases are low in signal on T2 W image and may have a "halo" of increased signal on the T2 W image.[1]
  - It is usually multifocal.

Essential Facts about Benign Notochordal Cell Tumor

- Incidentally detected lesions of the spine.
- Rare, benign tumor of notochordal cell origin.[13,14,15]
- Typically found in the midline of the vertebra near the basivertebral plexus.
- CT/X-ray appearance: BNCT shows mild osteosclerosis (ill defined, high density) without trabecular destruction.
- MRI appearance: Well defined and low in signal on T1 W images but have very high signal on T2 W images. There is no enhancement with gadolinium-based contrast agents (GBCA) or extension beyond the confines of the vertebral body.[14]
- Although controversial in that some surgeons would still recommend biopsy, a number of cases have been followed conservatively with repeat imaging.[15]
- The presence of cortical breakthrough, enhancement, or increased uptake of radio tracer on bone scan is concerning for a chordoma and surgical consultation is necessary.[14,15]

33.10 Key Point Summary

- A solitary sclerotic lesion that has a "spiculated" border, no evidence of a T2-bright halo on MRI, and is extremely dense is most likely a bone island.
- Bone scans may be helpful in that although bone islands may be warm, a cold bone scan virtually excludes osteoblastic metastatic disease.
- Prostate cancer in the male and breast cancer in the female are the most common primary malignancies to result in osteoblastic metastatic disease.
- Benign notochordal cell tumors have a very characteristic appearance. They are usually centered within the vertebral bodies, and most often are slightly sclerotic. They are very well defined, nonenhancing, hyperintense on T2 W and hypointense on T1 W images. Management is controversial due to concern about the relationship with chordoma and difficulty in making a definitive distinction between these two related entities both radiographically and pathologically.

References

[1] Schweitzer ME, Levine C, Mitchell DG, Gannon FH, Gomella LG. Bull's-eyes and halos: useful MR discriminators of osseous metastases. Radiology. 1993; 188(1):249–252

[2] Ulano A, Bredella MA, Burke P, et al. Distinguishing untreated osteoblastic metastases from enostoses using CT attenuation measurements. AJR Am J Roentgenol. 2016; 207(2):362–368

[3] Go RT, El-Khoury GY, Wehbe MA. Radionuclide bone image in growing and stable bone island. Skeletal Radiol. 1980; 5(1):15–18

[4] Brien EW, Mirra JM, Latanza L, Fedenko A, Luck J, Jr. Giant bone island of femur. Case report, literature review, and its distinction from low grade osteosarcoma. Skeletal Radiol. 1995; 24(7):546–550

[5] Hall FM, Goldberg RP, Davies JA, Fainsinger MH. Scintigraphic assessment of bone islands. Radiology. 1980; 135(3):737–742

[6] Roback DL. Tc-99m-MDP bone scintigraphy and "growing" bone islands: a report of two cases. Clin Nucl Med. 1980; 5(3):98–101

[7] Onitsuka H. Roentgenologic aspects of bone islands. Radiology. 1977; 123(3):607–612

[8] Haukaas S, Roervik J, Halvorsen OJ, Foelling M. When is bone scintigraphy necessary in the assessment of newly diagnosed, untreated prostate cancer? Br J Urol. 1997; 79(5):770–776

[9] Resnick D, Nemcek AA, Jr, Haghighi P. Spinal enostoses (bone islands). Radiology. 1983; 147(2):373–376

[10] Murphey MD, Andrews CL, Flemming DJ, Temple HT, Smith WS, Smirniotopoulos JG. From the archives of the AFIP. Primary tumors of the spine: radiologic pathologic correlation. Radiographics. 1996; 16(5):1131–1158

[11] Trombetti A, Noël E. Giant bone islands: a case with 31 years of follow-up. Joint Bone Spine. 2002; 69(1):81–84

[12] Smith J. Giant bone islands. Radiology. 1973; 107(1):35–36

[13] Yamaguchi T, Suzuki S, Ishiiwa H, Shimizu K, Ueda Y. Benign notochordal cell tumors: a comparative histological study of benign notochordal cell tumors, classic chordomas, and notochordal vestiges of fetal intervertebral discs. Am J Surg Pathol. 2004; 28(6):756–761

[14] Nishiguchi T, Mochizuki K, Ohsawa M, et al. Differentiating benign notochordal cell tumors from chordomas: radiographic features on MRI, CT, and tomography. AJR Am J Roentgenol. 2011; 196(3):644–650

[15] Iorgulescu JB, Laufer I, Hameed M, et al. Benign notochordal cell tumors of the spine: natural history of 8 patients with histologically confirmed lesions. Neurosurgery. 2013; 73(3):411–416

Section V

Extraspinal Incidental Findings

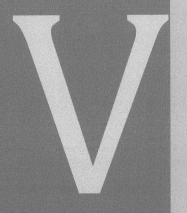

Introduction

Many neuroradiological examinations, particularly MR imaging of the lumbosacral (LS) spine, are likely to detect incidental findings (IFs) because the field of view includes many organs and vessels. Although incidental, as these findings are usually unrelated to the reason for the examination, their detection is extremely important. Quattrocchi et al found IFs present on LS spine MRI in 68.8% of patients. These findings were considered either indeterminate, therefore possibly needing further evaluation, or clinically significant in 17.6%.[1] A recent large, retrospective review of LS spine MRI demonstrated that renal IFs were the most common, followed by those involving the uterus and adnexa.[2]

In this section, we will show examples of important extraspinal findings to increase the radiologist's and clinician's awareness.

We will also give an overview of the management in each case that includes imaging strategies for the situation in which a potentially serious abnormality has been incompletely imaged on the lumbar spine MRI.

References

[1] Quattrocchi CC, Giona A, Di Martino AC, et al. Extra-spinal incidental findings at lumbar spine MRI in the general population: a large cohort study. Insights Imaging. 2013; 4(3):301–308

[2] Tuncel SA, Çaglı B, Tekataş A, Kırıcı MY, Ünlü E, Gençhellaç H. Extraspinal incidental findings on routine MRI of lumbar spine: prevalence and reporting rates in 1278 patients. Korean J Radiol. 2015; 16(4):866–873

34 Abdominal Aortic Aneurysm

Eduardo J. Matta, Steven S. Chua, Kaustubh G. Shiralkar, and Chakradhar R. Thupili

34.1 Case 1

34.1.1 History

A 75-year-old man presented with a 3-month history of left lower extremity L5 radiculopathy. He had a history of chronic mild lower back pain that had been stable for years. Pulses were equal in his lower extremities. An MRI of the lumbar spine without contrast was performed.

34.1.2 Imaging Findings

The noncontrast MRI of the lumbar spine reveals a partially visualized fusiform dilation of the abdominal aorta. On axial images (▶ Fig. 34.1b), it measures 3.4 cm in maximal caliber. On sagittal images (▶ Fig. 34.1a), the craniocaudal extent is approximately 8.0 cm.

34.1.3 Impression

An incidentally detected infrarenal abdominal aortic aneurysm (AAA) measuring 3.4 cm.

34.1.4 Additional Testing Needed and Rationale

Follow-up imaging is essential as AAAs have a risk of rupture that increases with caliber size. Further, AAAs are typically asymptomatic and may continue to enlarge without significant symptoms.[1]

Follow-up imaging time interval: The American College of Radiology (ACR) Incidental Findings Committee II has developed specific recommendations for the imaging follow-up of patients with incidentally detected AAAs.

Modality options for AAA cross-sectional imaging evaluation and follow-up are as follow:

- ACR Incidental Findings Committee II does not specifically endorse a modality for follow-up; however, most other recommendations in the past have relied on ultrasound,[2,3,4] which has near 100% sensitivity and is the least expensive modality.
- CT and MR provide the most detail and are most accurate.
- If there are any suspicious findings on ultrasound or clinical examination, further characterization may be obtained with a more detailed CT angiogram.
- MR angiography may also be considered for more detailed characterization.

34.1.5 Management Decision

In this case, it was recommended to the referring doctor that an abdominal ultrasound to evaluate the infrarenal AAA be performed in 3 years.

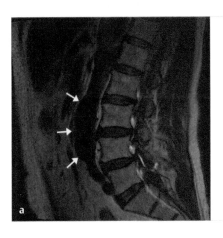 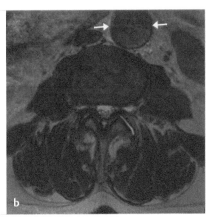

Fig. 34.1 Sagittal **(a)** and axial **(b)** T1-weighted images of the lumbar spine demonstrate a fusiform aneurysm of the infrarenal abdominal aorta (*yellow arrows*).

34.2 Case 2

34.2.1 History

A 59-year-old man presented with mild, chronic lower back pain that had been stable for several years. The pain was worse in the evenings and improved with rest. Physical examination was within normal limits and lower extremity pulses were equal. An MRI of the lumbar spine without contrast was performed. Images are shown below.

34.2.2 Imaging Findings

The noncontrast MRI of the lumbar spine reveals a partially visualized fusiform dilation of the abdominal aorta and the right iliac artery. The localization image (▸ Fig. 34.2a) shows the anterior aspect of the aneurysm better than other images, which have saturation bands that partially obscure the aorta (▸ Fig. 34.2b). On axial images, the aneurysm measures 4.6 cm in maximal caliber. On sagittal images, the craniocaudal extent is approximately 7.5 cm. The right iliac artery is 2.5 cm, also dilated (▸ Fig. 34.2d).

34.2.3 Impression

A large, 4.6-cm infrarenal AAA and 2.5-cm right iliac artery aneurysm with uncertain relationship to the patient's lower back pain. As lower back pain was mild, mechanical in nature, and unchanged in severity for many years, the aneurysm was most likely incidental in nature.

34.2.4 Additional Evaluation Needed and Rationale

Because of the large size, this aneurysm is at a higher risk of rupture, and requires a shorter follow-up (see ▸ Table 34.1). Further, the risk is such that it is prudent to establish a referral with a vascular surgeon, especially with the history of lower back pain.

In addition, this patient also has an incidentally found 2.5-cm right iliac artery aneurysm.

Iliac artery aneurysms are defined as greater than 1.5 times the normal iliac artery diameter or greater than 2.5 cm in diameter.

Follow-up imaging time interval: The ACR Incidental Findings Committee II also has criteria for follow-up of iliac artery aneurysms (▸ Table 34.2).

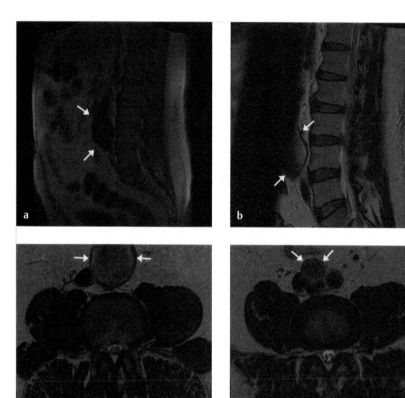

Fig. 34.2 Localization image **(a)**, sagittal T2-weighted image **(b)**, and axial T2-weighted images **(c, d)** of the lumbar spine.

Table 34.1 Abdominal aortic aneurysm: follow-up, expansion rate, and risk of rupture

Aortic diameter	Follow-up interval	Average annual expansion	Absolute lifetime risk of rupture	Comments
2.5–2.9 cm	5 y			May consider surveillance for at-risk patients[a]
3.0–3.4 cm	3 y	0.1–0.4 cm		Caliber of ≥3.0 considered aneurysmal
3.5–3.9 cm	2 y	0.1–0.4 cm		
4.0–4.4 cm	1 y	0.3–0.5 cm		
4.5–4.9 cm	6 mo	0.3–0.5 cm		Consider vascular/endovascular referral
5.0–6.0 cm	3–6 mo	0.3–0.5 cm	20–40%	Consider vascular/endovascular referral
6.0–7.0 cm		0.7–0.8 cm	40–50%	Consider vascular/endovascular referral

Source: Adapted from Khosa et al[2] and Keisler and Carter.[3]

[a]Risk factors include atherosclerosis, cerebrovascular disease, coronary artery disease, first-degree relative with AAA, history of other vascular aneurysms, hypercholesterolemia, hypertension, male sex, obesity, older age, or tobacco use.

Table 34.2 Iliac artery aneurysm follow-up guidelines

Iliac artery diameter (cm)	Follow-up interval
2.5–2.9	Tend to expand slowly; no specific follow-up interval given
3.0–3.5	Initial 6-mo follow-up, then, annual follow-up if unchanged
>3.5	Consider vascular/endovascular therapy

Source: Adapted from Khosa et al.[2]

34.2.5 Management Decision

In this case, at minimum, a follow-up ultrasound should be performed in 6 months and vascular/endovascular referral should also be considered (see ▶ Table 34.1; recommendation for follow-up interval for AAA is based on size). No specific follow-up for the iliac artery aneurysm is suggested, but attention to this may be paid in follow-up examinations for AAA surveillance should the surgeon consider the aneurysm incidental and not elect intervention.

34.3 Differential Diagnosis

The appearance of AAAs is essentially pathognomonic, but some differential considerations of alternative diagnoses and types of aneurysm remain and are listed in ▶ Table 34.3.

34.4 Diagnostic Imaging Pearls and Pitfalls

- An AAA should have a fusiform shape with smooth transition.
- A saccular aneurysm should prompt further investigation into alternative diagnoses, such as pseudoaneurysms or mycotic aneurysms.
- Wall thrombus and peripheral wall calcification may be present. Irregular wall thrombus should prompt close inspection for ulcerated plaque. Similarly, if calcification is present centrally, an aortic dissection should be excluded.
- Erosion of adjacent vertebral bodies may be seen due to sustained pulsation of the dilated aorta.
- Draping of the aorta over the adjacent vertebrae may indicate a contained rupture/pseudoaneurysm.
- Surrounding haziness or stranding of fat planes raises suspicion for infection or rupture.
- A crescent of hyperdensity on noncontrast CT, hyperintensity on T1-weighted image on MR or enhancement on either CT or MR may be seen with dissection or intraluminal hematoma.

Table 34.3 Differential diagnosis of abdominal aortic aneurysm (AAA)

Differential diagnosis	Comments
AAA	This is a true aneurysm, involving all layers of the aortic wall, and defined as dilation of the infrarenal aorta ≥ 3.0 cm, or as aortic dilation 1.5 times the normal diameter[2]
Pseudoaneurysm	This is a false aneurysm. Rather than dilation of layers, there is disruption of some layers with intraluminal blood usually contained by the adventitia or surrounding tissues. These are more commonly saccular and have a high risk of rupture[5]
Mycotic aneurysm	This is also a false aneurysm secondary to aortic wall disruption as a result of infection. Hematogenous spread of endocarditis, osteomyelitis, or psoas abscess may be culprits. As with other false aneurysms, there is a high risk of rupture. They can also more commonly be saccular, have lobulated contours and para-aortic inflammation[5]
Para-aortic fluid collection	Fluid collections surrounding the aorta, including hematoma, may mimic AAAs. Further, hematoma may accompany or be sequela of AAAs or pseudoaneurysms, in which case it may be a medical emergency[6]
Aortic dissection or intramural hematoma	This may be seen in isolation or in conjunction with AAAs, as a dissecting aneurysm. A dissection flap is diagnostic and should be sought for in all AAAs. Blood or hematoma may be seen in the false lumen between the intimal flap and the outer layers.[5] Central, rather than peripheral, calcification may also imply separation of the intimal layer from the aortic wall, as seen with dissection[7]
Para-aortic lymphadenopathy	Para-aortic lymphadenopathy may mimic AAAs when it presents as a conglomerate mass surrounding the aorta, most commonly in the setting of lymphoma. The aorta may be displaced anteriorly. Lobulated contour and soft-tissue appearance distinguish this entity from AAAs. Soft tissue may enhance if a contrast agent is administered[6]
Para-aortic tumor	Similar to para-aortic lymphadenopathy, para-aortic tumors, such as a retroperitoneal sarcoma, may mimic AAAs. As with lymphadenopathy, contour lobulation and soft-tissue appearance/enhancement may distinguish this from AAA[6]
Retroperitoneal fibrosis	Fibrosis surrounding the aorta may mimic AAAs, or para-aortic lymphadenopathy or tumor. In contrast to lymphadenopathy, the aorta is not raised anteriorly. If active inflammation or malignancy is present, high T2 signal intensity is expected, whereas low T2 signal is seen with abatement of inflammation[8]

Table 34.4 Key components of radiologist report

Maximal transaxial diameter

Approximate craniocaudal measurement

Description of craniocaudal extent (where aneurysm begins and ends relative to anatomic structures)

Shape of aneurysm (fusiform vs. saccular)

Involvement of other aortic branches

Complicating features: findings of rupture, dissection, or infection

Recommendations for follow-up as per ▶ Table 34.1

34.5 Essential Additional Information about Abdominal Aortic Aneurysms

- AAAs are most common below the renal arteries extending inferiorly to the aortic bifurcation and may be detected incidentally on lumbar MRI examinations.
- AAAs are defined as greater than 1.5 times the normal aortic diameter or greater than 3.0 cm in diameter.[2]
- Iliac artery aneurysms are defined as greater than 1.5 times the normal iliac artery diameter or greater than 2.5 cm in diameter.
- Aortic aneurysms are most commonly secondary to atherosclerosis and also develop as a result of cystic medial necrosis, vasculitis, infection, and injury.[8]
- Management, either surgical intervention or imaging follow-up, depends on size if incidental or the patient's development of symptoms.
- AAAs are associated with an independent risk of cardiovascular disease.
- AAAs are also associated with an increased risk of developing intracranial aneurysms (IA).[9] Although screening for AAAs in patients with IA has been suggested,[3,10] the opposite has not yet been recommended. That is, the role of screening for IA in patients with AAA has yet to be validated[9] (▶ Table 34.4).

34.6 Key Point Summary

As a general rule, smaller aneurysms should be followed up with imaging surveillance, whereas larger, complicated, or symptomatic ones should be referred for surgical or endovascular evaluation. The ACR Incidental Findings Committee II details specific recommendations for incidental findings of other vascular entities. These are summarized in ▶ Table 34.5.

Table 34.5 Management of incidental abdominal aortic aneurysms (AAAs) and other vascular findings

Incidental finding	Recommendations
AAA	See ▶ Table 34.1
Iliac Artery Aneurysms	See ▶ Table 34.2
Penetrating aortic ulcer	• Asymptomatic: annual follow-up • Symptomatic: consider surgical or endovascular intervention, or more frequent follow-up
Renal artery aneurysms	• 1.0–1.5 cm: follow-up every 1–2 y • >1.5 cm: consider surgical or endovascular therapy
Splenic Artery Aneurysms	• <2 cm: evaluate for risk factors such as rapidly increasing size, occurrence in women of childbearing age, cirrhosis, or symptoms that can be attributable to the aneurysm. Otherwise, yearly follow-up is recommended. Surveillance intervals of >1 y may be reasonable, depending on comorbidities and life expectancy • >2 cm: consider endovascular therapy
Visceral artery aneurysms	• >2 cm: treatment should be recommended • A lower threshold should be considered for nonatherosclerotic aneurysms
Pancreaticoduodenal artery aneurysms	These are felt to be at higher risk for rupture, and all should be considered for treatment

Source: Adapted from Khosa et al.[2]

References

[1] Gouliamos AD, Tsiganis T, Dimakakos P, Vlahos LJ. Screening for abdominal aortic aneurysms during routine lumbar CT scan: modification of the standard technique. Clin Imaging. 2004; 28(5):353–355

[2] Khosa F, Krinsky G, Macari M, Yucel EK, Berland LL. Managing incidental findings on abdominal and pelvic CT and MRI, Part 2: white paper of the ACR Incidental Findings Committee II on vascular findings. J Am Coll Radiol. 2013; 10(10):789–794

[3] Keisler B, Carter C. Abdominal aortic aneurysm. Am Fam Physician. 2015; 91(8):538–543

[4] Chaikof EL, Dalman RL, Eskandari MK, et al. The Society for Vascular Surgery practice guidelines on the care of patients with an abdominal aortic aneurysm. J Vasc Surg. 2018; 67(1):2–77.e2

[5] Anwer B. Interventional radiology. In: Elsayes KM, Oldham SA, eds. Introduction to Diagnostic Radiology. 1st ed. New York, NY: McGraw Hill; 2014: 492–493

[6] Ho SSM. Abdominal vessels. In: Ahuja AT, Griffith JF, Wong KT, et al, eds. Diagnostic Imaging Ultrasound. 1st ed. Manitoba, Canada: Amirsys; 2007:18–24

[7] Federle MP. Vascular disorders. In: Federle MP, Jeffrey RB, Woodward PJ, et al, eds. Diagnostic Imaging: Abdomen. 2nd ed. Manitoba, Canada: Amirsys; 2009:50–52

[8] Roberts D, Siegelman ESMR. Imaging and MR angiography of the aorta. In: Siegelman ES, Adusumilli S, Roberts D, et al., eds. Body MRI. 1st ed. Philadelphia, PA: Elsevier Saunders; 2005:487–494

[9] Rouchaud A, Brandt MD, Rydberg AM, et al. Prevalence of intracranial aneurysms in patients with aortic aneurysms. AJNR Am J Neuroradiol. 2016; 37(9):1664–1668

[10] Ball BZ, Jiang B, Mehndiratta P, et al. Screening individuals with intracranial aneurysms for abdominal aortic aneurysms is cost-effective based on estimated coprevalence. J Vasc Surg. 2016; 64(3):811–818.e3

35 Renal Mass

Steven S. Chua, Chakradhar R. Thupili, Eduardo J. Matta, and Kaustubh G. Shiralkar

35.1 Case 1

A 63-year-old woman presents with lower back and bilateral lower extremity pain. An MRI of the lumbar spine without contrast was performed to evaluate for radiculopathy.

35.1.1 Imaging Impression

An ill-defined right renal mass is incompletely evaluated in this noncontrast lumbar spine MR examination (▶ Fig. 35.1). The appearance is worrisome for malignancy and additional imaging is required.

35.1.2 Diagnostic Testing Needed

Given that an incompletely characterized right renal mass without diagnostic features of a simple cyst is visualized, additional imaging is required and a CT renal mass protocol was subsequently performed with findings compatible with a 6-cm right renal cell carcinoma (RCC) shown in ▶ Fig. 35.2.

35.1.3 Imaging Interpretation

A right expansile 6-cm arterially enhancing renal mass with washout compatible with an RCC.

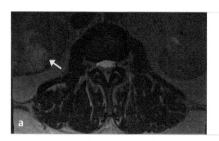
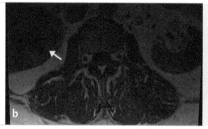

Fig. 35.1 T2-weighted **(a)** and T1-weighted **(b)** axial images of the lumbar spine demonstrate a heterogeneous to hyperintense T2 and a T1 isointense mass within the right kidney, partially seen (*yellow arrow*). The right renal mass is less apparent and more ill defined in the T1-weighted image.

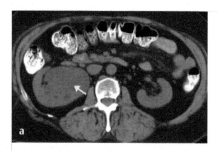
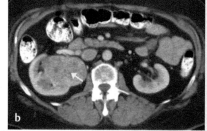
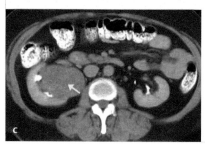
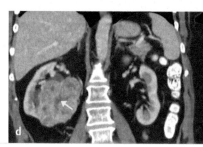

Fig. 35.2 A CT renal mass protocol demonstrates a right renal expansile 6-cm hypodense mass in the axial precontrast **(a)** image, which enhances in the axial **(b)** and coronal **(d)** nephrographic phase, showing mild washout in the axial excretory phase **(c)**, compatible with a renal cell carcinoma (RCC). The *yellow arrows* indicate the right RCC.

35.2 Case 2

An 80-year-old woman presents with back pain after a fall. MRI of the lumbar spine without contrast was performed for evaluation.

35.2.1 Imaging Impression

A left renal mass with high T1 and T2 signal is incompletely evaluated by the noncontrast lumbar spine MRI (▶ Fig. 35.3). As the signal intensity of this mass does not follow that of fluid, and it is incompletely imaged, additional imaging is required.

35.2.2 Additional Testing Needed

The finding of a left renal mass without imaging characteristics of a renal cyst on MRI (well-marginated and homogeneously high in signal on T2 and low in signal on T1 weighted images) requires additional imaging to exclude malignancy. If the lesion was detected on a lumbar spine CT without intravenous contrast, incomplete imaging, heterogeneity, or internal density measurements between 20 and 70 HU, it would require additional imaging. The ACR recommends CT scan with and without intravenous contrast or MRI pre- and postcontrast, especially if the lesion is < 1.5 cm.[1,2,3] Given that the lesion is T1 and T2 hyperintense, there is suggestion of a fat-containing lesion like an angiomyolipoma. If there had been a fat-saturated sequence (frequency selective), the presence of signal loss in the left renal lesion would be compatible with an angiomyolipoma with macroscopic fat. Angiomyolipomas can also contain microscopic fat, and loss of signal in the opposed-phase image in chemical shift MR will confirm that finding.

Unlike microscopic fat-containing RCCs, angiomyolipomas typically do not contain calcifications. Therefore, a fat-containing mass in the kidney without calcifications most likely represent an angiomyolipoma.

Fortunately, a CT with and without contrast was performed about 10 years prior to the MRI and that CT demonstrated a left renal fat-containing lesion with macroscopic fat without calcifications, compatible with a macroscopic fat-containing angiomyolipoma. On the other hand, a lesion with macroscopic fat and calcification within the kidney is highly suspicious for a RCC. No further imaging was necessary, given that the lesion was less than 4 cm. However, if that lesion were larger than 4 cm, there is a propensity for bleeding and the blood supply to these lesions are typically embolized, especially if a renal artery aneurysm is greater than 0.5 cm.[3,4]

35.2.3 Imaging Interpretation

Left renal lesion containing macroscopic fat, compatible with a 3.8-cm renal angiomyolipoma.

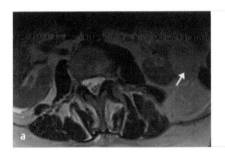
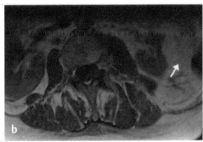

Fig. 35.3 T2-weighted **(a)** and T1-weighted **(b)** axial images of the lumbar spine demonstrate a T1 and T2 hyperintense left renal mass measuring about 3.8 cm.

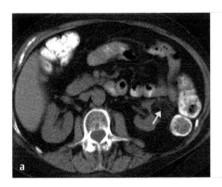
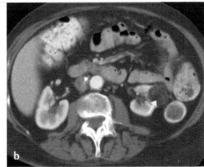

Fig. 35.4 A prior abdomen and pelvis CT performed for abdominal pain showed a macroscopic fat containing left renal lesion measuring about 3.8 cm in the precontrast phase **(a)**, with mild enhancement in the portal venous phase **(b)**. This left renal lesion is compatible with a lipid-rich angiomyolipoma. Given that the mass is less than 4 cm, no further follow-up is necessary.

35.3 Differential Diagnosis

Differential diagnosis (DDx) for lesions of the kidney are presented in ▶ Table 35.1.

Table 35.1 Differential diagnoses (DDx) of renal lesions[5,6]

DDx	Comments
Mass	This term usually refers to a solid lesion in the kidney and can range from primary renal cell carcinoma (RCC), urothelial cancer, lymphoma, and inflammatory myofibroblastic tumors to metastatic disease. Tumors that metastasize to the kidney include melanoma, solid tumors of the breast, lung, and gastrointestinal and genitourinary systems, More benign-appearing lesions of the kidney include angiomyolipomas and oncocytomas. Angiomyolipomas show macroscopic fat, which will demonstrate loss of signal in fat-saturated (frequency-selective) sequences on MR and may also show microscopic fat, which will demonstrate loss of signal in the opposed-phase sequences (chemical shift type II) in MR, and generally do not contain calcifications, unlike microscopic fat-containing RCCs, which can contain calcification. Oncocytomas may show a stellate scar and enhance avidly, with progressive enhancement.
Pseudotumor	Pseudotumors include hypertrophied columns of Bertin, an extension of the cortex into the medulla of the kidney, which enhance similar to renal parenchyma on all phases. In addition, the dromedary bulging from the interpolar region of the left kidney and fetal lobulations are also examples. No further follow-ups are required.
Focal infection	Focal pyelonephritis or intrarenal abscesses are also considerations for renal masses. Typically, if pyelonephritis or intrarenal abscesses were discovered on imaging, a follow-up scan after treatment with a CT abdomen and pelvis with contrast is performed.
Pseudoaneurysm	Pseudoaneurysm of the renal artery or renal vein can have masslike appearance in the kidney especially in noncontrast images. However, on contrast imaging, these lesions follow the enhancement profile of the vessels.
Cyst	This structure is the most common lesion of the kidney. Cysts can range from benign to complex, classified by the Bosniak criteria[7] on CT or MR imaging. Benign cysts can be simple with fluid, contain varying amounts of proteinaceous or hemorrhage components to minimally complex with septations and thin calcifications, to complex with thickened irregular septations with enhancing nodularities to cystic renal cell carcinoma. Please see Table 35.2 for more details.
Renal sinus cyst	This term refers to cysts found in the renal sinus and include parapelvic cyst (cyst extending from the renal parenchyma into the renal hilum) vs. peripelvic cyst (lymphatic cysts extending from the hilum into the renal cortex), and can mimic hydronephrosis. An excretory phase with contrast in the renal collecting systems can show that hydronephrosis is not present with these cysts not opacifying with contrast as they are not connected to the collecting system.
Calyceal diverticulum	A calyceal diverticulum extends from and is connected to the renal collecting system and will opacify with contrast in the excretory phase of a contrast-enhanced CT/MR examination. Frequently, milk of calcium or calcium deposits can be found in this herniated sac.

35.4 Diagnostic Pitfalls and Pearls

- On noncontrast MR imaging of the lumbar spine, portions of the kidneys are frequently best seen in the axial images due to the coned down nature of the MR technique to present a small field of view to evaluate the spine. If localizer images or coronal images are available, the kidneys or presence of renal masses can also be seen. An expanded field of view in the coronal plane in lumbar spine MR may allow better visualization of the kidneys and identification of other incidental findings.[8] The sagittal images are frequently too coned down to allow for evaluation of the kidneys in this configuration.

- Renal lesions with internal attenuation between 20 and 70 HU on noncontrast enhanced CT are considered indeterminate and requires further workup by CT/MR renal mass protocol.[3] Without contrast, it can be very difficult to distinguish between benign (oncocytomas, lipid poor angiomyolipomas, pseudolesions, mildly complex cysts) and malignant entities (solid or cystic RCCs or metastatic lesions).

- The smaller the renal mass (< 1 cm), the greater chance that the lesion is benign (oncocytomas, lipid poor angiomyolipomas) or indolent nonaggressive RCCs.[9,10]

- Clear cell RCCs are the most common subtype, and could be heterogeneous, with nodularity on noncontrast CT and heterogeneous to slightly T2 hyperintense on MRI.[3]

- The papillary subtype can be confused with complex renal cystic lesions or cystic RCCs.[9,11]

- Angiomyolipomas typically display attenuation of < −10 HU on noncontrast CT[12] and possess both macroscopic and microscopic fat and typically do not contain calcifications, unlike microscopic fat-containing RCCs, which only rarely contain macroscopic fat but do possess calcification.[9]

- Lipid-poor angiomyolipomas tend to be hyperdense on noncontrast-enhanced CT and can be hypointense on T2-weighted MR imaging and enhance homogenously.[13]

- Oncocytomas can possess central stellate scar and enhance avidly with washout.

- MR imaging possesses superior soft-tissue contrast and can be a good problem-solving tool with the use of subtraction imaging to assess for enhancement in lesions with intrinsic T1 hyperintensity in noncontrast images. Also, MRI is useful in instances where there is pseudoenhancement on CT due to volume averaging or beam-hardening artifacts.

- CT imaging allows for the detection of calcifications in the solid renal lesions, but is inferior compared to MR imaging to detect for enhancement in these lesions. MR can be utilized in these situations to better access for enhancement.

35.5 Essential Facts about Renal Masses Detected Incidentally on MRI

MR imaging features of renal masses:
- Fluid density cysts (≤ 20 HU) on CT or MR or hyperdense cysts (≥ 70 HU) corresponding to proteinaceous/hemorrhagic cysts require no further follow-up.[14,15] Lesions between 20 and 70 HU on nonenhanced CT merit follow-up by CT/MR renal mass protocol as it is difficult to distinguish between benign

and malignant lesions on the basis of nonenhanced CT.[3,6,16] The smaller the renal mass (< 1 cm), the higher the propensity for it being a benign lesion (oncocytoma or lipid poor angiomyolipoma) or an indolent neoplastic lesion (RCC). The larger the renal lesion, the greater chance of it being a malignant mass (RCC).[9,10]

- Solid RCCs are more aggressive than cystic RCCs, which tend to be more indolent.[9,11,15,17]

- Management of incidentally detected solid renal lesions is based on the 2010 ACR white paper,[11] and with updated criteria from the 2018 ACR white paper[3] using contrast-enhanced CT/MR renal mass protocol, which are documented in ▶ Table 35.2.

- Clear cell subtype of RCC is the most common type and typically demonstrates avid enhancement and washout in the delayed phases. They can be slightly T2 hyperintense on MRI.[3]

- Papillary RCCs do not enhance as avidly as clear cell RCCs. The papillary subtype can be confused with atypical complex renal cysts and cystic RCCs.[9,11]

- Enhancement of a renal lesion on CT is defined as an increase attenuation of > 20 HU compared to noncontrast exam, whereas no enhancement is defined as less than 10 HU increase and indeterminate enhancement is defined as between 11 and 20 HU increase.[3,6]

- Fat-containing RCCs can possess microscopic fat and calcifications and rarely macroscopic fat.

- Angiomyolipomas possess macroscopic fat with attenuation of < −10 HU on noncontrast CT,[12] where loss of signal in the frequency selected fat-saturated sequences is seen, and microscopic fat, where loss of signal in the opposed-phase sequences (chemical shift artifact type II) is detected and typically without calcifications.[9] No further follow-up unless symptomatic, > 4 cm, and with vascular aneurysm > 0.5 cm.[3,4]

- Lipid poor angiomyolipomas can appear hyperdense on noncontrast CT and T2 hypointense on MRI, and demonstrates homogeneous enhancement and can be difficult to differentiate from RCC, where tissue diagnosis may be necessary.[1,13]

- Oncocytomas can present as lesions with stellate scars, which demonstrate avid enhancement with washout. However, the scar is not always present and can be confused with malignant lesions, necessitating tissue diagnosis for a more definite diagnosis.

Key components of radiology report:
- Size of mass.
- T1 and T2 signal intensities of the mass.
- Presence of lymphadenopathy or invasive nature.
- Enhancing characteristics if contrast was given.

Management of incidentally identified renal lesions by MR imaging:
- Well-defined renal cystic lesions up to 20 HU (hypodense cyst) and 70 HU or higher in attenuation (hyperdense cyst) require no further follow-up. T2 hyperintense well-defined cysts with CSF signal and without nodularity or complex septations also require no further follow-up.[3,9,11,13,14]
- Renal lesions with macroscopic fat (-10 HU or less) without calcifications are favored to represent angiomyolipomas.[3,4] If < 4 cm and asymptomatic, no further follow-up. If > 4 cm or symptomatic, prophylactic treatment.

Table 35.2 Management of renal masses as determined by CT/MR renal mass protocol and differential diagnoses as adapted from Silvermann et al[9] and ACR white paper,[11] with updated criteria from ACR white paper[3]

Size of mass	Too small to characterize (TSTC)	<1 cm (very small)	1–4 cm (small)	>4 cm (large)
Probable diagnosis	Renal cell carcinoma, oncocytoma, angiomyolipoma	Renal cell carcinoma, oncocytoma, angiomyolipoma	Renal cell carcinoma, provided scant fat on CT/MR	Renal cell carcinoma, provided scant fat on CT/MR
Differential diagnosis	Lipid poor angiomyolipoma (AML). Oncocytoma. Benign lesions, especially if small or very small lesions	Lipid poor AML. Oncocytoma. Benign lesions, especially if small or very small lesions	Lipid poor AML. Oncocytoma. Benign lesions, especially if small or very small lesions	Lipid poor AML. Oncocytoma
Management	General population: No further workup for benign cystic lesions.[a] If not benign, MR renal mass protocol preferred due to lesion size within 6 months.[b] These TSTC lesions are felt to be indolent neoplastic or insignificant lesions. However, if growth and change in morphology, follow-up MR renal mass protocol until 1 cm.[c] Limited life/comorbidities: MRI surveillance until 1 cm. If growth, follow-up MRI, biopsy, or surgery depending on comorbidities	General population: No further workup for benign cystic lesions.[a] If not benign, MR renal mass protocol preferred due to lesion size at 6–12 months for 5 years.[b] If stable, likely not clinical significant and no further follow-up.[d] If growth and morphology change,[c] refer for management and consider biopsy if lesion is hyperattenuating on CT or hypointense on T2 as this could represent lipid poor AML. Limited life/comorbidities: MRI surveillance until 1 cm. If growth, follow-up MRI, biopsy, or surgery depending on comorbidities	General population: No further workup for benign cyst. If not benign, MR/CT renal mass protocol, surgery or biopsy if lesion is hyperattenuating on CT or hypointense on T2 as this could represent lipid poor AML. AMLs < 4 cm, no workup. Symptomatic AMLs regardless of size, urology consult. AMLs > 4 cm or those with aneurysms > 0.5 cm, prophylactic treatment. Limited life/comorbidities: MR/CT surveillance, biopsy, or surgery based on comorbidities	General population: No further workup for benign cyst. If not benign, surgery or biopsy if lesion is hyperattenuating on CT or T2 hypointense on MRI as this could represent lipid poor AML. AML < 4 cm, no workup. Symptomatic AMLs regardless of size, urology consult. AML > 4 cm or those with aneurysms > 0.5 cm, prophylactic treatment. Limited life/comorbidities: MR/CT surveillance, biopsy or surgery based on comorbidities and life expectancies

[a]If lesion is homogeneous and visually lower attenuation than renal parenchyma on all phases or higher attenuation than nonenhanced parenchyma, it is likely a benign cystic lesion not needing further workup.
[b]MR renal mass protocol is preferred for evaluating small renal lesions < 1.5 cm due to superior contrast enhancement and lack of pseudoenhancement.
[c]Growth is defined as > 4 mm increase/year and morphological change is defined as changes in contour, attenuation, or number of septations.
[d]Stable is defined as < 3 mm growth/year average for 5 years.

- Renal lesions with attenuation between 20 and 70 HU on noncontrast CT and that do not display T2 hyperintensity are indeterminate (solid or complex cystic lesions) on MR and merit further evaluation with contrast CT/MR renal mass protocol and should be managed per ACR white papers.[3,11]
- The smaller the solid renal lesion, the higher chance the lesion is benign and/or indolent neoplastic lesion.[9,10]
- Most renal lesions less than 1 cm are benign or indolent if neoplastic, with low malignant potential. Cystic RCCs are also less aggressive than solid RCCs.[3,9,11,15,17]
- Renal lesions less than 1.5 cm are felt to be benign or indolent malignancies,[18] whereas lesions > 4 cm are 90% malignant.[19]
- The white paper criteria for management of incidentally discovered renal masses (2010) and updated criteria from the 2018 ACR white paper,[3] based on further evaluation on CT/MR renal mass protocol are given in ▶ Table 35.2. This criteria applies to incidental renal lesions found in general population adults >18 years of age without medical or genetic conditions that predispose to renal malignancies.[3]

References

[1] O'Connor SD, Pickhardt PJ, Kim DH, Oliva MR, Silverman SG. Incidental finding of renal masses at unenhanced CT: prevalence and analysis of features for guiding management. AJR Am J Roentgenol. 2011; 197(1):139–145

[2] Pooler BD, Pickhardt PJ, O'Connor SD, Bruce RJ, Patel SR, Nakada SY. Renal cell carcinoma: attenuation values on unenhanced CT. AJR Am J Roentgenol. 2012; 198(5):1115–1120

[3] Herts BR, Silverman SG, Hindman NM, et al. Management of the incidental renal mass on CT: a white paper of the ACR incidental findings committee. J Am Coll Radiol 2018;15(2):264–273

[4] Dickinson M, Ruckle H, Beaghler M, Hadley HR. Renal angiomyolipoma: optimal treatment based on size and symptoms. Clin Nephrol. 1998; 49(5):281–286

[5] Wood CG, III, Stromberg LJ, III, Harmath CB, et al. CT and MR imaging for evaluation of cystic renal lesions and diseases. Radiographics. 2015; 35(1):125–141

[6] Mazzioti S, Cicero G, D'Angelo T, et al. Imaging and management of incidental renal lesions. Hindawi Biomed Res Int. 2017; 2017

[7] Bosniak MA. The current radiological approach to renal cysts. Radiology 1986;158(1):1–10

[8] Maxwell AWP, Keating DP, Nickerson JP. Incidental abdominopelvic findings on expanded field-of-view lumbar spinal MRI: frequency, clinical importance, and concordance in interpretation by neuroimaging and body imaging radiologists. Clin Radiol. 2015; 70(2):161–167

[9] Silverman SG, Israel GM, Herts BR, Richie JP. Management of the incidental renal mass. Radiology. 2008; 249(1):16–31

[10] Frank I, Blute ML, Cheville JC, Lohse CM, Weaver AL, Zincke H. Solid renal tumors: an analysis of pathological features related to tumor size. J Urol 2003;170(6 Pt 1):2217–2220

[11] Berland LL, Silverman SG, Gore RM, et al. Managing incidental findings on abdominal CT: white paper of the ACR incidental findings committee. J Am Coll Radiol. 2010; 7(10):754–773

[12] Simpson E, Patel U. Diagnosis of angiomyolipoma using computed tomography-region of interest < or =−10 HU or 4 adjacent pixels < or =−10 HU are recommended as the diagnostic thresholds. Clin Radiol 2006;61(5):410–416

[13] Silverman SG, Gan YU, Mortele KJ, Tuncali K, Cibas ES. Renal masses in the adult patient: the role of percutaneous biopsy. Radiology 2006;240(1):6–22

[14] Heilbrun ME, Remer EM, Casalino DD, et al. ACR Appropriateness Criteria indeterminate renal mass. J Am Coll Radiol. 2015; 12(4):333–341

[15] Silverman SG, Israel GM, Trinh Q-D. Incompletely characterized incidental renal masses: emerging data support conservative management. Radiology. 2015; 275(1):28–42

[16] Sasaguri K, Takahashi N. CT and MR imaging for solid renal mass characterization. Eur J Radiol. 2018; 99:40–54

[17] Han KR, Janzen NK, McWhorter VC, et al. Cystic renal cell carcinoma: biology and clinical behavior. Urol Oncol 2004;22(5):410–414

[18] Hindman NM. Approach to very small (< 1.5 cm) cystic renal lesions: ignore, observe, or treat? AJR Am J Roentgenol. 2015; 204(6):1182–1189

[19] Umbreit EC, Shimko MS, Childs MA, et al. Metastatic potential of a renal mass according to original tumour size at presentation. BJU Int 2012;109(2): 190–194, discussion 194

36 Renal Cyst

Steven S. Chua, Chakradhar R. Thupili, Kaustubh G. Shiralkar, and Eduardo J. Matta

36.1 Case Presentation

A 71-year-old man presents with lower back pain. An MRI of the lumbar spine without contrast was performed to evaluate for radiculopathy (▶ Fig. 36.1; also see ▶ Table 36.1).

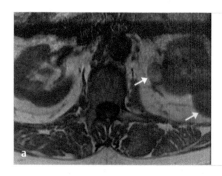 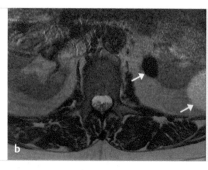

Fig. 36.1 T1-weighted **(a)** and T2-weighted **(b)** axial images of the lumbar spine demonstrate renal cystic lesions at the level of the mid to inferior pole of the left kidney. A slightly T1 intermediate to hyperintense left inferomedial 2-cm renal cyst (*white arrow* in **a**) is T2 hypointense (*white arrow* in **b**) in the left kidney. A T1 hypointense left inferoposterior renal cyst partially seen (*yellow arrow* in **a**) is T2 hyperintense (*yellow arrow* in **b**).

Table 36.1 Differential diagnosis for cystic lesions of the kidney[1]

Differential diagnosis	Comments
Cyst	This structure is the most common lesion of the kidney. Cysts can range from benign to complex, classified by the Bosniak criteria,[2,3,4] by CT or MR. Benign cysts can be simple with fluid, contain varying amounts of proteinaceous or hemorrhage components, to minimally complex with septations and thin calcifications, to complex with thickened irregular septations with enhancing nodularities to cystic renal cell carcinoma
Renal sinus cyst	This term refers to cysts found in the renal sinus and include parapelvic cyst (cyst extending from the renal parenchyma into the renal hilum) vs. peripelvic cyst (lymphatic cysts extending from the hilum into the renal cortex), and can mimic hydronephrosis. An excretory phase with contrast in the renal collecting systems can show that hydronephrosis is not present with these cysts not opacifying with contrast as they are not connected to the collecting system
Calyceal diverticulum	A calyceal diverticulum extends from and is connected to the renal collecting system and will opacify with contrast in the excretory phase of a contrast-enhanced CT/MR examination. Frequently, milk of calcium or calcium deposits can be found in this herniated sac
Mass	This term usually refers to a solid lesion in the kidney and can range from primary renal cell carcinoma (RCC), urothelial cancer, lymphoma, and inflammatory myofibroblastic tumors to metastatic disease. Tumors that metastasize to the kidney include melanoma and solid tumors of the breast, lung, and gastrointestinal and genitourinary systems. More benign-appearing lesions of the kidney include angiomyolipomas and oncocytomas. Angiomyolipomas show macroscopic fat, which will demonstrate loss of signal in fat-saturated sequences and may also show microscopic fat, which will demonstrate loss of signal in the in- and opposed-phase sequences, and generally do not contain calcifications, unlike fat-containing RCCs, which can contain calcification. Oncocytomas may show a stellate scar and enhance avidly
Pseudotumor	Pseudotumors include hypertrophied columns of Bertin, an extension of the cortex into the medulla of the kidney, which enhance similar to renal parenchyma on all phases. In addition, the dromedary bulging from the interpolar region of the left kidney and fetal lobulations are also examples. No further follow-up are required
Focal infection	Focal pyelonephritis or intrarenal abscesses are also considerations for renal masses. Typically, if pyelonephritis or intrarenal abscesses were discovered on imaging, a follow-up scan after treatment with a CT abdomen and pelvis with contrast is performed
Pseudoaneurysm	Pseudoaneurysm of the renal artery or renal vein can have masslike appearance in the kidney especially in noncontrast images. However, on contrast imaging, these lesions follow the enhancement profile of the vessels

36.2 Diagnostic Testing Needed

When renal cysts are identified in lumbar spine MRI without contrast, they may be further evaluated with renal ultrasound, or renal mass protocol CT/MR, depending on their complexity and size. Ideally, if prior imaging is available, comparison can be helpful to determine stability versus changes. Fluid density cysts that are T2 hyperintense and T1 hypointense are most certainly benign and require no further follow-up especially if these are less than 1 cm, and follow fluid signal like cerebrospinal fluid (CSF) on T2 and T1 sequences,[5] have no solid components, and have well-defined borders. Fluid density cysts greater than 1 cm or those lesions that are partially imaged can be evaluated by renal ultrasound. Lesions without fluid signal or lesions on MRI that are greater than 1 cm can be evaluated by CT/MR renal mass protocol.[5,6]

On nonenhanced CT, homogenous lesions with internal attenuation less than 20 HU (simple cyst) or greater than 70 HU (hemorrhagic cysts) are considered benign and require no further follow-up, but if the lesions have internal attenuation of between 20 and 70 HU, they are deemed indeterminate and require further workup.[7,8] Studies have shown that homogeneous renal lesions greater than 70 HU on nonenhanced CT have a greater than 99.9% of being a hemorrhagic cyst than renal cell carcinoma.[9] This is pertinent as renal cysts can be seen on noncontrast CT of the lumbar spine.

Because the patient had a history of treated lung cancer, a PET/CT was performed to evaluate for the presence of residual disease and a CT abdomen and pelvis with contrast was performed for abdominal pain. Typically, PET/CT examinations are not performed to evaluate renal cysts, but in our patient's case, the PET/CT examination was useful because it allowed for comparison of the renal cysts. Therefore, the left renal cysts seen on this MRI study can then be compared to these studies.

Given that the left inferomedial cyst was hyperdense in the noncontrast image (*white arrow* in ▶ Fig. 36.2a) and was T1 hyperintense and T2 hypointense, this structure is most likely a proteinaceous/hemorrhagic cyst and requires no further follow-up. Similarly, the T2 hyperintense and T1 hypointense nonenhancing fluid density inferoposterior cyst is a simple cyst, and requires no further follow-up.

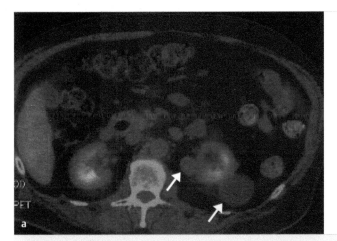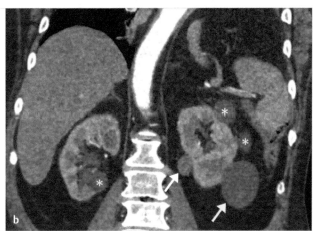

Fig. 36.2 A previous PET/CT fusion axial image of the abdomen **(a)** at the same level as the prior lumbar spine MRI and a recent contrast-enhanced CT image of the abdomen **(b)** demonstrate the presence of a hyperdense cyst in the left kidney (*white arrow* in **a** and **b**), corresponding to the previous T1 hyperintense and T2 hypointense cyst (*white arrow* in ▶ Fig. 36.1a,b) and a hypodense cyst (*yellow arrow* in **a** and **b**) corresponding to the previous T1 hypointense and T2 hyperintense cyst (*yellow arrow* in ▶ Fig. 36.1a,b) in the left kidney. Image **(b)** also demonstrates a few fluid density nonenhancing cysts (marked by *yellow asterisks*) in the bilateral kidneys. None of the left renal cysts demonstrate fluorodeoxyglucose avidity.

36.3 Imaging Diagnosis

Left inferomedial mildly complex cyst is a proteinaceous/hemorrhagic cyst (Bosniak II), and no further follow-up is required. Left inferoposterior nonenhancing cyst is a simple fluid density cyst (Bosniak I), and no further follow-up is required. A few other simple-appearing fluid density cysts bilaterally (Bosniak I) also require no further follow-up. Higher Bosniak classifications, like IIF, III, and IV, require follow-up or surgery, and are also dependent on general population patients versus patients with limited life expectancies.[10,11] Please see ▶ Table 36.2 for more details.

MR imaging features of renal cysts:
- Renal cysts found in the kidney can display varying signal intensities based on their internal composition.
- Renal cysts are classified based on the Bosniak system[2] by CT or MRI and not on noncontrast ultrasound, because enhancement is a critical determinant in stratification. However, with the emerging use of contrast-enhanced ultrasound, an advanced technique that utilizes microbubble contrast injection, which allows depiction of a lesion's enhancement profile without any risk of nephrotoxicity, and with better familiarization of this technique, future classification schemes could include this modality, given that contrast-enhanced ultrasound has been adopted to stratify

Table 36.2 Management Guidelines for Bosniak II–IV lesions based on ACR Appropriateness Criterion[10]

Classification	Imaging characteristics	Management: general	Management: limited
I (simple) Malignant risk: 0%	Thin hairline walls Fluid density (< 20 HU) No solid components No calcifications No septations No enhancement	No follow-up Benign cyst, especially if cyst < 1 cm	No follow-up Benign cyst
II (minimally complex) Malignant risk: 0%	Few thin septa with or without perceptible enhancement Fluid density or hyperdensity < 3 cm (proteinaceous 20–40 HU cyst can appear anechoic on ultrasound; hemorrhagic > 70 HU cyst can show internal debris) and is partially exophytic No solid components Thin or slightly thickened calcifications No enhancement	No follow-up Benign cyst	No follow-up Benign cyst
IIF (mildly complex) Malignant risk: 5%	Multiple thin septa with or without perceptible enhancement Fluid density or hyperdensity > 3 cm (proteinaceous 20–40 HU; hemorrhagic > 70 HU) No solid components Slightly thickened and nodular calcifications No enhancement Cyst occupies most of intrarenal location	Follow-up for 5 years with 6–12 month CT/MR renal mass protocol, then yearly Evaluate for morphologic changes: Septations Enhancing nodularity If changes -> surgery	If changes occur with increased septations or enhancement, should undergo surgery. Follow-up for 5 years with 6–12 month CT/MR renal mass protocol, then yearly Evaluate for morphologic changes: Septations Enhancing nodularity If changes occur with increased septations or enhancement, should undergo surgery or f/u based on life expectancy **Renal cystic lesions that are < 1.5 cm and cannot be defined as simple cysts may not require further assessment based on limited life expectancies or multiple comorbidities**
III (moderately complex) Malignant risk: 50–55%	Thickened septa with measureable enhancement Presence or absence of calcifications	Surgery[a]	Surgery[a] or follow-up[b] for 5 years with 6–12 month CT/MR renal mass protocol, then yearly, based on life expectancy
IV (cystic RCC) Malignant risk: 100%	Thickened septa with measureable enhancement Enhancing soft-tissue component Presence or absence of calcifications	Surgery[a]	Surgery[a] or follow-up[b] for 5 years with 6–12 month CT/MR renal mass protocol, then yearly, based on life expectancy

Source: Adapted from Berland et al.[10]

[a]Open, laparoscopic, or partial nephrectomy can provide tissue diagnosis. Open, laparoscopic, or percutaneous ablation procedures if available can be performed but biopsy needed for tissue diagnosis. Long-term results (5–10 years) of ablation not yet known.

[b]Follow-up is based on life expectancy or comorbidities; study by Smith et al[11] also supported findings that Bosniak IIF and III lesions can be followed up in these individuals.

hepatic lesions under the LI-RADS (Liver Imaging Report and Data System) v2017. Indeed, there have been studies comparing contrast ultrasound to contrast-enhanced CT/MR in classifying renal lesions,[12,13] showing promise in this technology.

- Simple renal cysts with fluid density signal similar to CSF or gallbladder lumen are T2 hyperintense and T1 hypointense, demonstrate no solid components, have well-defined borders, and require no further follow-up.[5] Indeed, a recent study using only T2-weighted images in lumbar spine MR studies suggested that renal T2 hyperintense cysts similar to CSF intensity without internal septations or nodularity may not require follow-up.[14]
- A hemorrhagic/proteinaceous cyst will show intrinsic T1 hyperintensity and T2 hypointensity. MR subtraction images if available can be helpful to assess if a hyperintense cyst seen on the contrast-enhanced MR examination is truly enhancing —an enhancing cyst will remain hyperintense in the subtracted images, while a cyst with intrinsic proteinaceous/hemorrhagic components and is nonenhancing will appear hypointense in the subtracted images. In the absence of enhancement or solid nodularity, these do not require further follow-up.
- Renal cysts can contain internal septations or wall calcifications and may be seen in T2 sequences. However, the presence of internal septations without enhancement does not upgrade a cystic lesion based on the Bosniak system (described below).[2]
- In contrast-enhanced MR images, cysts with enhancing solid nodules are concerning for malignancy. Enhancement is an important determinant for malignancy.[5,16]

Key components of radiology report:
- Size of cyst.
- T1 and T2 signal intensities of the cyst.
- Presence of solid nodularities or septations if present.
- Enhancing characteristics if contrast was given.

36.4 Diagnostic Pitfalls and Pearls

- On MR imaging of the lumbar spine, portions of the kidneys are frequently best seen in the axial images due to the coned down nature of the MR technique to present a small field of view to evaluate the spine. If localizer images or coronal images are available, the kidneys or presence of renal cysts can also be seen. The sagittal images are frequently too coned down to allow for evaluation of the kidneys in this configuration.
- Renal cysts less than 1 cm with fluid density similar to CSF and gallbladder seen on initial noncontrast MRI, display no solid nodularity, and have well-defined borders are simple cysts (Bosniak I) and require no further workup or follow-up.[16] For simple-appearing cysts greater than 1 cm or partially seen on the initial noncontrast MRI, ultrasound can be helpful for further evaluation. Recent results appear to suggest that T2 hyperintensity should be weighted more than size as criteria for follow-up based on retrospective evaluation.[14] However, further prospective studies may be required to ensure application to larger populations, and relying on just the lumbar spine T2 images can be problematic, without T1 images, as the MR techniques, artifacts generated, and the

ability to have the whole renal cyst(s) imaged and evaluated could confound interpretation. Nonetheless, this study shows promise and can help reduce the need for follow-up studies when results can be applied more universally.

- Mildly complex cysts (other than those with fluid density) can display T1 hyperintensity and T2 hypointensity and may represent proteinaceous/hemorrhagic cysts but may also contain small solid components based on initial noncontrast MR imaging. Therefore, these cysts are considered indeterminate and further imaging with CT/MR renal mass protocol can be helpful to exclude malignancy.[5]
- In noncontrast CT lumbar spine images, fluid density cysts (≤ 20 HU) less than 1 cm, or hyperdense hemorrhagic cysts (≥ 70 HU), no further follow-up is necessary.
- In indeterminate cysts that are greater than 1 cm with internal attenuation (between 20 and 70 HU) and that could represent proteinaceous cysts, with possible solid components, further characterization with CT/MR renal mass protocol can be helpful.
- Limitations of CT renal mass protocol include volume averaging if thick slices were used (5 mm), and pseudoenhancement especially for smaller cystic lesions due to volume averaging, which can confound interpretation and thin sections (1.5– 2.5 mm) can be helpful. However, CT is better for characterization of calcifications, which can be seen in RCC. However, for dense calcifications, which may obscure any enhancement or does not permit accurate evaluation of the cyst's internal composition, MR is the preferred modality.
- Limitations of MR renal mass protocol include increased sensitivity of detecting septations within cysts in T2 sequences, which can erroneously be upgraded in the Bosniak system[2] and the sensitivity of MR to motion and breathing.[16] However, MR offers superior soft-tissue contrast if performed optimally, can evaluate the internal components of a lesion better than CT, and does not suffer from pseudoenhancement. Additionally, with the use of properly registered subtraction imaging, intrinsic enhancement can be determined.

36.5 Management of Incidentally Identified Renal Cysts by MR Imaging

- The most common renal lesion is the renal cyst and with the use of increased imaging, more incidental renal lesions are identified. This is especially true with advancing age as more renal lesions are seen in the elderly.
- Most renal lesions less than 1 cm are benign or indolent if neoplastic, with low malignant potential. Cystic RCCs are also less aggressive than solid RCCs.[15]
- Renal lesions less than 1.5 cm are felt to be benign or indolent malignancies and limited data are available to guide the management of these lesions.[15]
- The Bosniak system has been created to manage incidentally identified renal lesions in the general population and in those with limited life comorbidities but not in those already with RCC. The classification of cystic lesions based on the Bosniak system,[2] imaging characteristics, and management as proposed by the ACR Appropriate Criteria and others are summarized in ▶ Table 36.2.[10]

References

[1] Wood CG, III, Stromberg LJ, III, Harmath CB, et al. CT and MR imaging for evaluation of cystic renal lesions and diseases. Radiographics. 2015; 35(1): 125–141

[2] Bosniak MA. The current radiological approach to renal cysts. Radiology. 1986; 158(1):1–10

[3] Bosniak MA. The small (less than or equal to 3.0 cm) renal parenchymal tumor: detection, diagnosis, and controversies. Radiology. 1991; 179(2): 307–317

[4] Bosniak MA, Rofsky NM. Problems in the detection and characterization of small renal masses. Radiology. 1996; 200(1):286–287

[5] Silverman SG, Israel GM, Trinh Q-D. Incompletely characterized incidental renal masses: emerging data support conservative management. Radiology. 2015; 275(1):28–42

[6] Mazzioti S, Cicero G, D'Angelo T, et al. Imaging and management of incidental renal lesions. Hindawi Biomed Res Int. 2017; 2017

[7] O'Connor SD, Pickhardt PJ, Kim DH, Oliva MR, Silverman SG. Incidental finding of renal masses at unenhanced CT: prevalence and analysis of features for guiding management. AJR Am J Roentgenol. 2011; 197(1):139–145

[8] Pooler BD, Pickhardt PJ, O'Connor SD, Bruce RJ, Patel SR, Nakada SY. Renal cell carcinoma: attenuation values on unenhanced CT. AJR Am J Roentgenol. 2012; 198(5):1115–1120

[9] Jonisch AI, Rubinowitz AN, Mutalik PG, Israel GM. Can high-attenuation renal cysts be differentiated from renal cell carcinoma at unenhanced CT? Radiology. 2007; 243(2):445–450

[10] Berland LL, Silverman SG, Gore RM, et al. Managing incidental findings on abdominal CT: white paper of the ACR incidental findings committee. J Am Coll Radiol. 2010; 7(10):754–773

[11] Smith AD, Remer EM, Cox KL, et al. Bosniak category IIF and III cystic renal lesions: outcomes and associations. Radiology. 2012; 262(1):152–160

[12] Quaia E, Bertolotto M, Cioffi V, et al. Comparison of contrast-enhanced sonography with unenhanced sonography and contrast-enhanced CT in the diagnosis of malignancy in complex cystic renal masses. AJR Am J Roentgenol. 2008; 191(4):1239–1249

[13] Graumann O, Osther SS, Karstoft J, Hørlyck A, Osther PJ. Bosniak classification system: a prospective comparison of CT, contrast-enhanced US, and MR for categorizing complex renal cystic masses. Acta Radiol. 2016; 57(11): 1409–1417

[14] Nelson SM, Oettel DJ, Lisanti CJ, Schwope RB, Timpone VM. Incidental renal lesions on lumbar spine MRI: who needs follow-up? AJR Am J Roentgenol. 2019; 212(1):130–134

[15] Hindman NM. Approach to very small (< 1.5 cm) cystic renal lesions: ignore, observe, or treat? AJR Am J Roentgenol. 2015; 204(6):1182–1189

[16] Israel GM, Hindman N, Bosniak MA. Evaluation of cystic renal masses: comparison of CT and MR imaging by using the Bosniak classification system. Radiology. 2004; 231(2):365–371

[17] Herts BR, Silverman SG, Hindman NM, et al. Management of the incidental renal mass on CT: A white paper of the ACR incidental findings committee. J Am Coll Radiol. 2018; 15(21):264–273

37 Thyroid Mass

Steven S. Chua, Eduardo J. Matta, Kaustubh G. Shiralkar, and Chakradhar R. Thupili

37.1 Case 1

A 49-year-old woman presents with left arm weakness. MRI of the cervical spine without contrast was performed to evaluate for possible cervical nerve root compression (▶ Fig. 37.1).

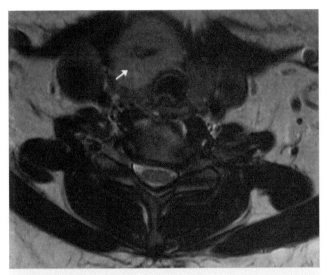

Fig. 37.1 T2-weighted axial image of the cervical spine demonstrates a T2 hyperintense lesion (*yellow arrow*) within the right thyroid lobe, extending through the midline into the isthmus. This lesion measures about 5 cm in maximum dimension.

37.1.1 Imaging Impression

Incidentally detected, 5-cm solid mass in the right lobe of the thyroid gland, which is incompletely imaged on this cervical spine MRI (▶ Fig. 37.2).

37.1.2 Additional Testing Needed: Thyroid Ultrasound

Given that thyroid nodules can have variable signal characteristics depending on their composition and that most MRIs of the cervical spine are not optimized for an accurate diagnosis, thyroid nodules meeting the criteria for size and age based on the ACR Appropriateness Criteria (>1 cm for individuals younger than 35 years and >1.5 cm for individuals older than 35 years without history of thyroid cancer or symptomatic thyroid disease)[1] are often further evaluated by thyroid ultrasound. Please see ▶ Table 37.3 for more details. Thyroid ultrasound can provide a higher resolution method to better evaluate the nodules to determine the need for fine needle aspiration (FNA). The thyroid ultrasound is shown in ▶ Fig. 37.3.

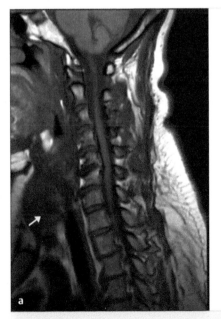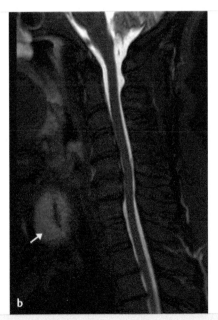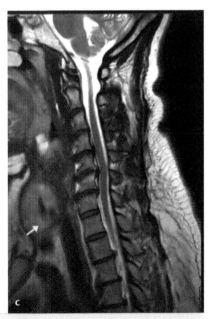

Fig. 37.2 Sagittal images of the cervical spine. The previously visualized right thyroid lesion is again depicted as isointense in the T1-weighted image **(a)**, hyperintense in the short tau inversion recovery (STIR) image **(b)**, and hyperintense in the T2 image **(c)**.

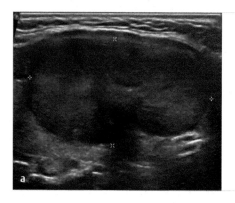 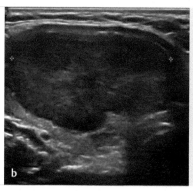

Fig. 37.3 Gray scale images of the right thyroid lobe were obtained in the longitudinal **(a)** and transverse **(b)** planes and demonstrated a 4.6 × 2.4 × 4 cm solid-appearing, hypoechoic, slightly lobulated nodule without significant internal punctate echogenic foci, wider-than-tall nodule, corresponding to the nodule seen on the prior MRI of the cervical spine.

Table 37.1 TI-RADS v2017 scoring criteria and imaging attributes and points (pts)

Composition	Echogenicity	Shape	Margin	Echogenic foci
Cystic (0 pts)	Anechoic (0 pts)	Wider than tall (0 pts)	Smooth (0 pts)	None (0 pts)
Spongiform (0 pts)	Hyperechoic (1 pt)	Taller than tall (0 pts)	Ill-defined (0 pts)	Comet-tail (0 pts)
Mixed (1 pt)	Isoechoic (1 pt)		Lobulated (2 pts)	Macrocalcification/coarse (1 pt)
Solid (2 pts)	Hypoechoic (2 pts)		Extrathyroidal (3 pts)	Peripheral/rim calcifications (2 pts)
Cannot determine (2 pts)	Very hypoechoic (3 pts)		Cannot determine (1 pt)	Punctate/microcalcification (3 pts)
	Cannot determine (1 pt)			

Source: Adapted from Tessler et al.[2]

Note: Nodule characteristics are evaluated based on five imaging attributes of composition, echogenicity, shape, margin, and echogenic foci based on the TI-RADS v2017 criteria.

37.1.3 Imaging Interpretation

Incidentally detected 4.6-cm thyroid mass is solid, hypoechoic without internal echogenic foci, wider than tall, and fairly well marginated with a slightly lobulated contour.

Based on TI-RADS v2017 criteria,[2] the thyroid nodule scores a total of 6 points and is considered moderately suspicious, meeting the criteria for FNA.

The TI-RADS (Thyroid Imaging Reporting and Data System) v2017[2] grades nodules based on five criteria: nodule composition, nodule border, nodule shape, presence of echogenic foci, and nodule echogenicity; it also assigns points and stratifies nodules to benign (0 points), not suspicious (1–2 points), mildly suspicious (3 points), moderately suspicious (4–6 points), and highly suspicious (≥ 7 points). Please see ▶ Table 37.1 for more details.

Management: ultrasound-guided FNA.

FNA results: adenomatous nodule without malignant features.

37.2 Case 2

A 73-year-old man with back pain. MRI of the entire spine was ordered for evaluation (▶ Fig. 37.4).

37.2.1 Imaging Impression

Incidentally detected 4-cm, solid thyroid isthmus mass and left cervical lymphadenopathy are worrisome for thyroid malignancy with metastatic disease.

37.2.2 Additional Testing Needed

A thyroid ultrasound is the next appropriate examination as it will allow better characterization of the mass and assist with possible FNA.

Thyroid ultrasound is shown below in ▶ Fig. 37.5.

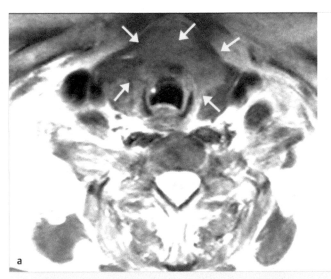
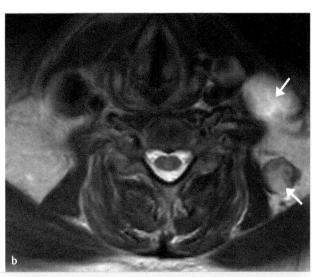

Fig. 37.4 T2-weighted axial image of the spine demonstrates irregular T2 intermediate thyroid isthmus mass, measuring about 4 cm with bulging borders, worrisome for malignancy (*yellow arrows* in **a**). Axial T2-weighted image of the cervical spine at the level of the vocal cords (**b**) demonstrates enlarged intermediate to hyperintense left supraclavicular lymph nodes (*white arrows*).

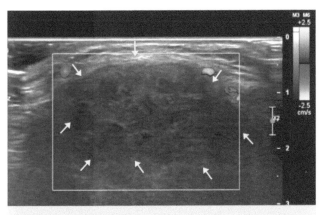

Fig. 37.5 Transverse image of a solid-appearing hypoechoic isthmus nodule measuring about 4 cm demonstrates mild extrathyroidal extension without significant punctate echogenic foci, and is wider than tall.

Table 37.2 Differential diagnosis (DDx) of thyroid lesions

DDx	Comments
Nodule	This is the most common lesion of the thyroid gland. Nodules can have variable signal on MRI, depending on the composition of the nodule. A nodule can be cystic, mixed solid-cystic, or solid. Solid nodules can enhance. Nodules can be benign or malignant
Mass	This usually refers to a solid lesion in the thyroid gland, which can manifest as solid nodules (primary thyroid cancer) or metastases (rare), and have variable signal on MRI depending on the composition. Most common thyroid cancer is papillary thyroid cancer, with microcalcifications (psammoma bodies) and follicular thyroid cancer. Medullary thyroid cancer can have coarse calcifications. Anaplastic thyroid cancer is rare. Metastases to the thyroid gland can come from head and neck cancers, breast, lung, GI tract, and kidney
Thyroglossal duct cyst	This is a cystic lesion that is usually found in the midline of the neck and extends from the foramen cecum of the tongue toward the thyroid gland and usually elevate upon tongue protrusion. Typically, this cystic lesion can have variable signal on MRI, typically T2 hyperintense, but can be mixed, if infected with debris
Branchial cleft cyst	These are congenital lesions that persist due to incomplete involution of the branchial cleft structures and are usually located in the lateral neck, along the path of the sternocleidomastoid muscle. These lesions can be T2 hyperintense or have variable signal if they contain proteinaceous components or are infected
Dermoid cyst	Usually T1 hyperintense cystic lesion in the subcutaneous tissue, and contains more than one germ layer, typically all three, and can have varying imaging signal characteristics depending on its composition. Frequently, hair, skin, fat, and cartilage can be found

37.2.3 Imaging Impression

This nodule scored a total of 7 points and was considered highly suspicious, and met the criteria for FNA (see ▶ Table 37.1) Features on ultrasound that favor malignancy include solid, very hypoechoic (appearing darker than the strap muscles on ultrasound) to hypoechoic (darker than the thyroid parenchyma), presence of microcalcifications, taller-than-wide configuration in the transverse plane, and irregular and bulging borders. Previously, internal vascularity was also one of the factors that portended malignancy, but is not one of the imaging attributes of the TI-RADS v2017 of the American College of Radiology (ACR) committee.[2]

Management: FNA of the nodule was not performed in this patient as they had multiple bony metastases that were detected on further workup.

An ultrasound-guided biopsy of a rib lesion yielded metastatic papillary thyroid cancer (▶ Table 37.2).

37.3 Diagnostic Pearls and Pitfalls

- Based on MR appearance, it is difficult to ascertain the benignity or malignant potential of a nodule, especially for benign versus intermediate-risk nodules.
- Nodules can show variable signal on MR based on composition and signal sequence utilized.
- MR does not have the resolution of thyroid ultrasound, which allows examination of the nodule's borders, presence of calcifications, and nodule composition to be discerned more accurately and clearly.
- High-grade malignant nodules tend to have bulging and irregular borders, and larger size, and can be suspected on MR and be confirmed by ultrasound.
- Always evaluate for the presence of enlarged or suspicious cervical lymph nodes (> 1.5 cm for jugulodigastric nodes and > 1 cm short axes for other cervical nodes; nodes with calcifications), which can favor malignancy.

37.4 Essential Facts about Thyroid Nodules Detected Incidentally on MRI

MR imaging features of thyroid nodules are as follows:
- Axial and sagittal MR images of the cervical spine are where thyroid nodules can be incidentally identified.
- Thyroid nodules are found within the thyroid gland.
- Nodules can have varying signal based on nodule composition (i.e., cystic, mixed solid and cystic, or solid).
- Nodules can demonstrate varying levels of enhancement.
- Nodules can contain calcifications, better seen on ultrasound or CT, and could show up as areas of signal void if the calcifications are large enough.
- Nodules that are irregular, with bulging borders and extend or invade into the neighboring tissue favor malignancy.

Key components of radiology report are the following:
- Size of the nodule.
- Location of the nodule.
- Signal characteristics of the nodule.
- If the nodule is contained within the thyroid gland or if there is extrathyroidal extension.

Management of incidentally identified nodules by MR imaging is as follows:
- Thyroid nodules are very common in the adult population, with at least 50% of the adult population having one or more nodules, often detected incidentally by MR, CT, PET/CT, or ultrasound.[3]
- Because of selection biases in studies, the range of malignancy of thyroid nodules identified incidentally on MR can range from 0 to 11%.[4]
- However, only less than 7% of all thyroid nodules evaluated on ultrasound are malignant[5] and hence the management of thyroid nodules is often difficult as there is a need to balance

Table 37.3 Criteria for further imaging of incidentally discovered thyroid nodules

Population	Nodule characteristics	Thyroid ultrasound imaging
Limited life	Suspicious or nonsuspicious	No
General < 35 years old	Suspicious	Yes
General < 35 years old	Nonsuspicious, < 1 cm	No
General < 35 years old	Nonsuspicious, > 1 cm	Yes
General > 35 years old	Suspicious	Yes
General > 35 years old	Nonsuspicious, < 1 cm	No
General > 35 years old	Nonsuspicious, > 1 cm	Yes

Source: Adapted from Hoang et al.[1]

between excessive follow-up imaging, FNAs, and surgeries to obtain definitive diagnoses versus missing a small amount of incidental thyroid cancers, which are often papillary thyroid cancer and indolent when small in size.[6]

- The ACR Appropriateness Criteria[1] were thus created to better manage thyroid nodules and are based on the suspicious nature of the thyroid nodules (i.e., abnormal or enlarged cervical nodes; > 1.5 cm for jugulodigastric and > 1 cm for other cervical nodes short axes; calcifications in the nodes), age of the patient (older or younger than 35 years), and size of the nodule incidentally identified on MR imaging. Considerations are also made to the general population versus individuals with limited life expectancies/multicomorbidities and do not apply to patients with increased risk of thyroid cancer, those with thyroid disease, and pediatric patients. These criteria are summarized as follows in ▶ Table 37.2.

References

[1] Hoang JK, Langer JE, Middleton WD, et al. Managing incidental thyroid nodules detected on imaging: white paper of the ACR Incidental Thyroid Findings Committee. J Am Coll Radiol. 2015; 12(2):143–150

[2] Tessler FN, Middleton WD, Grant EG, et al. ACR thyroid imaging, reporting and data system (TI-RADS): White paper of the ACR TI-RADS Committee. J Am Coll Radiol. 2017; 14(5):587–595

[3] Mortensen JD, Woolner LB, Bennett WA. Gross and microscopic findings in clinically normal thyroid glands. J Clin Endocrinol Metab. 1955; 15(10): 1270–1280

[4] Youserm DM, Huang T, Loevner LA, Langlotz CP. Clinical and economic impact of incidental thyroid lesions found with CT and MR. AJNR Am J Neuroradiol. 1997; 18(8):1423–1428

[5] Papini E, Guglielmi R, Bianchini A, et al. Risk of malignancy in nonpalpable thyroid nodules: predictive value of ultrasound and color-Doppler features. J Clin Endocrinol Metab. 2002; 87(5):1941–1946

[6] Bahl M, Sosa JA, Nelson RC, Hobbs HA, Wnuk NM, Hoang JK. Thyroid cancers incidentally detected at imaging in a 10-year period: How many cancers would be missed with use of the recommendations from the Society of Radiologists in Ultrasound? Radiology. 2014; 271:888–894

38 Adrenal Mass

Chakradhar R. Thupili, Steven S. Chua, Kaustubh G. Shiralkar, and Eduardo J. Matta

38.1 Case 1

A 77-year-old woman presents with pain in the thoracic spine and left lower quadrant abdominal pain. MRI of the thoracic spine was performed to evaluate the etiology of back pain (▶ Fig. 38.1).

38.1.1 Imaging Impression

Incidentally detected, right adrenal lesion on MRI, incompletely evaluated, and remains indeterminate.

38.1.2 Additional Testing Needed

A CT adrenal mass protocol consisting of precontrast, enhanced, and delayed phases is needed for complete evaluation of the right adrenal lesion, where the absolute washout of the adrenal lesion can be calculated. Alternatively, chemical shift MR sequences can also be formed to evaluate for the presence of microscopic fat in the adrenal lesion, with signal loss in the opposed-phase images. In our case, the clinician ordered a CT adrenal mass protocol to evaluate the right adrenal lesion (▶ Fig. 38.2).

38.1.3 Imaging Impression

The right adrenal nodule showed an attenuation of 5 HU in the precontrast image, 65 HU in the portal venous phase, and 25 HU in the delayed phase, and has a calculated absolute washout of 66.6%, consistent with a lipid-rich adenoma (please see formula below for absolute washout calculation). Indeed, when an adrenal lesion shows an attenuation of less than 10 HU in the precontrast phase, this finding has a greater than 98% specificity that the lesion is a lipid-rich adrenal adenoma, and in this case, a precontrast image would have been sufficient to diagnose the right adrenal lesion as a lipid-rich adenoma.

However, should an adrenal nodule show an attenuation of greater than 10 HU on the precontrast phase, the lesion is considered indeterminate, as there is overlap between a lipid-poor adenoma (about 30% of all adenomas) with other more sinister adrenal lesions like malignancy, metastases, and pheochromocytomas. In such an instance, a CT adrenal mass protocol is then performed, which consists of a precontrast, 1-minute (post) postcontrast, and 15-minute delayed (delay) phase used to ascertain if that adrenal lesion demonstrates washout kinetics characteristic of an adenoma. Adrenal washout can either be calculated as absolute percentage washout (APW) or as relative percentage washout (RPW) if only enhanced and delayed CT images are available. The formulas for absolute washout (APW) and relative washout (RPW) are as follows:

$$\text{Absolute washout} = \frac{\text{Post} - \text{Delayed}}{\text{Post} - \text{Pre}} \times 100\%$$

$$\text{Relative washout} = \frac{\text{Post} - \text{Delayed}}{\text{Post}} \times 100\%$$

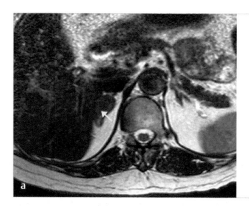
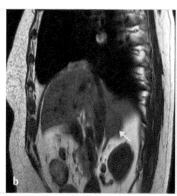

Fig. 38.1 Axial T2-weighted **(a)** and sagittal T2-weighted **(b)** images show the right adrenal nodule (*yellow arrow*) with intermediate signal intensity.

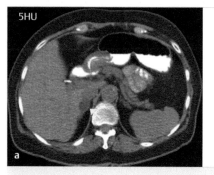
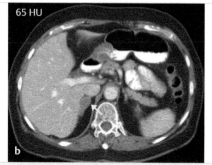
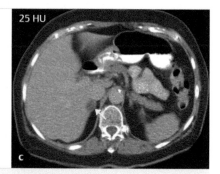

Fig. 38.2 A CT adrenal mass protocol was performed consisting of a precontrast **(a)**, portal venous **(b)**, and delayed **(c)** phases, which re-demonstrated a right adrenal nodule (*arrows*). The attenuation of the right adrenal nodule was 5 HU in the precontrast phase, 65 HU in the portal venous phase, and 25 HU in the delayed phase, demonstrating an absolute washout of 66.6%, consistent with a lipid-rich adrenal adenoma.

For example, if the absolute washout is greater than 60%, then this classifies the adrenal lesion as a benign adenoma. If the relative washout is greater than 40%, then this classifies the adrenal lesion as a benign adenoma.

Alternatively, a chemical shift MR protocol utilizing T1-weighted in- and opposed-phase imaging can also be performed to look for microscopic fat in the adrenal lesion. A region of interest is selected over the adrenal lesion and the arbitrary attenuation units compared between the in- and opposed-phase images. A loss of signal greater than 20% in the opposed-phase image would indicate the presence of microscopic fat in the adrenal nodule, consistent with a lipid-rich adenoma. In the event that the chemical shift MR method is inconclusive, a CT adrenal mass protocol should be performed to allow better quantification.

Management: No further imaging is required for this adrenal adenoma. As there was no clinical evidence of adrenal hyperfunction, this patient was diagnosed with an incidentally detected, nonfunctioning adrenal adenoma.

38.2 Case 2

A 76-year-old man presents with low back pain extending to the right side. MRI of the lumbar spine was performed to investigate the etiology of patient's back pain (▶ Fig. 38.3).

38.2.1 Imaging Impression

Incidentally identified left adrenal lesion with high T2 signal, suggestive of fluid component but not conclusive.

38.2.2 Additional Testing Needed

A CT abdomen and pelvis with contrast was performed to evaluate the left adrenal lesion (▶ Fig. 38.4).

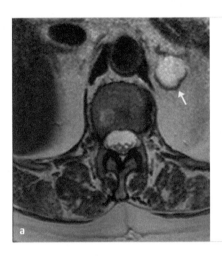
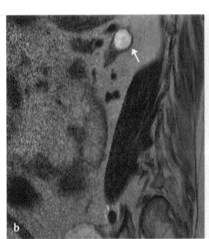

Fig. 38.3 Axial (a) and sagittal (b) T2-weighted images show left adrenal lesion with high T2 signal intensity (*yellow arrow*).

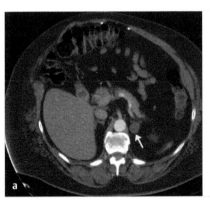
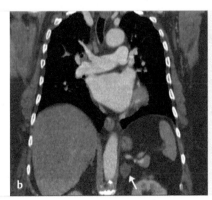

Fig. 38.4 Axial (a) and coronal (b) contrast-enhanced CT images show a nonenhancing left adrenal lesion, with fluid density, consistent with cyst (*yellow arrow*).

38.2.3 Imaging Impression

The finding of an adrenal lesion with high T2 signal is not diagnostic of an adrenal cyst as a pheochromocytoma can also have high T2 signal. However, a CT with contrast demonstrates fluid density and no enhancement of an adrenal lesion is consistent with an adrenal cyst, requiring no further follow-up. In the case of a pheochromocytoma, the patient may be symptomatic, demonstrate high levels of metanephrines in the urine, and on imaging will show enhancement on contrast CT/MR, unlike the lack of enhancement in an adrenal cyst.

Management: Benign adrenal cyst requiring no further follow-up or workup.

38.3 Case 3

A 77-year-old woman presents with paraspinous lumbar pain posttrauma. A noncontrast CT was performed to evaluate etiology of pain (▶ Fig. 38.5).

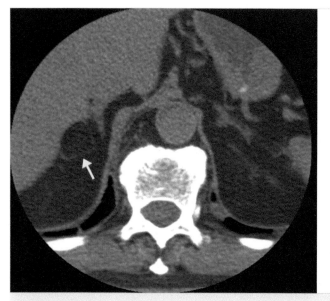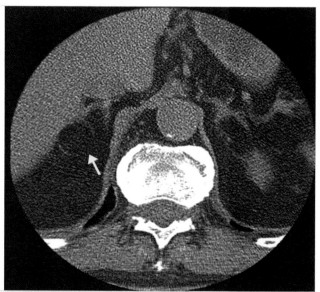

Fig. 38.5 (a, b) Axial noncontrast CT demonstrates a right adrenal lesion with attenuation similar to the adjacent retroperitoneal fat consistent with an adrenal myelolipoma (*yellow arrow*).

Table 38.1 Differential diagnosis (DDx) for adrenal nodules

DDx	Comments
Adenoma	This is the most common incidental lesion of the adrenal gland and represents up to 75% of lesions seen on CT. Adenomas are typically well-defined, round, or oval small lesions that measure less than 3 cm and are often homogeneous in attenuation. Up to 70% contain intracellular or microscopic lipids. A CT attenuation of 10 HU or less has a specificity of 98% for the diagnosis of lipid-rich adenoma. Chemical shift MR imaging can distinguish adenomas by looking for microscopic fat by loss of signal intensity (> 20%) in out-of-phase images in comparison with in-phase images.
Myelolipoma	Myelolipomas are benign adrenal lesions containing macroscopic fat. On CT imaging, macroscopic fat similar in attenuation to the adjacent retroperitoneal fat is seen. On MR imaging, the lesion is bright on both T1- and T2-weighted imaging and hypointense on fat suppression. On T1-weighted opposed-phase images, India ink artifact can be seen at the fat–water interface, but there is no loss of signal in the opposed-phase images.
Cyst	This is a cystic adrenal lesion that has an attenuation between –10 and 20 HU on CT and is hypointense on T1-weighted imaging and hyperintense on T2-weighted imaging. Sometimes thin nonenhancing septations may be present.
Pheochromocytoma	These lesions arise from chromaffin cells and most (90%) of them are benign. On CT imaging, these lesions have soft-tissue attenuation but tend to be hypervascular with intense arterial-phase enhancement. On MR imaging, most pheochromocytomas are hyperintense on T2-weighted imaging and are described as light-bulb bright and demonstrate avid enhancement with contrast administration.
Hemorrhage	Adrenal hemorrhages are asymptomatic, but can present with flank pain. In acute hemorrhage, the appearance depends on time of imaging with an attenuation value ranging from 50 to 90 HU on noncontrast CT. MR appearance of the hemorrhage depends on the age of the blood products.
Malignancy	Malignant adrenal lesions like adrenocortical carcinomas tend to be larger (> 4 cm) at presentation and are heterogeneous with necrosis and irregular margins. Metastases are uncommon as an incidental finding without a known primary malignancy. Metastases to the adrenal glands arise from lung cancer, colorectal cancer, breast, pancreatic, renal cell carcinoma, and melanoma.

38.3.1 Imaging Impression

An incidental macroscopic fat-containing right adrenal lesion consistent with an adrenal myelolipoma was detected. This adrenal lesion would be expected to demonstrate signal loss in the frequency selective fat saturation MR sequences due to the presence of macroscopic fat.

Management: Benign macroscopic fat-containing adrenal myelolipoma. As the lesion measured <4 cm and the patient had no evidence of endocrine dysfunction, no further follow-up or treatment was advised in absence of development of symptoms (▶ Table 38.1).

38.4 Diagnostic Pearls and Pitfalls

- Because of the coned-in images and the type of MR sequences used in many thoracic or lumbar spine MR images, it may not always be possible to confidently characterize an adrenal incidentaloma (AI), and further imaging is often required.
- Adrenal adenomas, the most common adrenal lesion for the most part (> 70%), contain microscopic or intracellular fat and this can be confirmed with chemical shift MR imaging where there is a loss of signal of greater than 20% in the opposed-phase images and on noncontrast CT show an attenuation of < 10 HU with greater than 98% specificity.
- Adrenal lesions that show an attenuation greater than 10 HU in noncontrast CT remain indeterminate as these can be lipid-poor adenomas and other more sinister lesions. A CT adrenal mass protocol needs to be performed to characterize the washout characteristics of this lesion.

- Adrenal lesions that demonstrate greater than 60% absolute washout and greater than 40% relative washout are favored to represent adrenal adenomas.
- An adrenal lesion with high T2 signal on MR imaging may represent a cyst or a possible pheochromocytoma. A noncontrast CT or contrast CT will show the cyst to be of fluid density without enhancement, while a pheochromocytoma will show soft-tissue attenuation and enhance, with delayed washout.
- A large adrenal lesion (generally > 4 cm) with irregular border and heterogeneous enhancement is favored to represent malignancies like adrenocortical carcinoma.
- Though rare, metastases to the adrenal glands do occur and are usually associated with known primary malignancies.

38.5 Essential Facts about Adrenal Incidentalomas Detected on MRI

Incidence of AIs:

- AIs are very common and are usually 1 cm or larger and are typically discovered during imaging studies performed for unrelated reasons excluding malignancy workup.
- Adrenal glands are common sites for primary benign and malignant tumors and metastases. Incidental nodules are seen in approximately 4 to 7% of abdominal CT scans and increase in frequency with increasing patient age.
- Most incidentally discovered adrenal masses are benign and the purpose of the diagnostic imaging is to differentiate benign lesions from those that require follow-up or further treatment.

Table 38.2 Benign and malignant adrenal lesions

Benign adrenal lesions	Malignant adrenal lesions
Adenoma (contains microscopic fat)	Adrenocortical carcinoma (> 4 cm)
Hemorrhage	Metastases
Cyst	Pheochromocytoma (larger ones)
Myelolipoma (contains macroscopic fat)	
Pheochromocytoma (smaller ones)	

- Adrenal lesions that are larger, irregular, contain necrosis, and demonstrate interval growth favor malignancy. ▶ Table 38.2 denotes benign versus malignant adrenal lesions.

Imaging features of adrenal incidentalomas:
- Suspicious features for malignancy include large size (> 4 cm), interval growth, heterogeneity, irregular margins, and necrosis (i.e., adrenocortical carcinomas, large pheochromocytomas, and metastases).
- CT can differentiate most adenomas from nonadenomas using the APW or RPW as adenomas tend to enhance earlier and stronger and also wash out earlier and to a greater degree than nonadenomas.
- An adrenal lesion that displays less than 10 HU and is homogenous on a nonenhanced CT has a greater than 98% specificity of being a lipid-rich adenoma (about 70% contain microscopic fat), and requires no further follow-up. On chemical shift MR imaging, an adenoma will show greater than 20% signal loss in the opposed-phase image when compared to the in-phase image, indicating the presence of microscopic fat.
- An adrenal lesion with greater than 10 HU can be a lipid-poor adenoma (30% of adenomas) or other nonadenomas like pheochromocytoma, metastases, or adrenocortical carcinoma.
- An adrenal lesion that demonstrates greater than 60% absolute washout and greater than 40% relative washout is a lipid-poor adrenal adenoma.

- Lesions that demonstrate less than 60% absolute washout or less than 40% relative washout are indeterminate and further endocrinology workup is needed.
- Adrenal lesion with large amount of macroscopic fat is diagnostic of an adrenal myelolipoma, and on nonenhanced CT, the attenuation should be ≤ 10 HU and on MR fat-saturated sequences, there will be signal loss.
- Adrenal cysts (rare) and pseudocysts (uncommon) are of fluid density (0–20 HU) on CT and T2 hyperintense on MR and these lesions do not enhance.
- Adrenal hemorrhage tends to have higher attenuation on CT, and a prior history of trauma or anticoagulation can be helpful information. MR imaging has variable signal intensities on T1- and T2-weighted imaging and do not enhance.
- If a lesion cannot be diagnosed as one of the above benign entities, pheochromocytoma, adrenal cortical carcinoma, and metastasis should be excluded and a history of malignancy should be sought.
- On imaging, pheochromocytomas have a variable appearance but tend to be hypervascular, with avid arterial-phase enhancement. On MR, these lesions can demonstrate T2 hyperintensity.
- Adrenocortical carcinomas tend to be large, usually measuring greater than 4 cm. In addition, tumor margins tend to be irregular, and central necrosis and hemorrhage are common, particularly when the tumor is larger than 6 cm.
- Metastases can be variable in appearance.

Key components of radiology report:
- Size of the adrenal nodule.
- Location of the nodule.
- Signal characteristics of the nodule.
- If further workup is required for the nodule.

In 2010, the ACR published a white paper, which included a flow chart on the management of incidental adrenal nodule findings that is summarized and shown in ▶ Fig. 38.6.

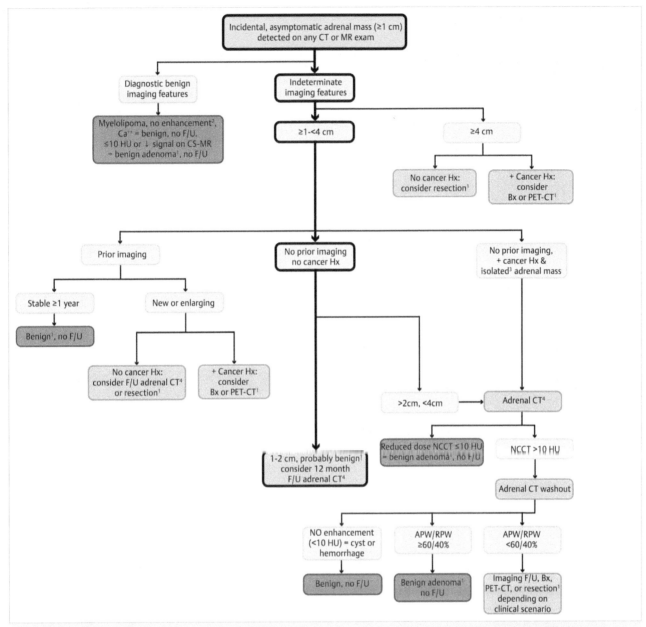

Fig. 38.6 Management and imaging features of adrenal incidentalomas.[0] (Reproduced with permission from the American College of Radiology: Mayo-Smith WW, Song JH, Boland GL, et al. Management of incidental adrenal masses: A white paper of the ACR incidental findings committee. J Am Coll Radiol 2017;14(8):1038–1044.)

38.6 Key Point Summary

- Incidentally detect adrenal lesions do not always represent metastatic disease.
- There are many benign adrenal lesions that require no further follow-up:
  - Adenoma.
  - Cyst.
  - Myelolipoma.
  - Hemorrhage.
- Indeterminate lesions (1–4 cm) are managed based on the presence of prior imaging, stability, and history of cancer, and these details are shown in ► Fig. 38.6 and also briefly described below.
- Prior imaging available:
  - If lesions have been stable for more than 1 year, these are favored to be benign and no further follow-up is required.
  - If lesions are new or enlarging, then they are resected if there is no cancer history and biopsied or undergo PET/CT for further evaluation if there is cancer history.
- No prior imaging available:
  - If lesions are 1–2 cm, and there is no cancer history, these lesions are probably benign and follow-up imaging in 1 year to document stability is performed.
  - If lesions are 2 to 4 cm, and there is no cancer history, a CT adrenal mass protocol is performed to ascertain if they could be adenomas, at which point no further follow-up is needed. However, if they are not adenomas, then biopsy, resection, or PET/CT imaging can be performed depending on the clinical scenario.
  - If isolated adrenal lesion is found and there is cancer history and no prior imaging, a CT adrenal mass protocol is performed. If the lesion is an adenoma, no further follow-up is required. If not an adenoma, resection, biopsy, or further PET/CT imaging is performed as warranted.
- Indeterminate lesions (>4 cm) can be resected if there is no cancer history or biopsied or undergo PET/CT for further evaluation.

Suggested Readings

Allen BC, Francis IR. Adrenal imaging and intervention. Radiol Clin North Am. 2015; 53(5):1021–1035

Kapoor A, Morris T, Rebello R. Guidelines for the management of the incidentally discovered adrenal mass. Can Urol Assoc J. 2011; 5(4):241–247

Mayo-Smith WW, Song JH, Boland GL, et al. Management of incidental adrenal masses: a white paper of the ACR Incidental Findings Committee. J Am Coll Radiol. 2017; 14(8):1038–1044

Willatt J, Chong S, Ruma JA, Kuriakose J. Incidental adrenal nodules and masses: the imaging approach. Int J Endocrinol. 2015; 2015:410185

39 Retroperitoneal Lymph Nodes

Kaustubh G. Shiralkar, Eduardo J. Matta, Steven S. Chua, and Chakradhar R. Thupili

39.1 Case 1

39.1.1 History

A 67-year-old woman presents with chronic back pain. MRI of the sacrum with and without intravenous (IV) contrast was performed to evaluate for possible nerve root compression (▶ Fig. 39.1).

39.1.2 Most Likely Imaging Diagnosis for Case 1

Case 1 demonstrates enlarged iliac chain lymph nodes incidentally detected at sacral MRI. Review of the patient's prior CT demonstrates that these nodes have been stable (▶ Fig. 39.2). Given the stability over 1 year, this is considered a benign finding and no further follow-up is required.

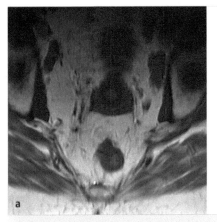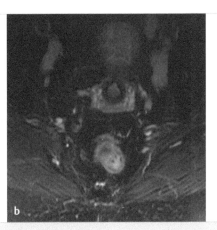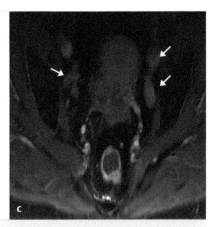

Fig. 39.1 T1-weighted nonfat saturation **(a)**, T2-weighted fat saturation **(b)**, and postcontrast T1-weighted fat saturation **(c)** axial images demonstrate bilateral enlarged lymph nodes within the iliac chain (arrows). These nodes are enlarged measuring up to 2 cm in short-axis diameter. There is homogeneous enhancement without evidence of necrosis.

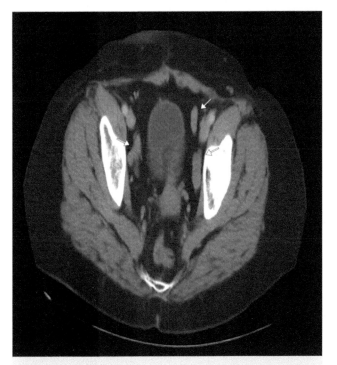

Fig. 39.2 Axial CT images approximately a year earlier showed stable size of the lymph nodes (arrows). There was no history of malignancy or other condition that might cause the lymph node enlargement.

39.2 Case 2

39.2.1 History

A 67-year-old man presents with worsening back pain and known history of lung cancer.

39.2.2 Most Likely Imaging Diagnosis for Case 2

Case 2 demonstrates retroperitoneal adenopathy in the setting of disseminated metastatic disease.

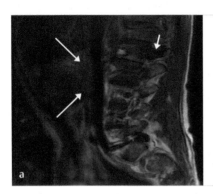 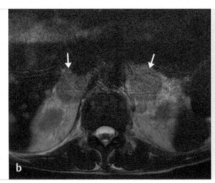

Fig. 39.3 T2-weighted sagittal image **(a)** demonstrates enlarged para-aortic lymph nodes only seen on sagittal images (*long arrows*). Also note the bone metastasis in the T12 pedicle (*short arrow*). Axial T2-weighted image **(b)** demonstrates bilateral adrenal masses (*arrows*) in keeping with the patient's known metastatic disease.

Differential diagnosis and imaging pitfalls	Comments
Metastatic disease/lymphoma	Lymphoma is often symmetric and will displace adjacent vascular structures (aorta, inferior vena cava [IVC]). Metastases tend to be more asymmetric and heterogeneous and there may be a known history of primary malignancy
Sarcoma	Liposarcoma is the most common sarcoma in the retroperitoneum. Look for areas of fat signal or fat attenuation within the large retroperitoneal mass
Retroperitoneal hemorrhage	May be due to underlying coagulopathy or ruptured aortic aneurysm High-attenuation fluid dissects along the fascial planes
IVC duplication/anomalies or collateral vessels	Tubular in shape like a vessel; flow voids or venous enhancement pattern may be visible
Retroperitoneal fibrosis	Ill-defined mass or soft-tissue thickening encasing lower aorta, IVC, and ureters without displacement or mass effect. However, it often causes medial ureteral deviation and obstruction

39.3 Differential Considerations and Diagnostic Checklist

- Ascertain whether the finding in question is truly an enlarged lymph node and/or abnormal.
- Confirm that the lesion is not arising from another retroperitoneal organ such as the kidney, adrenals, or pancreas. In these instances, it may be helpful to look for mass effect on an adjacent retroperitoneal structure like the aorta or IVC.
- Lymphoma classically displaces vascular structures such as the IVC and aorta anteriorly and rarely obstructs the ureters. In contrast, retroperitoneal fibrosis encases vascular structures without mass effect and often causes ureteral obstruction.
- It is critical to check multiple planes and use multiplanar reformats as the abnormality may be only seen on one or two planes (i.e., localizer sequence or sagittal on MR spine).
- Normal structures can simulate lymph node enlargement. Common pitfalls include the following:
  - Small bowel loops in close proximity to the retroperitoneum can mimic nodal disease.
  - Normal, prominent ovaries can simulate external iliac nodal enlargement.
  - Aberrant vessels can be mistaken for lymphadenopathy especially on noncontrast imaging. Normal anatomic variants such as a left-sided IVC or duplicated IVC may simulate nodal disease. Prominent cistern chyli can also simulate retrocrural nodal enlargement.
  - Postoperative hematomas, abscesses, and lymphoceles can all simulate nodal disease.

39.4 Additional Essential Information Regarding Incidentally Detected "Lymphadenopathy"

39.4.1 Definitions and Key Facts

- Lymphadenopathy refers to any pathology of lymph nodes and not necessarily just an increase in nodal size.
- Lymphadenopathy can include abnormal number of nodes or derangement of internal architecture (e.g., cystic or necrotic nodes).
- Increased size and/or abnormal internal architecture of lymph nodes does not necessarily imply neoplastic disease. Lymphadenopathy may represent various infectious, inflammatory, autoimmune, or idiopathic conditions.

- Reactive nodes are a healthy response and do not imply pathology of the node itself.

39.4.2 Imaging and Workup

- Normal lymph nodes are well demonstrated on CT. They are ovoid and soft-tissue density often with a central fatty hilum.
- On MRI, lymph nodes are typically isointense to muscle on T1-weighted imaging and isointense or mildly hyperintense on T2-weighted imaging.
- Normal nodes usually enhance homogenously and avidly with IV contrast on both CT and MR imaging.
- It is often difficult to differentiate normal from abnormal lymph nodes with cross-sectional imaging. However, certain morphologic features can be helpful to distinguish between the two.
- ACR white paper recommendations utilize a lymph node's size, shape, attenuation/signal, enhancement, and number as features.[1,2]
- Short-axis diameter of ≥ 1 cm in the retroperitoneum is recommended to discriminate between normal-sized and enlarged nodes.
- Since normal-sized nodes may also harbor disease, lymph node architecture and number should be also assessed.
- Marked enhancement or lack of enhancement (necrosis) is considered abnormal.
- A cluster of ≥ 3 lymph nodes in a single nodal station or a cluster of ≥ 2 lymph nodes in ≥ 2 regions (i.e., gastrohepatic ligament, retroperitoneum, and mesentery) may be considered suspicious.
- If a patient has an abnormal number or appearance of lymph nodes, and clinical and laboratory abnormalities suggest a possible lymphoproliferative disorder or known history of malignancy, an image-guided biopsy of an accessible, representative lymph node is recommended.
- For an incidental nodal finding in a patient who has a condition that is unlikely to cause adenopathy, correlation with patient's history and clinical scenario is recommended. Any relevant prior imaging should be reviewed and if the abnormal lymph node(s) has been unchanged for a period of 1 year, the finding may be considered stable and benign with no further follow-up recommended. Otherwise, a short-term follow-up CT or MRI is recommended in about 3 months.

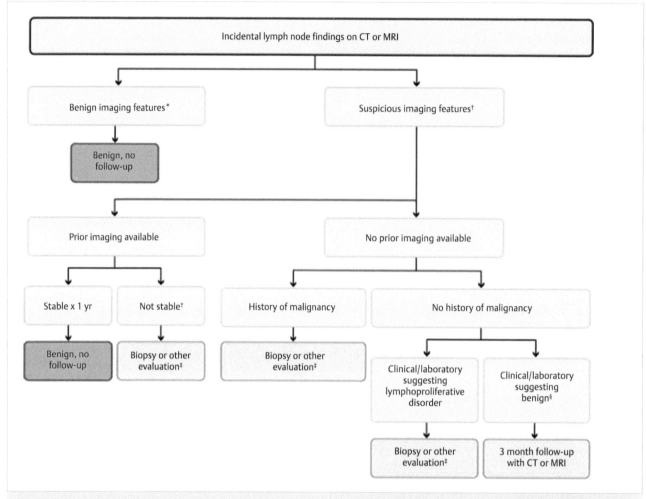

Fig. 39.4 Benign imaging features: normal short-axis diameter (< 1 cm in retroperitoneum), normal architecture (elongated, fatty hilum), normal enhancement, and normal node number. †Abnormal imaging features: enlarged short-axis diameter (≥ 1 cm in retroperitoneum), architecture (round, indistinct hilum), enhancement (necrosis/hypervascular), increased number (cluster of ≥ 3 lymph nodes in single nodal station or cluster of ≥ 2 lymph nodes in ≥ 2 regions).
‡Nonneoplastic disease: for example, infection, inflammation, connective tissue.
§Other evaluation (PET/CT, nuclear scintigraphy [MIBG], endoscopic ultrasound). (Use of the ACR flowchart of workup and management of Incidentally Detected Lymph nodes, from Heller MT, Harisinghani M, Neitlich JD, Yeghiayan P, Berland LL. Managing Incidental findings on abdominal and pelvic CT and MRI. Part 3: white paper of the ACR incidental findings committee II on splenic and nodal findings. J Am Coll 2013;10(11):833–839. Reproduced with permission from the American College of Radiology.)

39.5 Key Point Summary

- Most incidental nodal findings are nonspecific, but benign.
- Accurate identification of malignant lymph nodes is a major challenge in diagnostic radiology.
- Careful assessment of nodal morphology and correlation with patient's history and prior imaging can better indicate whether the node is abnormal and if further workup is needed.
- If a patient has abnormal lymph nodes, but no overt clinical or laboratory abnormalities suggesting a lymphoproliferative disorder, a short-term follow-up CT or MRI is recommended in 3 months.
- If an abnormal lymph node or nodal group(s) is unchanged for a period of 1 year, the finding may be considered benign.

References

[1] Heller MT, Harisinghani M, Neitlich JD, Yeghiayan P, Berland LL. Managing incidental findings on abdominal and pelvic CT and MRI. Part 3: white paper

of the ACR Incidental Findings Committee II on splenic and nodal findings. J Am Coll. 2013; 10(11):833–839

[2] Patel MD, Ascher SM, Paspulati RM, et al. Managing incidental findings on abdominal and pelvic CT and MRI, part 1: white paper of the ACR Incidental Findings Committee II on adnexal findings. J Am Coll Radiol. 2013; 10(9): 675–681

Suggested Readings

Baumgarten DA. Adnexal masses: ignore, follow, or treat. In: Sandrasegan K, Menias CO, eds. Oncologic Imaging: From Diagnosis to Cure. Leesburg, VA: American Roentgen Ray Society; 2016

Calgüneri M, Oztürk MA, Ozbalkan Z, et al. Frequency of lymphadenopathy in rheumatoid arthritis and systemic lupus erythematosus. J Int Med Res. 2003; 31(4): 345–349

Ganeshalingam S, Koh D-M. Nodal staging. Cancer Imaging. 2009; 9(1):104–111

George V, Tammisetti VS, Surabhi VR, Shanbhogue AK. Chronic fibrosing conditions in abdominal imaging. Radiographics. 2013; 33(4):1053–1080

40 Incidental Pelvic Mass

Kaustubh G. Shiralkar, Eduardo J. Matta, Steven S. Chua, and Chakradhar R. Thupili

40.1 Case Presentation

A 39-year-old woman presented with lower back pain for which an MRI of the lumbar spine without intravenous (IV) contrast was performed (▶ Fig. 40.1).

40.2 Imaging Findings and Impression

The MRI images demonstrate an incidentally detected, partially visualized multilocular cystic left adnexal mass with slightly thickened septations (*arrows* in ▶ Fig. 40.1). The abnormality is at the edge of the field of view and incompletely characterized on this examination. Benign physiologic ovarian/corpus luteal cysts are the most common cystic lesions in young, premenopausal women. In this case, however, the size and presence of septations warrant further workup and complete imaging.

40.2.1 Additional Testing Needed

- A pelvic ultrasound with transabdominal and transvaginal imaging is the first modality to work up a uterine or adnexal lesion (▶ Fig. 40.2).
- Cross-sectional imaging with CT and/or MRI with contrast can also be utilized in more complex cases and for problem-solving if ultrasound is inconclusive.

40.2.2 Pelvic Ultrasound Findings and Impression

Pelvic ultrasound examination done approximately 12 weeks later demonstrates a 9-cm large multilocular cystic mass with thickened septations. No internal vascularity is demonstrated. Findings are concerning for cystic ovarian neoplasm; therefore, referral to gynecologist was made. Due to size (> 7 cm), persistence on follow-up imaging, and internal complexity, the lesion was excised.

Follow-up: The patient underwent a left oophorectomy and final pathology revealed a serous cystadenoma.

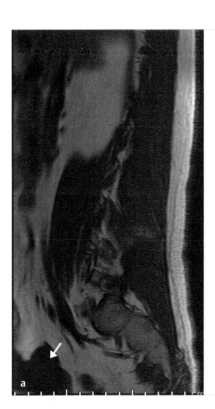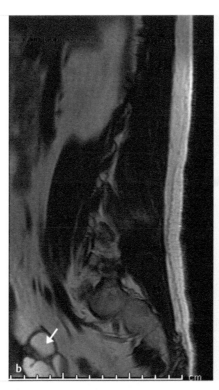

Fig. 40.1 Sagittal T1-weighted image **(a)** and sagittal T2-weighted image **(b)** from a lumbar spine MRI without contrast.

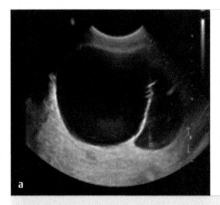 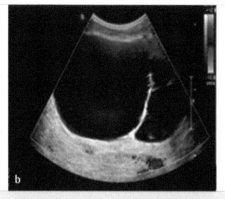 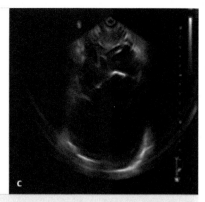

Fig. 40.2 Sagittal transabdominal (TA) ultrasound image of the left adnexa **(a)**, sagittal TA image with color of the left adnexa **(b)**, and transverse transvaginal image **(c)**.

40.3 Essential Information regarding Ovarian Serous Cystadenomas

- Ovarian serous cystadenoma is a benign lesion classified as epithelial ovarian neoplasm and often indistinguishable from functional ovarian cysts on imaging.
- It can be encountered at any age, but peak incidence is typically in the fourth and fifth decades of life.
- It accounts for 25% of all benign ovarian neoplasms and 10 to 20% are bilateral.
- Key in distinguishing it from a physiologic ovarian cyst is its size (average of 10 cm) and persistence on follow-up examinations (most important differentiating factor).
- It can be multilocular with septations, but will usually not have internal vascularity within the septation or solid component such as mural nodules. The best initial imaging tool for characterization is ultrasound (▶ Table 40.1).

Table 40.1 Differential diagnosis of commonly detected adnexal masses

Differential diagnosis	Comments
Physiologic ovarian/ para-ovarian cyst	Thin wall with lack of complex features such as thick septations or mural nodules; a hemorrhagic cyst may mimic a solid lesion but usually resolves with short-term follow-up
Corpus luteal cyst	Characteristic rim enhancement or vascularity
Ovarian cystic neoplasm	Complex multilocular with solid mural nodules and septations; often will enhance
Endometrioma	Solid or complex fluid density with nonspecific CT appearance; may have characteristic T2-"shading" and T1 bright signal due to intrinsic blood products on MR
Hydrosalpinx	May mimic ovarian cyst but tubular in shape and para-ovarian location
Dermoid cyst	Fat attenuation on CT and variable calcium; increased T1 and T2 signal with loss of signal on fat saturation images on MR due to macroscopic fat content
Uterine leiomyoma	Subserosal or pedunculated leiomyomas may mimic solid adnexal/ovarian lesions; Look for uterine origin on CT/MRI; Generally low T2 signal on MR and may have calcifications on CT.
Bowel loop	Use multiplanar reformats on CT or multiple planes on MR if available to differentiate from fluid-filled small bowel loops
Bladder diverticulum	Large bladder diverticulum or ureterocele can mimic a cystic adnexal lesion; look for connection to bladder or ureter

40.4 Essential Information about Incidental Pelvic Masses Detected on Lumbosacral MRI or CT

The normal imaging appearance (see ▶ Fig. 40.3a,b):

- Normal premenopausal ovary on CT is an oval soft-tissue density structure typically located in or near the iliac fossa and can be traced to the gonadal vessels (see ▶ Fig. 40.3a).
- Normal premenopausal ovary on MR is of homogenous low to intermediate signal on T1-weighted imaging, and has dark stroma and follicles of varying sizes on T2-weighted imaging (see ▶ Fig. 40.3b).
- Normal postmenopausal ovary is smaller in size and is a predominantly solid structure on CT because of relative increase of stromal tissue and decrease in follicles with T1 and T2 hypointensity on MR. Thus, the normal ovary should not be mistaken for a pelvic mass.
- The ovary will enhance on both IV contrast-enhanced CT and MR, but less than the normal uterine myometrium.

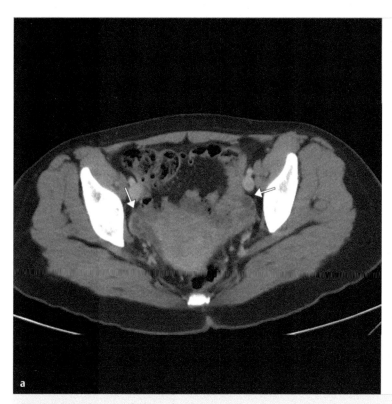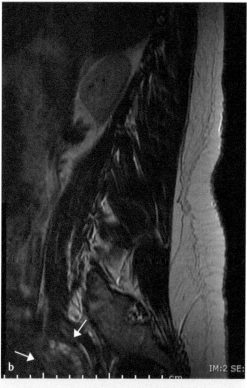

Fig. 40.3 Normal imaging findings of premenopausal ovaries are shown in this axial postcontrast CT of the pelvis **(a)** and parasagittal T2-weighted MR image from a lumbar spine MRI **(b)**.

The diagnostic approach to incidental pelvic findings on lumbo-sacral spine MRI (see ▶ Fig. 40.4)[1]:

- Pelvic ultrasound is recommended as the first, and usually, best test to attempt to determine the relationship of the mass to the ovary or organ of origin, which is of key importance.
- Ultrasound is also more accurate in characterizing the internal architecture of the lesion. Furthermore, the ability to identify small mural nodules on CT or unenhanced MRI has not been established.

- Follow-up ultrasound in premenopausal patents for simple or mildly complex cysts is in 6 to 12 weeks because the cyst may resolve or decrease in size on follow-up, thus obviating the need for further workup.
- Adnexal cysts in late menopause, larger mildly complex cysts (probably benign), and cysts with solid components are initially worked up with prompt ultrasound.
- Stratifying an incidentally identified adnexal mass is typically based on the patient demographics, morphologic characteristics, and size of the mass.

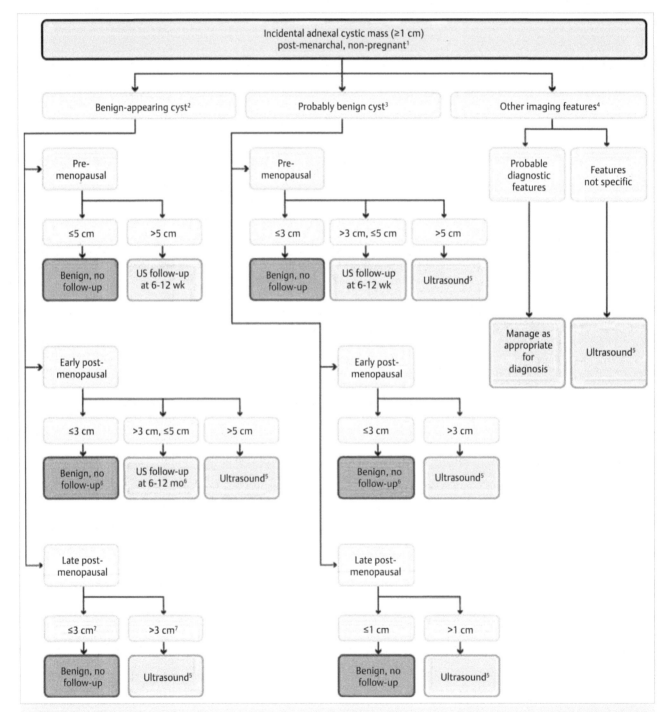

Fig. 40.4 Use of the ACR flowchart of workup and management of incidentally detected adnexal lesions. (Reproduced with permission from Patel MD, Ascher SM, Paspulati RM, et al. Managing incidental findings on abdominal and pelvic CT and MRI, part 1: white paper of the ACR Incidental Findings Committee II on adnexal findings. J Am Coll Radiol 2013;10(9):675–681.)

– Patient demographics:
  ○ If the patient's last menstrual period (LMP) is unknown, 50 years can be used as an arbitrary designation for early menopause and 55 years for late menopause.
  ○ If the LMP is known, "early" and "late" menopauses are defined as within 5 years and after 5 years of LMP, respectively.
– Lesion morphology:
  ○ Morphologic features and size are features of critical importance.
  ○ Simple cysts less than 10 cm in women of any age including postmenopausal patients are rarely malignant.
  ○ Mildly complex cysts or "probably benign" cysts, as stated by ACR Incidental Findings Committee II, may have angulated margins, not round or oval in shape, or incompletely/suboptimally imaged. Many incidentally detected pelvic lesions on neuroimaging will fall into this catagory.[0]
  ○ Other findings such as solid component, mural nodules, and thick septations are more concerning and will require more extensive workup.

40.5 Key Point Summary

- Increased use of cross-sectional imaging, improvement in image quality, and increasing legal concerns have led to increased detection of potentially important incidental findings. Although many adnexal lesions harbor little clinical significance, in some cases their detection may create the opportunity for early, potentially life-saving, treatment.
- When an incidentally identified adnexal lesion is detected, the first step is to determine whether the lesion is ovarian or extra-ovarian in nature.
- Risk stratification of the ovarian lesion and the need for further workup is then based on the size and complexity of the lesion, as well as the patient's age and menstrual status.
- Workhorse for initial characterization of an incidental adnexal mass is transabdominal and transvaginal pelvic ultrasound.

Reference

[1] Patel MD, Ascher SM, Paspulati RM, et al. Managing incidental findings on abdominal and pelvic CT and MRI, part 1: white paper of the ACR Incidental Findings Committee II on adnexal findings. J Am Coll Radiol. 2013; 10(9): 675–681

Suggested Readings

American Cancer Society (ACS). Cancer statistics center. ACS website. Available at: Ovary.cancerstatisticscenter.org/?_ga=1.203425104.1140738009.147 3004625#/cancer-site/Ovary

Maxwell AW, Keating DP, Nickerson JP. Incidental abdominopelvic findings on expanded field-of-view lumbar spinal MRI: frequency, clinical importance, and concordance in interpretation by neuroimaging and body imaging radiologists. Clin Radiol. 2015; 70(2):161–167

Modesitt SC, Pavlik EJ, Ueland FR, DePriest PD, Kryscio RJ, van Nagell JR, Jr. Risk of malignancy in unilocular ovarian cystic tumors less than 10 centimeters in diameter. Obstet Gynecol. 2003; 102(3):594–599

Spencer JA, Forstner R, Cunha TM, Kinkel K, ESUR Female Imaging Sub-Committee. ESUR guidelines for MR imaging of the sonographically indeterminate adnexal mass: an algorithmic approach. Eur Radiol. 2010; 20(1):25–35

Tuncel SA, Çaglı B, Tekataş A, Kırıcı MY, Ünlü E, Gençhellaç H. Extraspinal incidental findings on routine MRI of lumbar spine: prevalence and reporting rates in 1278 patients. Korean J Radiol. 2015; 16(4):866–873

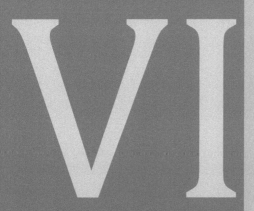

Section VI

Artifacts That May Obscure Pathology and Simulate Disease Entities

VI

Introduction

Artifact: *Any finding that appears in an image that is not present in the originally imaged object.*

Even though artifacts are by definition incidental findings, they have the potential to dangerously mimic pathologic processes, which may result in unnecessary additional testing and inappropriate treatment. One of the most important challenges in imaging interpretation is to recognize artifacts and work to eliminate them or, when not possible, to minimize their effects. Yet another error may occur when a suboptimal, artifact-degraded examination is summarily declared "nondiagnostic" and a partially masked, "real" pathologic finding is ignored.

Although artifacts may occur with all imaging modalities, we will focus on examples of some of the most troublesome CT angiography and beam-hardening artifacts (Chapter 41). Then, we will devote the remainder of this section to showing examples of artifacts that are specifically encountered on magnetic resonance imaging (MRI). Due to the complexity of MRI, an extensive variety of artifacts may occur, which are increasingly common and more difficult to recognize with the advent of parallel imaging and other advanced imaging techniques. MRI artifact cases will be presented in categories based on their etiology (Chapters 42, 43, and 44).

41 Computed Tomography Artifacts

Clark W. Sitton and Kaye D. Westmark

41.1 Computed Tomography Angiography

41.1.1 Case Presentation: CTA Artifacts Mimicking Carotid Artery Dissection

History: A 35-year-old man admitted to the neurosurgical service for management of a subdural hematoma suffered during motor vehicle collision. A CT angiography (CTA) of the neck was performed as routine screening based on the mechanism of the injury ▶ Fig. 41.1. The radiology report describes a dissection of the left carotid artery origin (see ▶ Table 41.1).

Imaging impression: Normal carotid bifurcation; the apparent filling defect is artifactual.

Cause: Artifactual hypodensity secondary to turbulence related to the carotid bifurcation, resulting in heterogeneous mixture of contrast and nonopacified blood.

Additional testing to consider in difficult cases:

- **Recommended:** Delayed contrast examination, such as routine contrast-enhanced CT of the neck. This admixture phenomenon is extremely transient and relates to the high speed of modern multidetector scanners.
- **Not recommended:** Two-dimensional time-of-flight MR angiography. If there is turbulence at the bulb significant enough to produce this artifact on CT, it will almost certainly produce a similar artifact on MRI, although the physics is completely different.

Other common phenomenon that may simulate acute dissection on CTA:

- **CT beam hardening artifact:** Streaklike artifact related to high-density material such as dental amalgam or other radiopaque foreign bodies as well as high-density contrast in the venous system. The resulting hypodense linear bands projected from the dense object traverse the vessel in the axial plane, resulting in linear filling defects on the reconstructed images, and sometimes a flaplike appearance may be present even on the source images.
- **Pulsation artifact:** Motion of the carotid artery during the CT acquisition results in the superimposition of the carotid density on adjacent structures, resulting in a Venn diagram type of overlap appearance on the axial image. This can then result in irregularity in the contour of the vessel lumen or the appearance of linear flaplike filling defects on reconstructed images. This primarily occurs in in two locations: at the thoracic junction, where the carotid artery pulsatility is more marked, and, in children and younger patients, in the internal carotid artery where it lies immediately adjacent to the internal jugular vein.
- **FMD:** Thickening of the vessel wall can result in a beaded, irregular appearance very similar to arterial dissection. Often bilateral, it can involve the vertebral arteries as well. It is important to recognize that FMD is associated with intracranial aneurysms and real dissections.

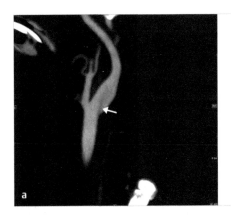

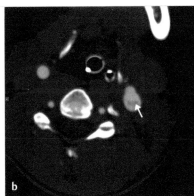

Fig. 41.1 Maximum-intensity projection (MIP) sagittal **(a)** and axial source **(b)** images from a CTA demonstrate a faint linear filling defect originating at the junction of the carotid bulb with the common carotid artery (*arrows*). On the axial images, the defect fails to make contact with the wall of the vessel.

Table 41.1 Differential diagnosis for flaplike filling defects at the origin of the internal carotid artery

Differential diagnosis	Comments
Flow/admixture artifact	Faintly seen linear or curvy linear area of reduced density originating at the posterior margin of the bulb and extending into the vessel lumen, often forming a curvilinear shape
Atherosclerotic dissection	Filling defect, surrounded by contrast, on contrast images and dynamic angiography with clear attachment to the vessel wall. Associated with atherosclerotic changes in the vessel walls such as calcification and irregularity
Traumatic dissection	Traumatic dissections of the internal carotid artery occur in two locations, between the origin and skull base, where this styloid ligament passes, and at or just beneath the skull base, where the artery is tethered by the carotid canal. Traumatic injuries elsewhere are extremely rare except in the case of penetrating trauma. Dissections will extend from the aortic arch into the common, and internal carotid arteries
Carotid web	1- to 2-mm-thick shelf of soft tissue arising from the posterior wall of the carotid not associated with atherosclerotic change

41.1.2 Companion Cases

Companion Case 1

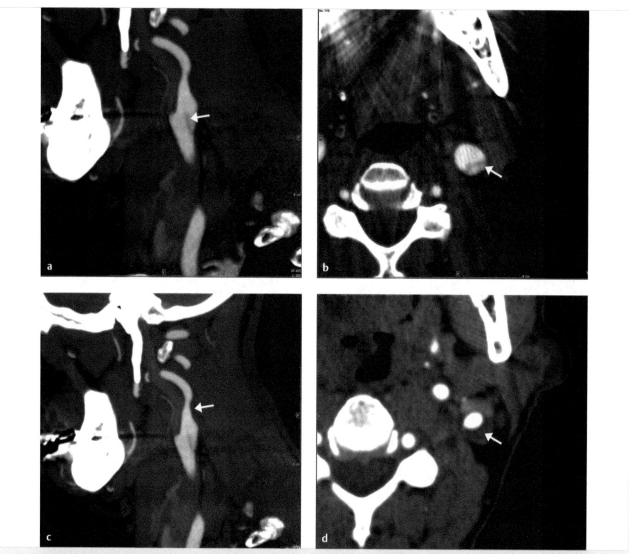

Fig. 41.2 A second case with similar artifactual findings at the carotid bifurcation presented for comparison. This patient had a left middle cerebral artery stroke and was being considered for endovascular therapy. **(a, b)** The artifactual filling defect (*arrows*). **(c, d)** The low-density atherosclerotic plaque (*arrows*), likely the actual culprit lesion.

Companion Case 2

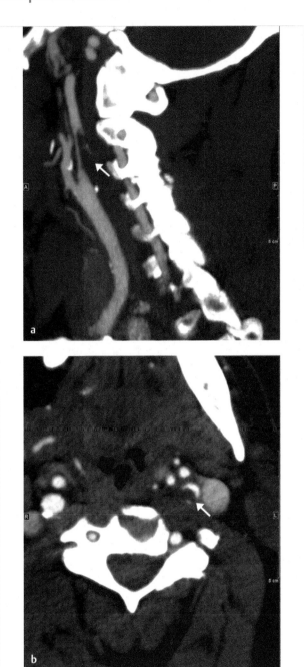

Fig. 41.3 (a, b) An intraluminal thrombus (*arrows*) adherent to an unstable atherosclerotic plaque extends from the calcified plaque wall distally into the arterial lumen, surrounded by contrast.

Companion Case 3

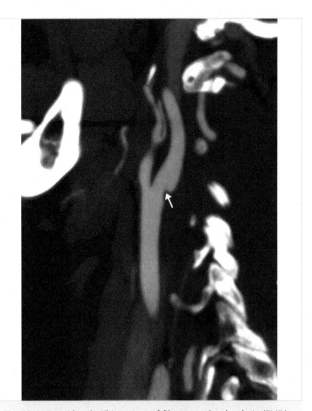

Fig. 41.4 Carotid web. This variant of fibromuscular dysplasia (FMD) arises from the posterior wall at the junction between the common carotid artery and the bulb, and produces a thin but dense flap of varying sizes. Females of Afro-Caribbean descent are the most affected, but the finding is seen in all populations. There is some correlation with microembolization, so anticoagulation may be indicated.

Companion Case 4

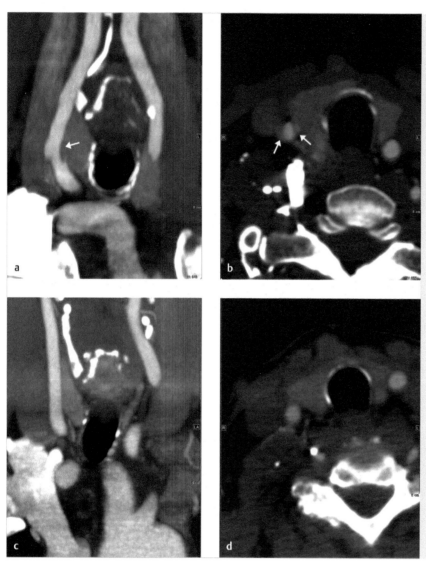

Fig. 41.5 This patient had a CT to follow up a vertebral artery dissection and this suspicious irregularity was identified in the right common carotid artery (*arrows* in **a** and **b**). Findings are typical for pulsation-related artifact. Note the Venn diagram appearance of the carotid in axial section on the right (**b**). A follow-up examination obtained a day later shows the vessel is normal (**c, d**).

Companion Case 5

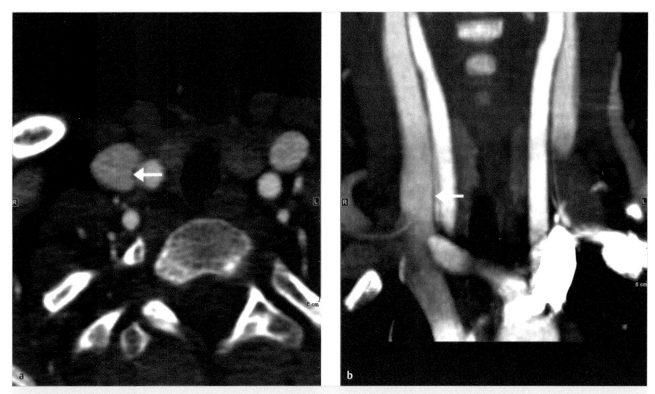

Fig. 41.6 These images show another example of pulsation artifact producing dissectionlike pseudo-flaps. In this case, the finding appears more linear and the Venn diagram appearance is not only apparent on the axial **(a)** but also on the coronal reconstruction **(b)**, as the margins of the jugular vein and carotid overlap.

Companion Case 6

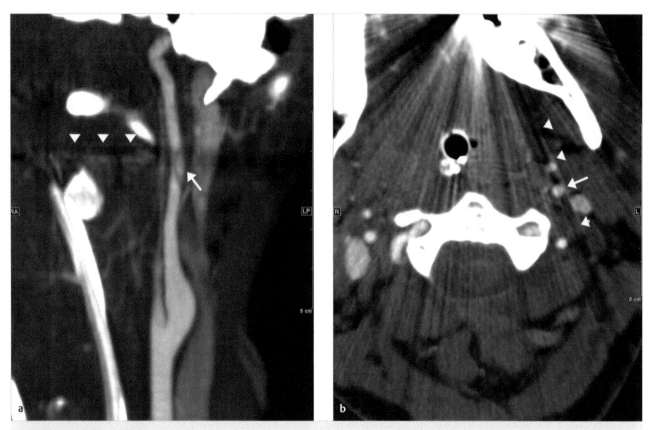

Fig. 41.7 Typical beam hardening artifact from dental amalgams. A flaplike defect is present within the internal carotid artery on the maximum-intensity reconstruction (*arrow* on **a**). Low-density linear streaks related to beam hardening (*arrowheads* in **b**) are better seen on the axial images, traversing an opacified artery and resulting in the artifactual defect. The same streak artifact can be perceived on the reconstructions as well, but is more subtle (*arrowheads* in **a**).

Companion Case 7

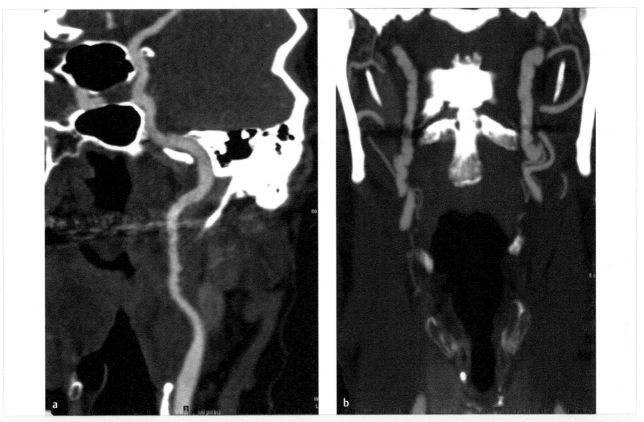

Fig. 41.8 FMD with the classic "string of beads appearance." There is an extensive, acute grade 1 dissection with non–flow limiting irregularity at the intersection of the internal carotid artery and the styloid ligament **(a)**. Note the bilateral involvement and sharp margins shown on the coronal reconstruction **(b)**.

41.1.3 Case Presentation: CTA Artifact Mimicking Partial Basilar Artery Thrombosis

History: A 65-year-old man underwent a circle of Willis CTA for evaluation of a possible transient ischemic attack.

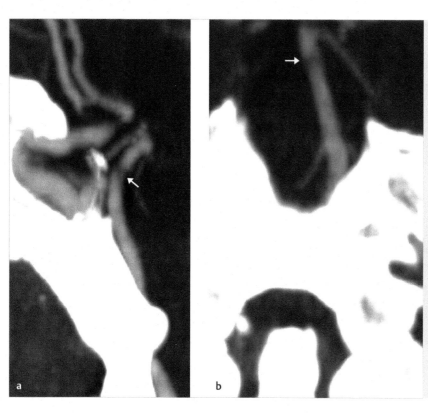

Fig. 41.9 Sagittal **(a)** and coronal **(b)** MIP reconstructions reveal an apparent filling defect (*arrows*) in the middle portion of the basilar artery. However, the lumen of the artery distal to this focal abnormality fills normally with contrast. Follow-up MRI of the brain did not reveal any associated abnormality (not shown).

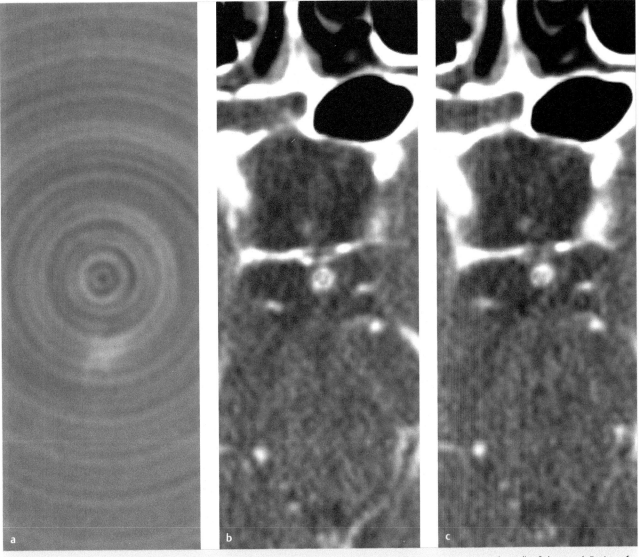

Fig. 41.10 (a–c) Close inspection of the source images reveals a focal intraluminal filling defect that does not contact the walls of the vessel. Review of the image with extremely wide windowing and low level (lung windowing) reveals a series of concentric rings located about the geometric isocenter of the scan field of view. These concentric rings are best seen utilizing lung windowing in the area immediately superior to the head where air is present.

It is important to correlate abnormalities on CTA with expected associated findings such as diminished distal flow or ischemic changes in the posterior circulation distribution.

Cause: Concentric ringlike artifacts are not uncommon with third-generation CT scanners and are due to a miscalibrated or defective detector element. They occur precisely in the center of the rotation and are best seen with a very wide window and low center level. If the low-attenuation central ring of the artifact falls precisely into an area of high attenuation, such as an enhancing vessel, an artifactual "filling defect" will be created.

Solution: The service engineer must calibrate or replace the defective detector element and the study should be repeated if possible.

Companion Case 1

History: Acute mental status change and sudden onset of hemi-body weakness. CTA was performed for the evaluation of a "stroke."

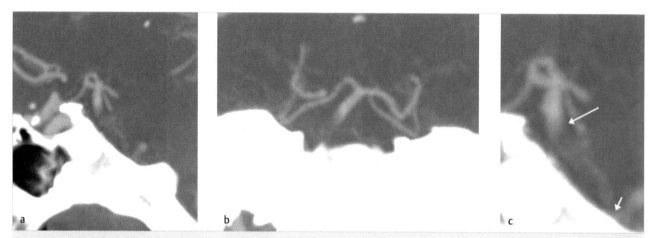

Fig. 41.11 (a–c) CTA sagittal **(a)** and coronal **(b)** reformatted images reveal occlusion of the proximal basilar artery at its origin with flow in the distal basilar artery resulting from anterior to posterior collateral flow through the posterior cerebral arteries. The segment in which there is no evidence of normal flow is indicated on a magnified sagittal reformatted image **(c)**. The *short arrow* indicates the junction of the normal vertebral artery into the proximal-most basilar artery, which is occluded immediately afterward. The *long arrow* indicates the flow reconstituted by collateral vessels in the more distal basilar artery.

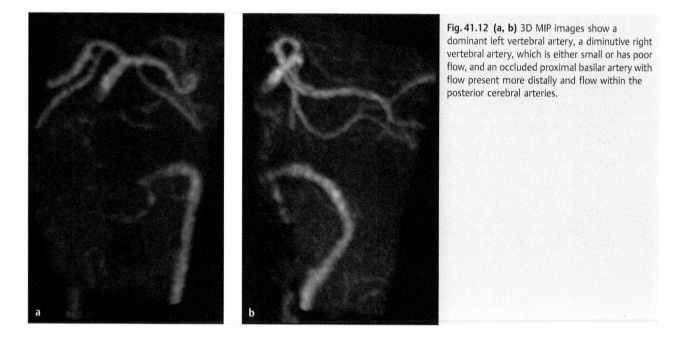

Fig. 41.12 (a, b) 3D MIP images show a dominant left vertebral artery, a diminutive right vertebral artery, which is either small or has poor flow, and an occluded proximal basilar artery with flow present more distally and flow within the posterior cerebral arteries.

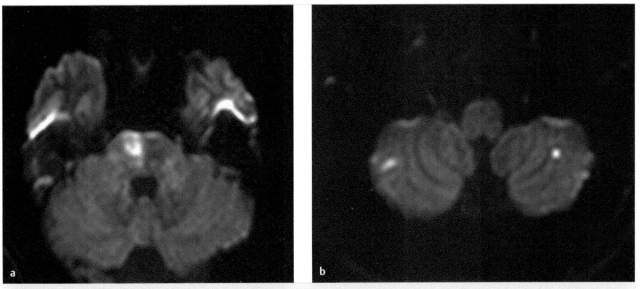

Fig. 41.13 (a, b) Diffusion-weighted images from a brain MR obtained later the same day reveals an acute right pontine infarction and smaller embolic infarctions scattered peripherally within the cerebellar hemispheres that have resulted from the partial basilar thrombosis.

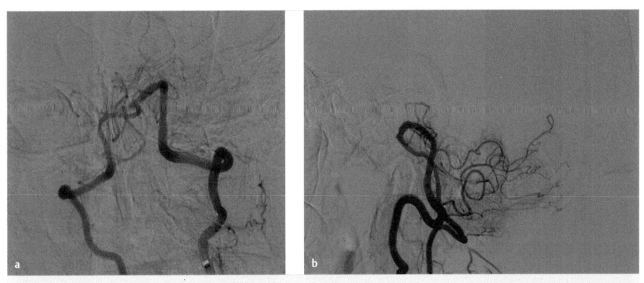

Fig. 41.14 (a, b) Anteroposterior and Lateral projections from a catheter angiography, left vertebral artery injection, reveal antegrade flow in the left vertebral artery with cross-filling into the very proximal-most part of the basilar artery and retrograde flow down the right vertebral artery. No flow is present within the basilar artery more distally with this vertebral injection.

41.2 Beam Hardening Artifact Mimics a Brain Tumor

History: A 30-year-old woman was referred for a brain MRI to further evaluate a mass in the left middle cranial fossa that was detected on a noncontrast head CT performed for headache (▶ Fig. 41.16).

Although on this single image the findings do appear worrisome for a hyperdense mass, it should be realized that if this were indeed a tumor, it would measure 2.5 cm × 1.7 cm × 0.3 cm, which is incompatible with an intra-axial mass as they have a more spherical growth pattern.

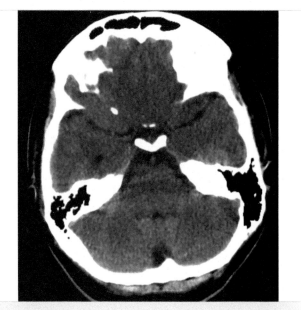

Fig. 41.15

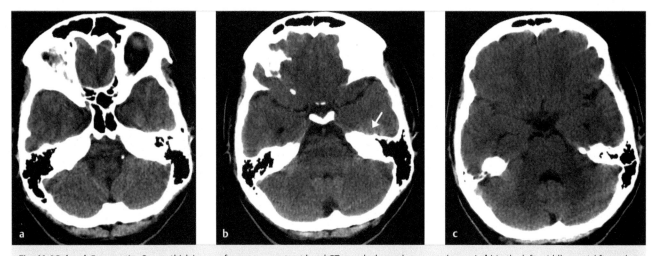

Fig. 41.16 (a–c) Consecutive 3-mm-thick images from a noncontrast head CT reveal a hyperdense area (*arrow* in **b**) in the left middle cranial fossa that measures 2.5 cm transverse by 1.7 cm anterior to posterior. The sylvian fissures are symmetric.

Imaging impression: Normal head CT. The finding of a possible mass is artifactual, which was confirmed by the subsequent MRI (▶ Fig. 41.17).

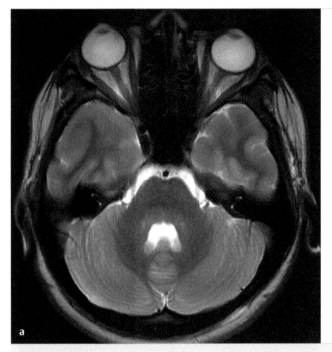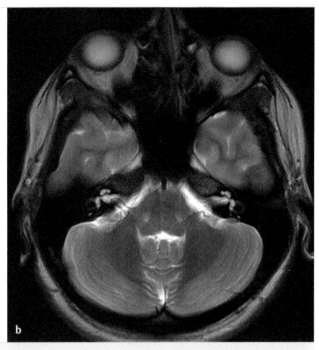

Fig. 41.17 (a, b)

Cause: Beam hardening-streak artifact on head CT arising from the dense petrous apices.

Solution: CT imaging is limited in the evaluation of the posterior fossa and brainstem for this reason. Dense skull base and petrous apices cause scatter of the CT beam and lead to areas of artifactually high and low density. Increasing the technique will decrease this artifact but also increase radiation dose. MRI is often required for further evaluation if the patient has symptoms referable to a posterior fossa/brainstem lesion.

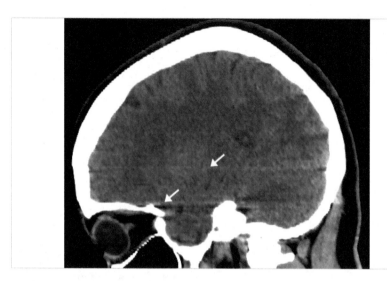

Fig. 41.18 Sagittal reconstruction of the head CT shows the linear artifact (*arrows*), arising from the dense petrous bone, extending through the middle cranial fossa.

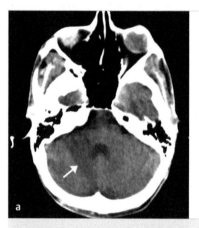 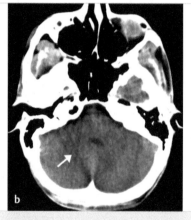 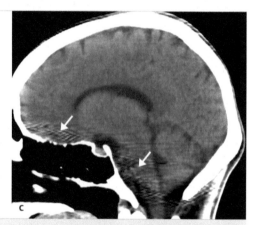

Fig. 41.19 **(a, b)** Axial images through the posterior fossa have linear areas (*arrows* in **a** and **b**) of marked hypodensity. The abrupt change, linear configuration, and crossing of normal anatomic boundaries as well as lack of any mass effect in the surrounding brain all help confirm the artifactual nature of this finding. **(c)** The sagittal reformation shows beam hardening and photon starvation artifact (*arrows*) severely affecting the posterior fossa and inferior frontal lobe adjacent to the skull base.

41.3 Ring Detector Artifact Simulates a Mass in the Basal Ganglia

History: A 4-year-old patient was transferred to a tertiary care hospital to further evaluate possible nonaccidental trauma. Soft-tissue swelling was present in the right occipital region and a possible 1-cm hemorrhage with surrounding edema was found in the right basal ganglia.

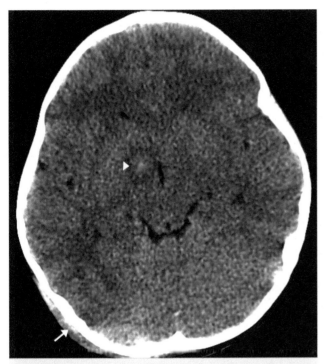

Fig. 41.20 Minimal soft-tissue (*arrow*) swelling is present overlying the right occipital region. A small hyperdensity is seen in the right basal ganglia with surrounding ring of hypodensity (see *arrowhead*). The findings were considered suspicious for an artifact due to complete lack of any mass effect on the surrounding brain and adjacent third ventricle despite the 1.5-cm-size "lesion." The head CT was repeated and was normal.

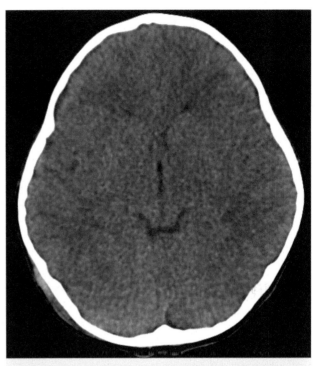

Fig. 41.21 Intracranially normal follow-up head CT performed later the same day with minimal overlying soft-tissue swelling again seen in the right occipital region.

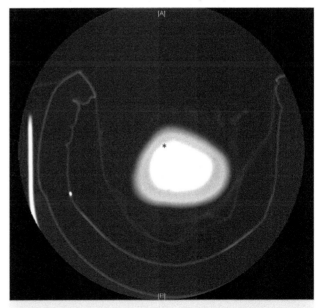

Fig. 41.22 Given the ringlike appearance of this abnormality, a ring detector artifact should be considered. If this is the cause, the ring artifact will always be located in the center of the field image even if the body part being imaged is off-center. Placing a cursor on the center of the ring artifact and scrolling up through the images above the head allowed clearer visualization of the circular field of view and revealed that the artifact was indeed centered.

Cause: Miscalibration or defect in one of the CT scanner detectors.

Solution: Call service for recalibration or replacement of the faulty detector.

Essential information regarding ring detector artifacts:

- Ring detector artifact on early generation scanners was usually very apparent and would appear as a concentric ring on virtually every image.

- With later generation scanners, which have an ever-increasing number of detectors, the failure of any one detector is much more difficult to detect. Rings do not appear on every image and can be subtler.

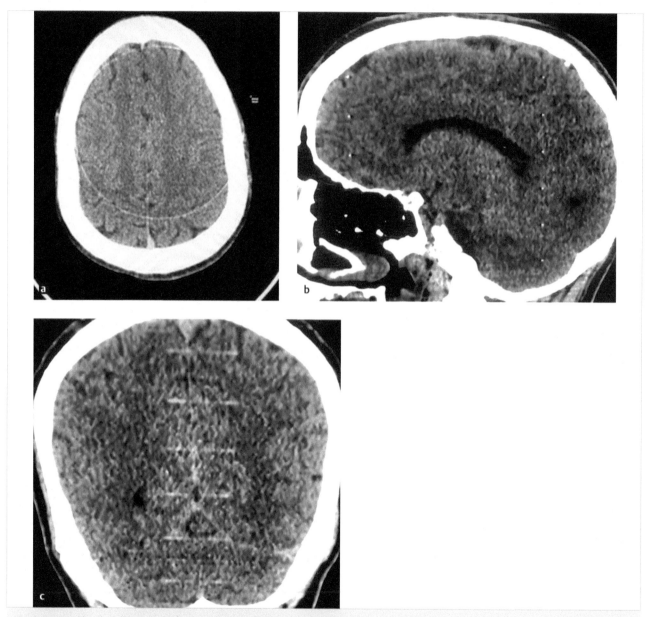

Fig. 41.23 Axial head CT **(a)** Image shows a hyperdense ring that is centered within the gantry but not necessarily the object being imaged as it may be off-center. The ring artifact was not present on every image as seen in the sagittal **(b)** and coronal **(c)** reformations.

42 MRI Patient-Related Motion Artifacts

Clark W. Sitton, Alexander B. Simonetta, and Kaye D. Westmark

42.1 Cerebrospinal Fluid Flow Artifacts

42.1.1 Case Presentation

Clinical History

A 50-year-old woman complains of mid-lower back pain. Her physical examination is normal.

Imaging Findings and Impression

There is a linear area of increased signal within the spinal cord on the short tau inversion recovery (STIR) sequence (*white arrows* in ▶ Fig. 42.1a) that is not present on neither the sagittal (▶ Fig. 42.1b) nor axial (▶ Fig. 42.1c) fast spin echo (FSE) T2-weighted images (T2WIs). This hyperintense central cord signal on the STIR image extends the entire length of the cord, does not taper superiorly, and does not expand the spinal cord.

In addition, multiple large, noncontiguous areas of decreased signal are seen in the CSF dorsal to the spinal cord on both the sagittal STIR (*blue arrows;* ▶ Fig. 42.1a) and FSE-T2WIs (*blue arrows;* ▶ Fig. 42.1b). Incidental note is made of a hemangioma in the body of L1 (*asterisk* in ▶ Fig. 42.1b).

Cause: Areas of decreased signal in the cerebrospinal fluid (CSF) are dorsal to the thoracic spinal cord in an area well known to experience turbulent CSF flow. Areas of signal loss in the CSF are bulky and noncontiguous rather than serpentine and are not closely applied to the pial surface of the cord. The linear area of increased signal seen within the spinal cord on the STIR sequence is not present in neither the sagittal FSE-T2WI nor the axial T2WI.

Diagnosis: These findings are artifactual and the spinal cord and canal are normal.

42.1.2 Differential Diagnosis

- Normal thoracic spine MR: Artifactual increased signal in spinal cord due to Gibbs' truncation artifact (TA) and artifactual decreased signal in CSF dorsal to thoracic cord due to turbulent CSF signal dephasing.
- Dural arteriovenous fistula (DAVF) with diffuse spinal cord edema: Linear, serpentine flow voids are closely applied to the pial surface of the spinal cord. Central area of increased signal in the spinal cord tapers superiorly and appears "cigar-like."
- Spinal cord infarction: Hyperacutely, despite even a severe clinical presentation of acute onset of back pain and paraplegia, the spinal cord may appear normal on T1 W and T2WIs

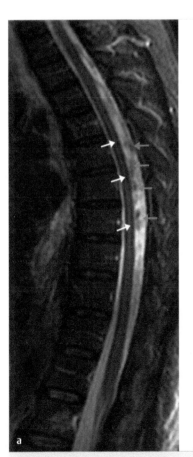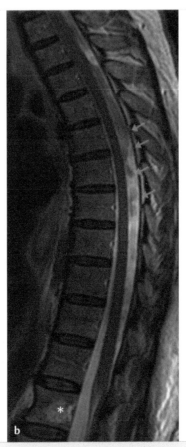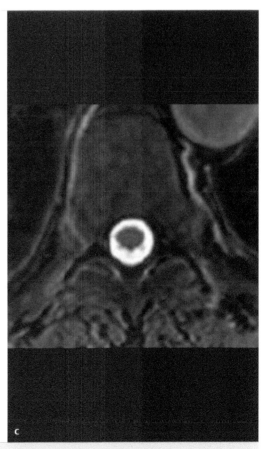

Fig. 42.1 Sagittal short tau inversion recovery (STIR) image **(a)** and sagittal **(b)** and axial **(c)** fast spin echo T2-weighted images of the thoracic spine.

but will have increased signal on diffusion-weighted images centrally by 8 to 12 hours. By 1 to 2 days, hyperintensity is seen centrally and affecting the anterior two-thirds of the spinal cord, usually in the thoracic region. By 1 week, the diffusion-weighted images will appear normal.[1]

- Persistent central canal: Normal finding often demonstrated on high-resolution MRI. This finding is present more often in younger patients. It appears as a linear area of hyperintensity on the T2 W sagittal images located precisely between the anterior one-third and posterior two-thirds of the spinal cord in the cervical and higher thoracic regions, moving more centrally nearer to the conus.[2] On axial images, it should be perfectly round and measure ≤ 2 mm (reported range 1–5 mm).[3] The surrounding spinal cord should be normal in course, caliber, and signal intensity. A symptomatic persistent central canal is a diagnosis of exclusion.

- Thoracic cord syringohydromyelia: Although the cavity will follow CSF in signal intensity, it is often more irregular in contour and larger than a simple persistent central canal. Contrast-enhanced MRI should be performed as some syrinxes are tumor associated. The posterior fossa should be examined for a Chiari malformation and the distal aspect of the cord should be examined to exclude the possibility of a tethered spinal cord associated with hydromyelia. In any patient with a possible syrinx, clinical correlation is very important to determine if they are symptomatic.[3]

42.1.3 Differential Diagnostic Pearls and Pitfalls

- Note if the area of decreased signal is bulky and noncontiguous in a region highly prone to turbulent CSF flow, that is, the dorsal thoracic region. These observations support artifactual flow-related CSF signal dephasing.

- Linear, serpentine, and contiguous flow voids, closely applied to the spinal cord, are more suspicious. Contrast enhancement is recommended for further evaluation.

- The gold standard test is spinal angiography, which may be required for confirmation and possible treatment in the cases in which a DAVF is suspected clinically.

42.1.4 Artifact Problem-Solving: Additional Evaluation Recommended in Difficult Cases

Possible signal abnormality in the spinal cord:
- Recommended: Evaluate cord signal on the axial T2WIs as no abnormal signal will be present if due to the Gibbs TA.
- Recommended: If high signal is seen within the spinal cord on the STIR sequence, compare to the higher resolution

sagittal FSE-T2WI as higher resolution sequences are much less prone to TAs.[4]
- Recommended: Increasing resolution and decreasing field of view (FOV) will reduce Gibbs TA.[4]
- Possibly recommended: Contrast-enhanced (CE) T1WI, CE-MRA and volumetric FSE-T2 W or steady-state gradient recalled echo (GRE) type sequences in the cases in which DAVF cannot be excluded as either there is true edema in the cord and the linear flow void areas are more serpentine and contiguous or clinical suspicion is high.

Possible abnormal flow voids versus CSF turbulent dephasing:
- Recommended: If linear, serpentine, and contiguous flow voids, closely applied to the spinal cord, the finding is more suspicious and contrast-enhanced T1 W sequence is recommended to evaluate for possible DAVF. Prior to obtaining the postgadolinium T1 W sequence, a dynamic, contrast-enhanced 3D MRA could also be acquired.[4,5]
- Recommended: A number of sequences are not as degraded by turbulent CSF flow artifacts as axial 2D FSE-T2 W imaging. GRE pulse sequences, which create images by gradient reversal rather than slice-selective radiofrequency (RF) pulse, are not affected by CSF flow artifacts. CSF should remain uniformly high in signal if normal. Volumetric (3D) heavily T2 W FSE type sequences also show much higher, uniform CSF signal that may assist in localizing the most likely site of a spinal DAVF.[6] Balanced steady-state GRE-type MRI sequences provide uniform, high signal within the CSF without signal loss due to turbulent dephasing.[4,7]
- Possibly recommended: The gold standard test to evaluate for DAVF is spinal angiography, which may be required for confirmation and possible treatment in the cases in which a DAVF is suspected clinically and routine MR imaging is highly suspicious.[8]

42.1.5 Essential Information:

Artifacts produced by CSF flow:
- FSE-T2 W and other spin echo–type sequences utilize a series of slice-selective RF pulses to create the image. Any substance moving through the imaging plane may lose signal due to flow-related dephasing as, although it may be "in plane" for the initial RF pulse, it has moved in location during the subsequent RF-refocusing pulse(s). This is why normal-flowing blood moving through the plane of imaging appears black.[4]
- GRE imaging sequences create images by gradient reversal rather than slice-selective RF pulses and are therefore not affected by CSF flow artifacts as signal is rephased by gradient reversal that is not slice selective. Therefore, this also explains why normal-flowing blood appears bright on GRE images.[4]

- Tarlov's cysts and intrathecal arachnoid cysts may appear "brighter" than the normal CSF on FSE-T2WIs within the thecal sac as the fluid within them is relatively stagnant. There is always some signal loss in CSF within the normal thecal sac due to normal pulsatile motion of the fluid.
- In an area of relative narrowing of the spinal canal dimensions, CSF may lose signal immediately distal to the constriction as its flow accelerates and there is increased turbulent dephasing. This phenomenon accounts for CSF flow-related signal loss in the fourth ventricle just inferior to the cerebral aqueduct on sagittal T2WI of the posterior fossa as well as triangular areas of signal loss in the CSF in the lateral recesses of the cervical spine on axial FSE-T2WIs.

The Gibbs truncation artifact:

- Pitfall: On spine images, it may create a false appearance of abnormal signal throughout the spinal cord, a pseudosyrinx.
- Appearance: Series of alternating high- and low-signal lines present within the image that are parallel to an area of normal anatomy that has an abrupt high-signal/low-signal interface. The artifact is most commonly seen on STIR images, which always have low signal-to-noise ratio because of suppression of virtually all signal except that which is coming from CSF (i.e., the bone marrow and subcutaneous fat signal that contributes to overall signal of the image has been completely suppressed). Lower field strength magnets will often make the situation even worse as they have inherently lower signal than high field strength magnets. Therefore, the low field strength magnet imaging protocols often employ a low matrix and low bandwidth to try and increase the signal-to-noise ratio on STIR imaging. Low matrix means that high-frequency information is not being collected, which is the source of the Gibbs TA.
- Typical locations: Inner table of the skull and CSF interface. Spinal cord and CSF interface.
- Cause: Abrupt transition from very high to very low signal over a very short distance is high-frequency information that must be collected during the MR imaging process in order to be accurately represented. In low-resolution imaging (the matrix is small and/or FOV is large), the collection of high-frequency data is much reduced. The data acquisition is basically "truncated," which results in the Gibbs TA, a periodic overshoot–undershoot in signal intensity immediately adjacent and parallel to a high-signal/low-signal interface.[4]

42.1.6 Companion Case

A 55-year-old man complains of progressive lower extremity weakness and now has trouble climbing stairs.

Imaging Findings and Impression

Numerous flow voids are present that appear punctate and serpentine and are closely applied to the pial surface of the spinal cord. The post contrast image (▶ Fig. 42.2b) shows abnormal enhancement of vessels that extend along the entire extent of the visualized spinal cord.

The T2WIs show edema centrally within the spinal cord and mild expansion of the cord in the second patient (▶ Fig. 42.2c). The edema, however, tapers superiorly and does not extend the entire length of the cord.

The following findings prove that this is a real abnormality rather than the Gibbs TA: lack of involvement of the entire spinal cord; no adjacent, alternating lines of high and low signal; tapering of the abnormal signal within the cord superiorly; subtle expansion of the spinal cord; association of the edema with abnormal flow voids in the subarachnoid space.

Furthermore, the patient had symptoms related to venous congestion and edema in the spinal cord, which are clearly not incidental findings.

Diagnosis: Spinal cord edema due to a DAVF.

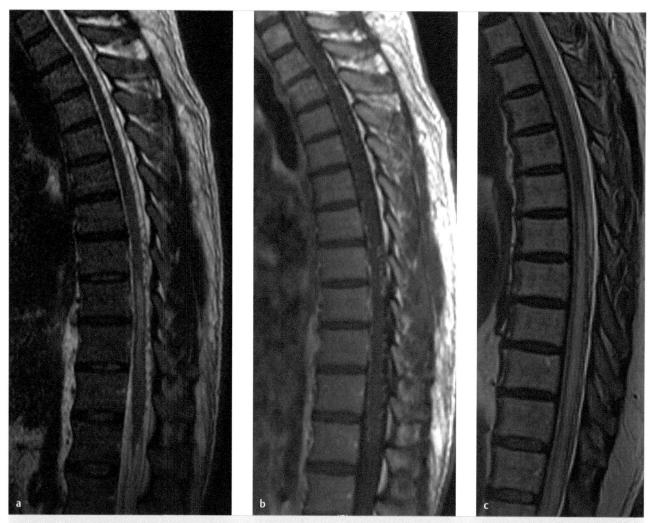

Fig. 42.2 Sagittal T2-weighted **(a)** and T1-weighted postcontrast **(b)** images of the companion case patient. A sagittal T2-weighted image **(c)** from a different patient with the same diagnosis.

42.2 Pulsatile Motion Artifact

42.2.1 Case Presentation

Imaging Findings

Axial T1WI reveals a perfectly round lesion within the L1 vertebral body in the region of the end plate (*asterisk* in ▶ Fig. 42.3).

Review of the axial T1WIs with a larger FOV and wider window reveals not only the round lesion within the vertebral body but also an identical lesion immediately anterior to the aorta (see *arrows* in ▶ Fig. 42.4a,b).

Review of the corresponding location on the sagittal T1WIs fails to identify any abnormality within the vertebral body (▶ Fig. 42.5).

Impression: Artifactual lesion created by aortic pulsations.

Cause: Phase-encoding pulsatile motion artifact.

Solution: Phase-encoding motion artifact has several solutions. However, it is most important to recognize the artifactual nature of the pseudo-lesions as often they do not obscure normal anatomy to the extent that the imaging sequence needs to be altered and repeated.

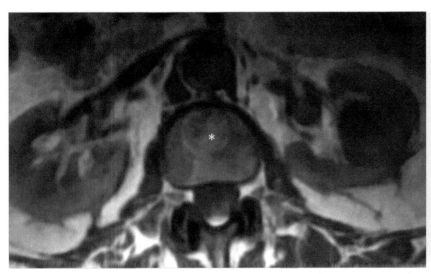

Fig. 42.3 Axial T1-weighted image from a lumbar spine MR of a patient who presents with chronic lower back pain. Interventional radiology consultation has been requested for possible biopsy of the lesion (*asterisk*) that could not be visualized on CT.

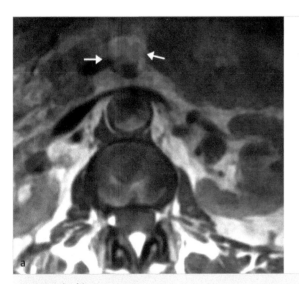
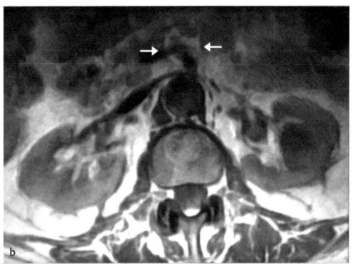

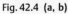

Fig. 42.4 (a, b)

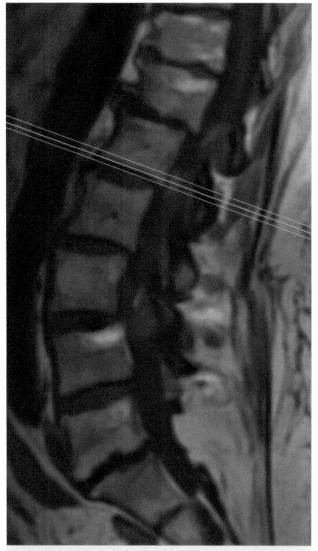

Fig. 42.5

42.2.2 Artifact Problem-Solving: Additional Evaluation or Sequence Modifications Recommended in Difficult Cases

The following techniques may be utilized to decrease or eliminate phase-encoding artifact:

- Swap phase and frequency-encoding directions to result in the phase-encoding motion artifact running in the direction in which it creates the least problem (i.e., running phase right to left for the orbits so that patient eye motion blurs the image in a right-to-left manner rather than obscuring view of the orbital apices).

- Cardiac or pulse-oximeter gating of the acquisition of phase-encoding information.
- Placing saturation bands over the vessels to eliminate signal coming from them.
- Placing saturation bands below the imaging plane to decrease the signal within the arterial blood flowing into the plane. This will also decrease intravascular high signal in the first slice of a series of images (i.e., entry slice phenomenon).
- Gradient moment nulling: Flow compensation gradients may be applied (i.e., flow comp) that help rephase signal within flowing blood and therefore help eliminate the phase error that results in spatial misregistration.
- Utilize the shortest possible imaging sequences (i.e., echo planar type imaging; parallel imaging techniques).
- Utilize special sequences that alter the phase-encoding direction and increase segmentation in a manner that does not allow accumulation of phase error due to either magnetic field inhomogeneity or in-plane motion artifact.

42.2.3 Essential Information: Motion Artifact on MRI Creating Pseudo-Lesions

- Motion artifact occurs in the phase-encoding direction because of the significantly longer amount of time it takes to collect phase change information in comparison to the time needed for frequency encoding, which occurs so quickly that it is unaffected by physiologic motion.
- Phase-encoding motion artifact, if due to random patient motion, will appear as distortion and blurring of the image. If the motion is periodic, such as arterial pulsation in the aorta, discrete "ghosts" of the vessel will appear with their spacing inversely related to the frequency of the pulsation.
- A well-known artifact occurs when aortic pulsation creates a round pseudo-lesion within the vertebral body.
- Widening the window may help identify additional ghosts that occur equally spaced throughout the image and extend beyond normal anatomic boundaries.
- Expect phase-encoding ghosts to occur in a periodic fashion, in line with pulsatile vasculature. Typical locations, in addition to the aorta, include the posterior fossa from the transverse sinus and the brain parenchyma adjacent to the internal cerebral veins/vein of Galen, as well as lateral to the cavernous sinuses, due to the cavernous segments of the carotid arteries.
- It is important to attempt to confirm enhancing lesions in multiple planes when a possible lesion is in line with an area known to be affected by phase-encoding "ghosts." However, it is important to know that if the images were obtained by reformation of a 3D acquisition, the artifact will be present in all three planes. A second, uniplanar, orthogonal acquisition may be necessary.

42.2.4 Companion Case

CSF pulsation into the fourth ventricle on FLAIR results in "ghosting" artifact (see ▸ Fig. 42.6).

Imaging Finding

Axial FLAIR images at the level of the medulla (▸ Fig. 42.6a) and pons (▸ Fig. 42.6b) reveal high signal intensity of the CSF within the fourth ventricle and "lesions" within the cerebellar hemispheres bilaterally (▸ Fig. 42.6a) and the posterolateral aspect of both middle cerebellar peduncles (▸ Fig. 42.6b). Inspection of the image at a wider window reveals similar appearing high-signal "lesions" are also present in the temporal bones (*arrows* in ▸ Fig. 42.6c).

Impression: Pulsation of the high-signal CSF into the fourth ventricle creating artifactual "ghosts."

Cause: The FLAIR sequence suppresses CSF signal with a slice-selective 180-degree RF pulse, followed by a 90-degree RF pulse, which is precisely timed to coincide with the point in the T1 recovery of fluid at which it is crossing the null point. Rapid motion of CSF through the imaging plane not only interferes with it receiving the inversion pulse (because it is slice selective) but also creates a ghosting artifact as motion occurring during the acquisition of the phase-encoding information leads to errors in spatial localization in the phase-encoding direction. Typically, these "ghosts" occur in a periodic fashion, in line with the fourth ventricular focus of high signal. Viewing images at a wider window assists in confirming the artifactual nature of these ghosts as they may be seen to extend beyond normal anatomic boundaries. Similar artifacts in the posterior fossa often occur on postcontrast T1WIs due to the motion of flowing blood within the transverse and sigmoid sinuses.

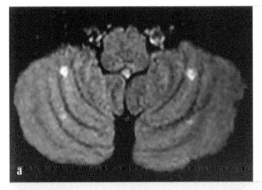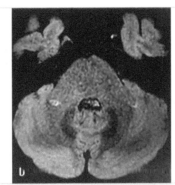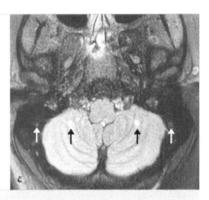

Fig. 42.6 (a–c)

42.3 Slow Flow in Vessels Creating Artifacts on MRI

42.3.1 Case Presentation

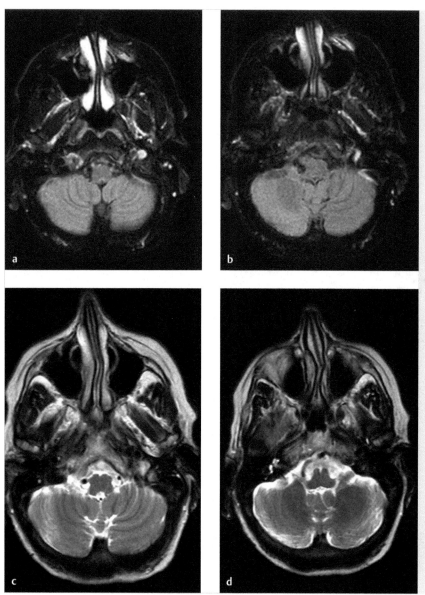

Fig. 42.7 Axial fluid-attenuated inversion recovery (FLAIR) **(a, b)** and T2-weighted **(c, d)** images at the level of the sigmoid sinus and jugular foramen.

History

A 57-year-old woman with persistent daily headache was referred by her primary care physician for a brain MRI without contrast. The radiologist noted: "T2 hyperintensity in the left sigmoid sinus and jugular foramen, which could represent venous sinus thrombosis or a mass lesion. Follow-up recommended."

Diagnosis: Normal skull base. Artifactual high signal in sigmoid sinus and jugular bulb due to slow-flowing blood (see ▶ Table 42.1 for the differential diagnosis; also see ▶ Figs. 42.8 and 42.9).

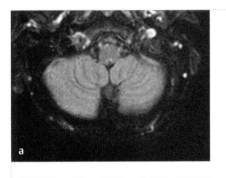
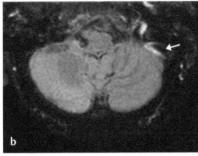
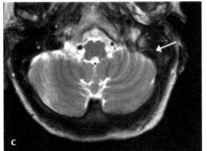
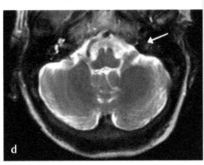

Fig. 42.8 (a–d) On both the fluid-attenuated inversion recovery (FLAIR) sequence and T2-weighted images (T2WIs), there is signal hyperintensity within the left jugular foramen (*long arrow*). On the T2WIs, there is dark signal intensity within the sigmoid sinus. On the FLAIR images, there is bright signal intensity within the sigmoid (*short arrow*). The jugular foramen appears to be normal in size and configuration and the adjacent mastoid and petrous apex are normal.

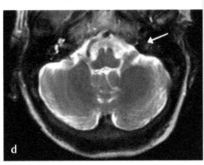

Fig. 42.9 CT of the head with intravenous contrast demonstrates normal opacification of the jugular vein and sigmoid sinus and a normal-sized jugular foramen. There is no evidence of mass lesion or thrombosis, which further confirms the artifactual nature of this incidental finding.

Table 42.1 Differential diagnosis for lesions of the jugular foramen

DDx	Comments
• Artifactual increased signal due to slow-flowing blood	T2 or FLAIR hyperintense signal in otherwise normal-appearing jugular foramen. Foramen appears normal on CT angiography and contrast-enhanced MRI examination. T2 signal may vary based on the imaging plane.
• Glomus tumor of the jugular foramen	Enhancing mass with bony erosion on CT. Salt-and-pepper appearance on T2WIs. Secondary to flow voids within the mass.
• Schwannoma	Homogeneously enhancing mass, bright on T2, with smooth bony remodeling/expansion of the jugular foramen on CT.
• Skull base metastasis	Variably enhancing variable T2 signal mass with bony erosion. Restricted diffusion
• Sigmoid sinus thrombosis	Filling defect, surrounded by contrast on post contrast-enhanced images and dynamic CT angiography. No bony abnormality. Hyperdense on noncontrast CT scan.

42.3.2 Differential Diagnostic Pearls

There are several clues that you are dealing with slow flow and not a thrombosis or lesion on a non–contrast enhanced MRI:

- T2 images are much more likely to have a flow void, so if there is a flow void on T2, the vessel is patent.
- Flow phenomenon is very often based on the plane of section, so if you can see the vessel looking normal in the coronal plane, for instance, then it is probably normal.
- If you see pulsation artifacts related to the vessel, it probably has flow in it.
- Remember to look at the non-contrast CT if it is available. It can be very helpful. Often, putting together all the information from multiple modalities gives one the greatest confidence rather than relying on any one sequence or modality.

42.3.3 Artifact Problem-Solving: Additional Evaluation to Consider in Difficult Cases

- **Recommended:** Contrast-enhanced examination, either CT or MRI. MR venography performed as a first-pass contrast-enhanced examination can be very helpful in this regard and is the optimal examination for excluding venous sinus thrombosis with greatest sensitivity and specificity. Including a standard MRI of the brain with and without contrast is highly recommended.
- **Not recommended:** MR venography without contrast is a bad idea as slow flow will tend to cause a lack of signal and you will still get an ambiguous result.

- **Recommended:** Remember to look at the noncontrast CT if it is available. It can be very helpful.

42.3.4 Essential Facts: Artifacts Produced by Flowing Blood on MRI

- Flow on MRI can produce two different phenomena: flow void and flow-related enhancement.
- Flow-related enhancement is usually caused by unsaturated protons moving into a region where there is relative saturation so that the signal they give off is brighter than the surrounding tissue.
- It is common to see flow-related enhancement in arteries on T1 W GRE sequences such as SPGR, but it can also be seen on FLAIR and T2WIs under certain circumstances, especially when there is slow flow.
- Common sites for this occurrence in the venous system are in the sigmoid sinus, jugular vein, and transverse sinus, where there may be, especially in the supine position, very limited flow in one of the jugular veins due to changes in intrathoracic pressure or mechanics of the subclavian vein and interaction with the aorta. This phenomenon can also be seen in arterial vessels when there is a proximal occlusion and the vessels are being filled such as in acute stroke.
- We also see "enhancement" on FLAIR related to CSF pulsation (see Companion Case in Section 42.2).
- Other common sites for this phenomenon outside the CNS would be the femoral and pelvic veins.

42.3.5 Companion Cases

Companion Case 1: Jugular and Sigmoid Sinus Thrombosis

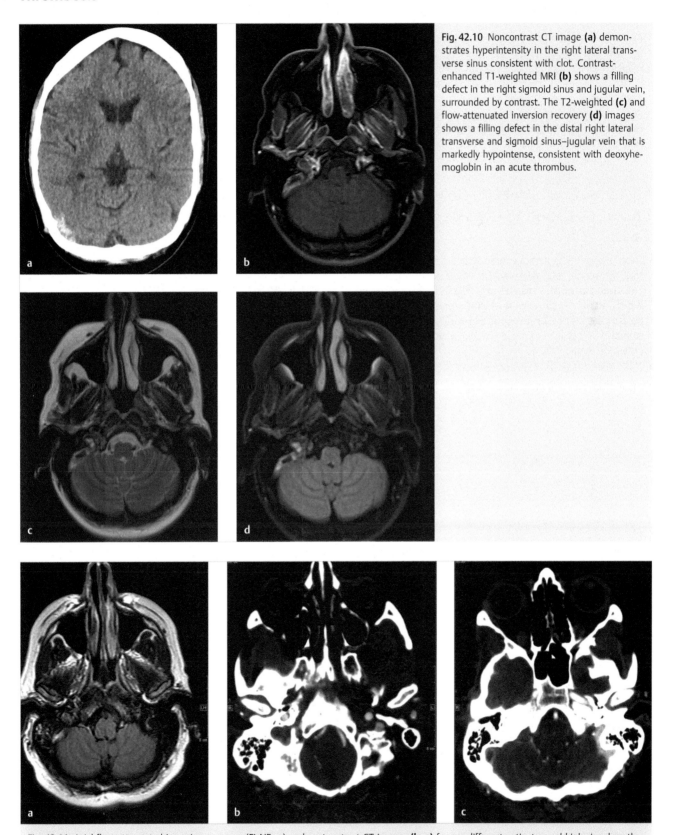

Fig. 42.10 Noncontrast CT image **(a)** demonstrates hyperintensity in the right lateral transverse sinus consistent with clot. Contrast-enhanced T1-weighted MRI **(b)** shows a filling defect in the right sigmoid sinus and jugular vein, surrounded by contrast. The T2-weighted **(c)** and flow-attenuated inversion recovery **(d)** images shows a filling defect in the distal right lateral transverse and sigmoid sinus–jugular vein that is markedly hypointense, consistent with deoxyhemoglobin in an acute thrombus.

Fig. 42.11 Axial flow-attenuated inversion recovery (FLAIR; **a**) and postcontrast CT images **(b, c)** from a different patient reveal high signal on the FLAIR image in the right transverse, sigmoid sinus, and jugular vein **(a)** and a filling defect demonstrated on CT angiography in the sigmoid sinus **(b)** and right transverse sinus **(c)** consistent with thrombus.

Companion Case 2: Skull Base Metastasis

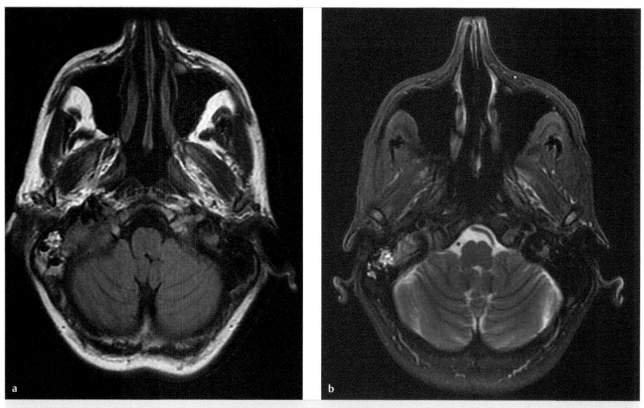

Fig. 42.12 Axial flow-attenuated inversion recovery **(a)** and fast spin echo T2-weighted **(b)** images reveal abnormal marrow signal in the temporal bone in which there is also a mastoid effusion. The jugular vein contains a flow void, but is small and anteriorly displaced in this patient with skull base metastasis.

Companion Case 3: Jugular Foramen Schwannoma

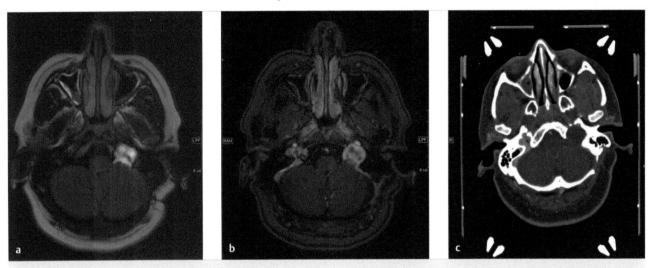

Fig. 42.13 Axial flow-attenuated inversion recovery **(a)** and postcontrast T1-weighted **(b)** images reveal a hyperintense, contrast-enhancing mass in the left jugular foramen, which smoothly expands the foramen. An arterial phase CT angiogram **(c)** does not show any enhancement. The CT demonstrates the smooth expansion of the jugular foramen by this schwannoma.

Companion Case 4: Glomus Jugulare Tumor

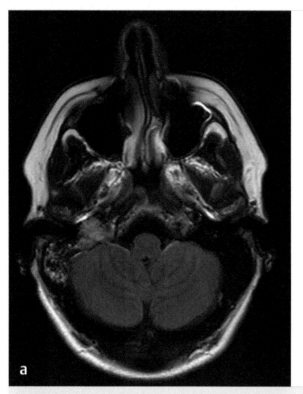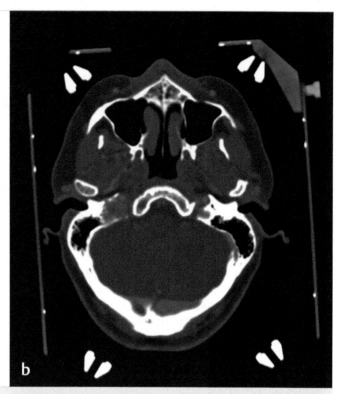

Fig. 42.14 Axial flow-attenuated inversion recovery (FLAIR) image **(a)** and contrast-enhanced CT scan **(b)** reveal hyperintense signal on the FLAIR image in the region of the right jugular foramen. Contrast-enhanced CT demonstrates an enhancing mass lesion associated with irregular bony erosion and expansion of the foramen consistent with a glomus tumor.

42.4 Random Patient Motion

42.4.1 Case Presentation

Imaging Finding

Axial FLAIR image of the brain (▶ Fig. 42.15) in a disoriented patient who had difficulty lying still for the examination shows evidence of patient motion. Curvilinear bands of alternating low- and high-signal intensity, which are partial replicas of the skull and subcutaneous fat, extend into the region of the brain and also outside of the head. This artifact partially obscures the patient's right subdural hematoma, as shown better on the CT scan in ▶ Fig. 42.16.

Possible solutions: Considerations include sedation, if medically possible, for patients who are unable to lie still for MR imaging. If sedation is contraindicated or is undesirable, especially in the pediatric population, "fast brain" protocols may be utilized, which significantly decrease imaging time, commonly to under 2 minutes. They typically employ ultrafast fast spin echo/turbo spin echo techniques to acquire T2WIs and echo planar techniques to obtain diffusion-weighted imaging (DWI) sequences and T2* images.

Parallel imaging techniques are now widely available and have significantly decreased imaging time by having multiple receiver coils, which are sensitive to only a portion of the body part being imaged, collecting a reduced number of phase-encoded signal. The signal from each coil is then recombined, based on the calculated sensitivity of each coil, which has the possibility of creating some very unusual motion and aliasing artifacts that are challenging to recognize (see Chapter 43, Companion Cases 1 and 2).

Motion artifact may be decreased by use of a special imaging sequence in which the direction of the phase-encoding gradients changes periodically throughout image acquisition. Rectangular, parallel blades of phase-encoding lines rotate and change direction periodically (PROPELLER: periodically rotated overlapping parallel lines with enhanced reconstruction) and are centered in the middle of k-space. This method of k-space data collection provides oversampling of the most important, central, region of k-space, which determines the signal-to-noise ratio and contrast within the image. Non-Cartesian, multisegmented collection of k-space data prevents accumulation of phase errors, especially those due to in-plane motion, and also increases imaging time and does not correct through plane motion. Propeller DWI has the additional value of mitigating the severe susceptibility artifact that occurs on DWI-type imaging in the posterior fossa near the skull base and petrous apices that may obscure small acute brainstem infarctions. It also has the specific clinical application for detection of middle ear region cholesteatomas, primary and recurrent, due to its improved visualization of the temporal bones on a diffusion-weighted sequence.[4]

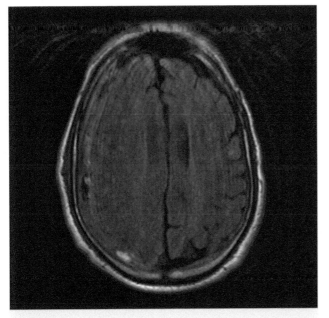

Fig. 42.15

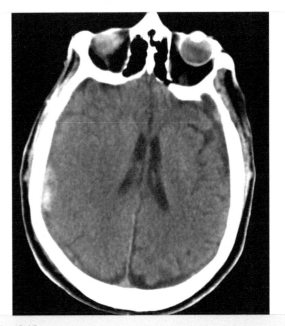

Fig. 42.16

Companion Case

Patient with a history of neck pain after a minor fall from a height of less than 5 feet undergoes a cervical spine CT. The patient's physical examination was normal.

Cause: Gross patient motion during the scan resulted in posterior repositioning of the patient's neck for the scan and subsequent artifactual malalignment on the sagittal reformation which simulated bilateral facet dislocation and anterior subluxation of C3 on C4. The scout images should always be reviewed when interpreting a CT scan. Source images should always be reviewed rather than relying on multiplanar reformations. Gross patient motion is best appreciated at air–soft-tissue interfaces on the sagittal reformations and should be confirmed on the axial source images. Even though this finding was obviously artifactual, the scan should be repeated if possible as motion artifact degrades the quality of the exam and may obscure real abnormalities.

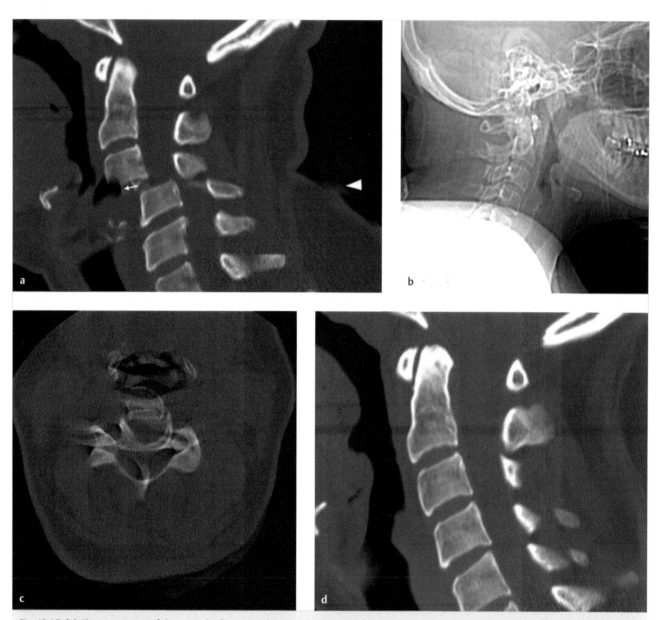

Fig. 42.17 **(a)** Close inspection of the sagittal reformation shows, in the exact axial plane of the apparent dislocation, nonanatomic malalignment of the tracheal air column (*white arrow*) and subcutaneous soft-tissue interface with air posterior to the neck (*white arrowhead*). **(b)** Review of the scout image for the cervical spine CT reveals normal alignment between C3 and C4. **(c)** Review of axial source images confirms severe patient motion was occurring at the moment the C3–C4 disc space level was being imaged. **(d)** Immediate repeat of the cervical spine CT reveals no abnormality and normal alignment.

References

[1] Küker W, Weller M, Klose U, Krapf H, Dichgans J, Nägele T. Diffusion-weighted MRI of spinal cord infarction. J Neurol. 2004; 251(7):818–824

[2] Petit-Lacour MC, Lasjaunias P, Iffenecker C, et al. Visibility of the central canal on MRI. Neuroradiology. 2000; 42(10):756–761

[3] Holly LT, Batzdorf U. Slitlike syrinx cavities: a persistent central canal. J Neurosurg. 2002; 97(2) Suppl:161–165

[4] Questions and Answers in MRI. Available at: www.mriquestions.com.

[5] Riccioli LA, Marliani AF, Ghedin P, Agati R, Leonardi M. CE-MR angiography at 3.0 T magnetic field in the study of spinal dural arteriovenous fistula. Preliminary results. Interv Neuroradiol. 2007; 13(1):13–18

[6] Kannath SK, Alampath P, Enakshy Rajan J, Thomas B, Sankara Sarma P, Tirur Raman K. Utility of 3D SPACE T2-weighted volumetric sequence in the localization of spinal dural arteriovenous fistula. J Neurosurg Spine. 2016; 25(1): 125–132

[7] Morris JM, Kaufmann TJ, Campeau NG, Cloft HJ, Lanzino G. Volumetric myelographic magnetic resonance imaging to localize difficult-to-find spinal dural arteriovenous fistulas. J Neurosurg Spine. 2011; 14(3):398–404

[8] Krings T, Geibprasert S. Spinal dural arteriovenous fistulas. AJNR Am J Neuroradiol. 2009; 30(4):639–648

43 Magnetic Susceptibility–Related Artifacts on MRI

Clark W. Sitton, Alexander B. Simonetta, and Kaye D. Westmark

43.1 General Magnetic Susceptibility–Related Artifacts

43.1.1 Case 1 Presentation

A patient with a history of ventriculoperitoneal shunt presents with a headache. After a lateral skull film was obtained to evaluate the shunt valve and type, a brain MRI was performed.

43.1.2 Imaging Findings

The lateral view of the skull reveals a Strata NSC valve (▶ Fig. 43.1).

The MR images (▶ Fig. 43.2) reveal marked loss of signal on these T2-weighted images (T2WIs) due to substantial dephasing of signal that results from magnetic susceptibility artifact generated by the metallic portion of the valve. The artifact is substantially worse on susceptibility weighted imaging (SWI; ▶ Fig. 43.2b) than it is on the fast spin echo (FSE) T2WIs (▶ Fig. 43.2a) due to multiple rephasing 180-degree radiofrequency (RF) pulses in the latter sequence, which refocuses spins that have been dephased. The fluid-attenuated inversion recovery (FLAIR) sequence images (▶ Fig. 43.2c) are particularly vulnerable to local field inhomogeneity as the 180-degree inversion pulse is slice and therefore frequency specific. Artifactual loss of cerebrospinal fluid (CSF) suppression adjacent to the posterior aspect of the right middle frontal gyrus (*arrow* in ▶ Fig. 43.2c) is seen some distance cranially from the shunt valve as the presence of the metallic valve exerts its influence on magnetic field homogeneity far beyond the images on which it is present.

Cause: Magnetic susceptibility artifact due to metallic shunt components.

43.1.3 Essential Facts about Magnetic Susceptibility Artifacts in MR Imaging (www.MRIquestions.com)

- The signal intensity of any given tissue depends upon many factors including proton density, T1 and T2 of the tissue, echo time (TE) and TR (repetition time) of the imaging sequence, and local magnetic field homogeneity.
- The signal intensity of tissues is markedly influenced by local magnetic field inhomogeneity especially on T2WIs that are of the gradient recalled echo (GRE) type of sequence as opposed to spin echo–type sequences.

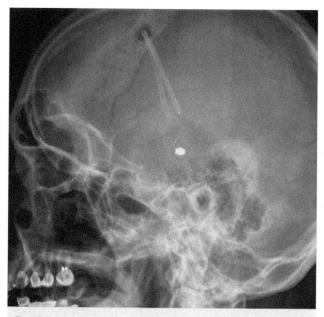

Fig. 43.1

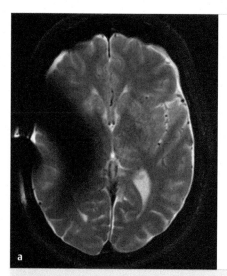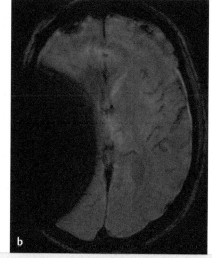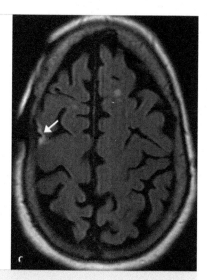

Fig. 43.2 (a–c)

- GRE, MPGR, SPGR, most echo planar, diffusion-weighted images (DWIs), and SWI are sequences that are particularly susceptible to loss of signal when there is an inhomogeneous magnetic field.
- Substances with unpaired electrons in their outer shell (deoxyhemoglobin, methemoglobin, ferritin, hemosiderin, Fe, Ni, Co) locally augment the magnetic field strength, which leads to field inhomogeneity and therefore a difference in frequency of the spin of protons. This leads not only to loss of phase, which means there will be a significant decrease in signal intensity on T2WIs, but also to incorrect spatial localization of signal. Misregistration of detected signal whose frequency has been altered by magnetic susceptibility artifact typically results in bright lines from signal "pile-up" and dark lines, due to signal being displaced.
- Bone–air or soft tissue/bone–air interfaces also distort the local magnetic field and result in similar artifacts.
- Although metal artifact may not be completely eliminated on MRI, the following techniques may reduce its effect:
  – View-angle tilting.
  – Using thinner slices.
  – Using higher bandwidth imaging.
  – Lower field strength magnet.
  – Using short tau inversion recovery (STIR) rather than chemical fat saturation techniques.
  – Use of FSE technique and avoidance of GRE-type imaging.

43.1.4 Companion Cases

Companion Case 1: The Use of Metal Suppression Techniques in MRI to Reduce Metal Artifacts

History

Brain MRI was obtained for the evaluation of headaches in a patient with a metallic pellet present in the ethmoid sinus.

Imaging Findings

Sagittal T1WI (▶ Fig. 43.3a) reveals substantial dephasing artifact that obliterates visualization of the paranasal sinuses even on the FSE-T2WIs (▶ Fig. 43.3b,c).

Sagittal T1WI (▶ Fig. 43.4**a**) from a different patient's brain MRI performed on the same magnet shows substantially worse artifact than that present in the first patient's images (▶ Fig. 43.3) due to a nonremovable dental appliance. However, use of metal

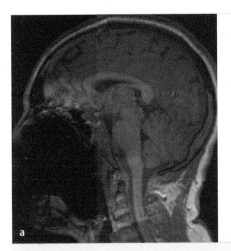
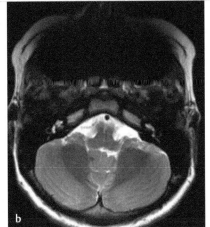
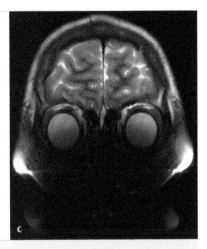

Fig. 43.3 (a–c)

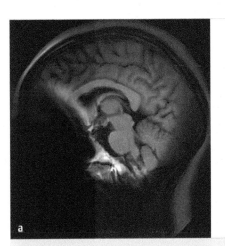
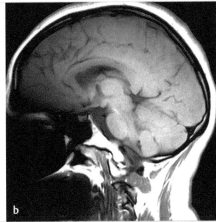
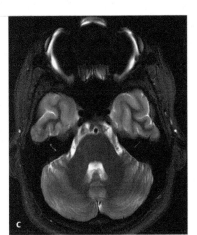

Fig. 43.4 (a–c)

suppression techniques dramatically reduces the metallic associated artifact on the repeat sagittal T1WI (▶ Fig. 43.4b) and also on the axial FSE-T2WI (▶ Fig. 43.4c).

Companion Case 2: Pigmented Cosmetics May Result in MRI Artifacts

History

Young woman's brain MRI plus special views of the orbits was ordered for a history of headache and blurred vision.

Imaging Findings

The MRI technologist noted magnetic susceptibility artifact present in association with the patient's eyelids on the brain MRI (▶ Fig. 43.5) prior to the orbit-specific images. The patient confirmed that, as she had indicated on the MRI screening form, she did not have either tattooed eyeliner or gold weights implanted for facial nerve injury. She was, however, wearing heavy purple eyeliner that she subsequently removed, and the scan was repeated showing elimination of this artifact (▶ Fig. 43.6a,b).

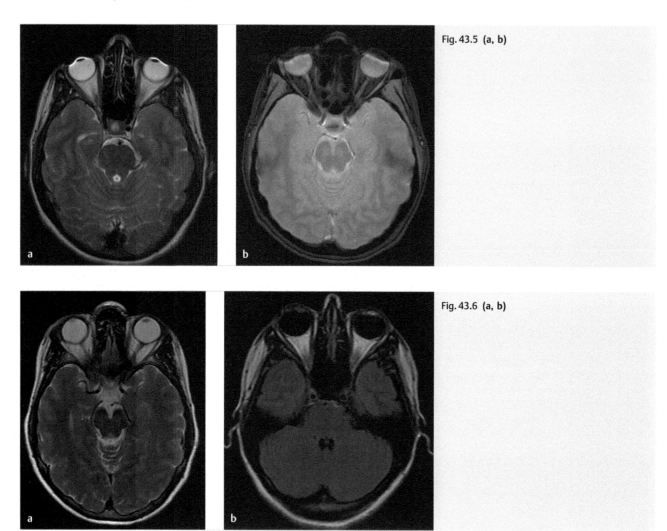

Fig. 43.5 (a, b)

Fig. 43.6 (a, b)

Companion Case 3: Large, Extensively Pneumatized Sinuses and Petrous Apices May Increase Bone–Soft Tissue/Air Interface Related Susceptibility Artifact

History

Brain MRI was obtained for possible microvascular ischemic disease in an older male patient.

Imaging Findings

Extensive signal abnormality is seen throughout the pons on the T2WIs (▶ Fig. 43.7a,b).

The DWIs were significantly distorted and evaluation was limited due to bilateral pneumatized petrous apices and a large, aerated sphenoid sinus. Distortion of the image occurs and appears to de-form the pons due to spatial misregistration (▶ Fig. 43.7c).

Companion Case 4: Prominent Calcification in the Falx Creates False-Positive Restricted Diffusion, Worrisome for "Acute Bilateral ACA Territory Infarction" on DWI

History

MRI was performed for episode of dizziness in an elderly patient (▶ Fig. 43.8).

Imaging Findings

The brain MRI was normal for age with the exception of high signal seen in the medial aspect of the superior frontal gyri bilaterally (*arrows* in ▶ Fig. 43.8) adjacent to the falx. The T2 and FLAIR images, however, were completely normal with the exception of very low signal seen in a thickened falx. The patient had a CT scan performed earlier the same day (▶ Fig. 43.9).

The noncontrast head CT (▶ Fig. 43.9) shows that prominent calcification accounts for the thickened, black falx on the MRI.

Review of the apparent diffusion coefficient (ADC) map from the brain MRI (▶ Fig. 43.10) reveals marked low signal in the region of the falcine calcification, but there was no evidence of decrease in signal in the frontal lobe cortex to suggest real restricted diffusion.

DWIs are typically created by spin echo, echo planar imaging with strong diffusion gradients. Echo planar imaging significantly decreases imaging time in order to "freeze" patient physiological motion but is extremely sensitive to magnetic field inhomogeneity, which can cause image distortion, loss of signal, and artifactual areas of high signal that have been spatially displaced. The region of the skull base is particularly affected due to air/soft tissue/bone interfaces, which create local magnetic field heterogeneity. In this case, the dense calcification of the falx next to the brain and CSF create artifactual high signal on the DWI within the adjacent frontal lobe cortex due to magnetic susceptibility artifact. As no true restriction of diffusion was present in the brain parenchyma, the ADC map did not show a corresponding decrease in signal within the cortex. The ADC calculations in regions of very low signal on the T2WI, in this case, the falcine calcification, are unreliable.[1]

In cases of acute ischemia due to infarction, extracellular water is trapped inside cells, which restricts the water molecules' ability to diffuse. This abnormal restriction of diffusion shows up as high signal on a DWI.

A well-known pitfall of DWI may occur because the images are inherently T2 weighted. Therefore, areas that are hyperintense on the T2WIs may "shine through" and create artifactual increase in signal on DWI that is not due to restricted diffusion within the tissue. Therefore, to accurately interpret increased signal on DWIs, the radiologist must correlate DWI findings with the ADC map.

Likewise, tissues with extremely low signal on T2WIs may create "T2 blackout" and falsely appear as regions of increased diffusion.[1]

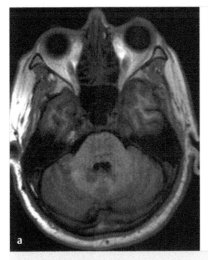 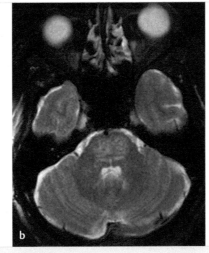 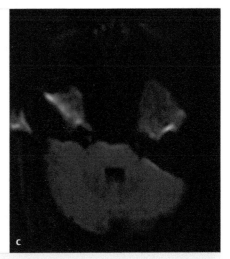

Fig. 43.7 (a–c) Companion Case 3.

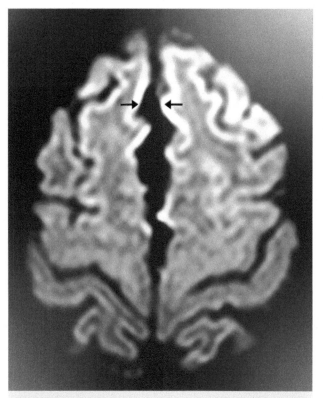

Fig. 43.8 Companion Case 4. Axial diffusion-weighted image.

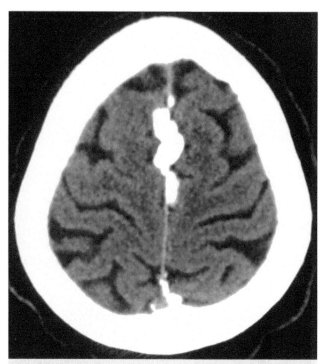

Fig. 43.9 Companion Case 4. Noncontrast head CT.

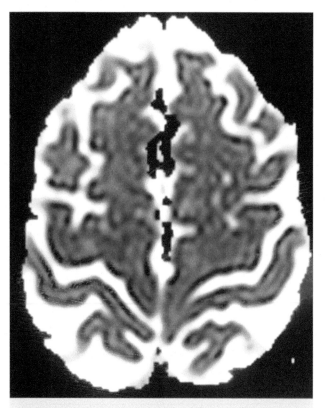

Fig. 43.10 Companion Case 4. Apparent diffusion coefficient map.

43.2 Vascular Stent Artifacts

43.2.1 History

This 58-year-old man is referred for further imaging evaluation with a history of transient left facial numbness and a history of carotid disease. Outside imaging report states there is severe stenosis or occlusion of the right internal carotid artery (ICA) (▶ Fig. 43.11).

43.2.2 Imaging Findings

Maximum intensity projection (MIP) of a 2D time-of-flight (TOF) MR angiography (MRA) demonstrates a complete lack of signal between the distal common carotid (*arrowhead* in ▶ Fig. 43.12) artery and the mid-ICA (*long arrow* in ▶ Fig. 43.12). There is also a gap between the common carotid artery and the external carotid artery (ECA; *short arrow* in ▶ Fig. 43.12).

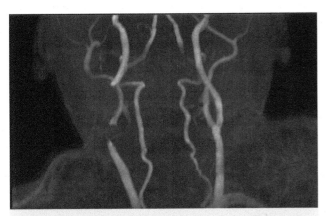

Fig. 43.11 Maximum intensity projection image from a 2D time-of-flight MR angiography.

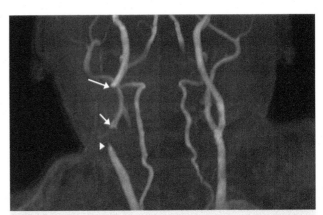

Fig. 43.12

43.2.3 Differential Diagnosis

- Artifact due to the presence of a carotid stent:
  - There is abrupt loss of signal at the proximal aspect of the stent, which reappears at the distal termination of the stent.
  - If robust flow signal is seen distal to the stent, it is almost certainly patent.
  - On axial images, the stent and its lumen demonstrate markedly decreased signal intensity on all pulse sequences.
  - Similar behavior is seen with intracranial stents and coils adjacent to the vessel lumen.
- Chronic carotid occlusion with backfilling of the ICA from the intracranial circulation:
  - Abrupt cutoff of the vessel lumen at the point of occlusion.
  - No significant distal signal in the ICA.
  - MRA of the head demonstrates very weak or absent signal in the carotid siphon and either weak or absent signal in the ipsilateral MCA distribution depending on the strength of intracranial collaterals.
- Severe carotid artery stenosis:
  - Stenosis of between 90 and 95% can produce apparent gaps in the MIP image of the carotid artery.
  - Careful inspection of the source images will generally reveal some signal in the residual lumen, and there is signal in ICA distal to the flow gap indicating patency.
  - There is never retrograde filling of the ICA on a 2D TOF MRI due to a traveling, superiorly placed saturation band.
  - If the stenosis is flow limiting, there may be decreased signal intensity in the ipsilateral intracranial MRA images.

43.2.4 Imaging Impression

Artifact related to carotid stenting. Robust signal within the vessel distal to the area of signal loss suggests that the stent is, in fact, patent.

Cause: Magnetic susceptibility artifact due to the presence of the stent.

Artifact Problem-Solving: Additional Testing to Consider

- **Recommended:** Contrast-enhanced CT examination. Contrast opacification can generally visualize the inner lumen of the stent if it is patent (▸ Fig. 43.13).
- **Not recommended:** MRI or MRA with contrast. Similar artifacts will be present.
- **Not recommended:** Doppler examination. Evaluation of flow within the stent lumen can be difficult secondary to luminal calcification and reflections from the stent itself.

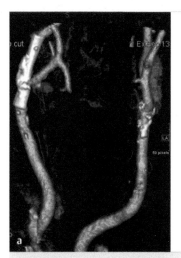 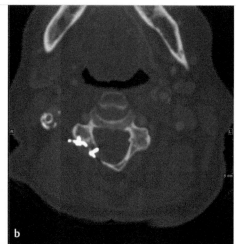 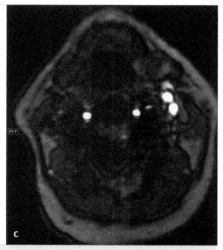

Fig. 43.13 Follow-up imaging using CT angiography was performed and illustrated the stent spanning the distal common carotid artery and extending into the proximal internal carotid artery. There is opacification of contrast in the stent lumen identified on axial images, and there is clearly continued flow through the stent into the external carotid artery origin. 3D reconstruction **(a)** demonstrates the stent location, corresponding exactly to the area of signal loss on the MRI. Axial reconstruction **(b)** demonstrates the stent inside the calcified vessel wall with opacification of the stent lumen by contrast. Cross-section from the MRI examination **(c)** reveals marked hypointensity related to susceptibility artifact in the region of the stent with complete loss of flow-related signal.

43.2.5 Essential Information regarding Stent-Related Artifacts

- Although most modern stents, aneurysm clips, and intravascular coils are MRI safe, they still create highly localized signal loss related to magnetic susceptibility effects.
- This is more exaggerated on gradient echo images, which form the basis for most MRA techniques, but can be seen to some degree on nearly every pulse sequence.
- The stent does not result in saturation of the spins, so signal intensity of the flow distal to the stent is less affected.

43.2.6 Common Artifactual Phenomenon Simulating Abnormalities on 2D TOF MRA

- Motion artifact: Projection images from either 2D MRA or CTA are made from stacks of axial images. Any motion of the artery occurring between slice acquisitions will result in irregularity of the vessel contour, sometimes appearing as a horizontal band of signal loss.
- In-plane flow: 2D TOF images are most sensitive to flow occurring perpendicular to the plane of imaging and least sensitive to in-plane flow. Flow occurring in the plane, in the x- or y-axis, rather than the z-axis, does not produce strong flow-related enhancement and thus appears as an area of signal loss. This is often apparent at the ICA origin, which is horizontal in orientation in relation to the common carotid artery. This also occurs in the vertebral arteries at the V2–V3 and V3–V4 junctions. This phenomenon is not observed on 3D TOF imaging or on contrast-enhanced MRA.
- Turbulent flow: Multidirectional or nonlaminar turbulent flow generated by vascular bifurcations and vessel kinking can produce signal loss on 2D TOF imaging, essentially related to in-plane flow within the vessel lumen, although the vessel itself is coursing perpendicular to the imaging plane. There is often a characteristic signet ring appearance on the source images with signal loss in the vessel lumen but signal preservation along the vessel margin where laminar flow is preserved. This artifact is eliminated by 3D TOF MRA and contrast-enhanced techniques.

43.2.7 Companion Cases

Companion Case 1: Chronic Carotid Artery Occlusion

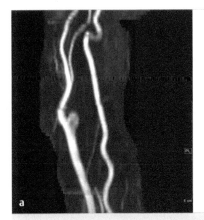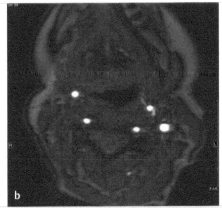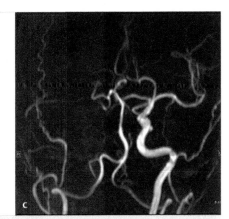

Fig. 43.14 (a–c) MRA reveals chronic occlusion of the carotid artery near its origin with turbulent flow in the stump and no distal flow on intracranial or extracranial imaging. Intracranial collaterals, if present, lack sufficient velocity to produce flow-related enhancement.

Companion Case 2: Critical Internal Carotid Artery Stenosis

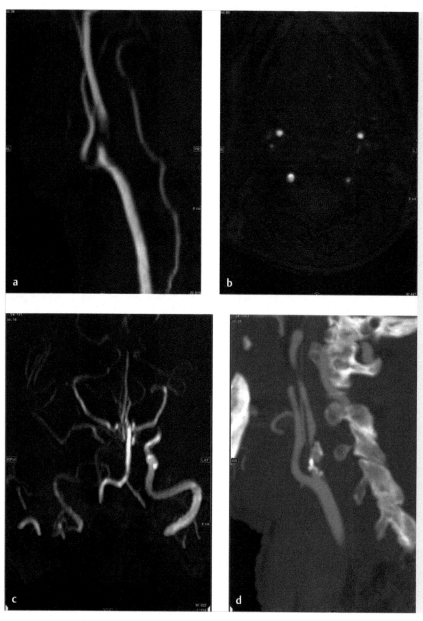

Fig. 43.15 Maximum intensity projection images of to the time-of-flight angiography **(a)** demonstrate a gap in the internal carotid artery (ICA) signal. Axial images from the same examination **(b)** demonstrate a tiny residual lumen. Intracranial 3D, flight MR angiography **(c)** reveals decreased flow velocity in the ICA with decreased signal intensity compared to the contralateral side. CT angiography **(d)** better demonstrates the anatomy of a complex plaque with critical stenosis and a submillimeter residual lumen.

Companion Case 3: Aneurysm Clip

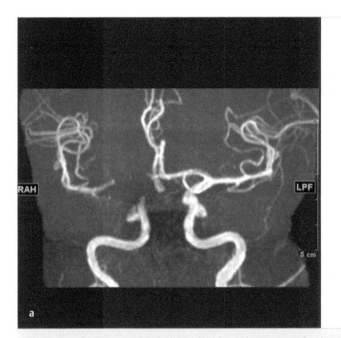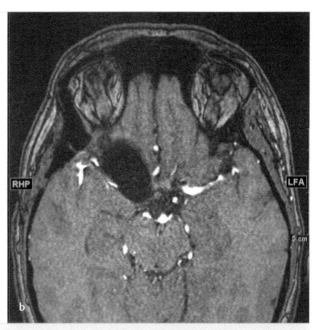

Fig. 43.16 (a, b) 3D time-of-flight MRA of the brain demonstrates focal signal loss secondary to an aneurysm clip. Note the complete loss of signal in the area on the source images, which creates an artifactual gap on the maximum intensity projection images.

Companion Case 4: Middle Cerebral Artery Stent

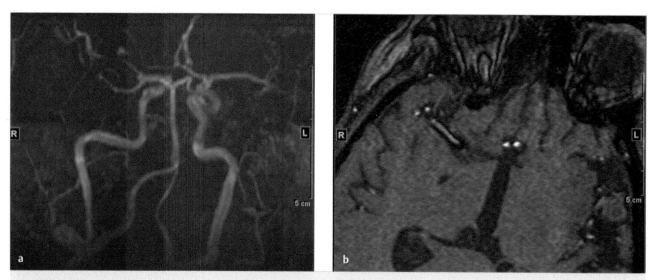

Fig. 43.17 (a, b) 3D time-of-flight MRA of the brain reveals signal loss in the region of the right middle cerebral artery where a stent is present. Note incomplete suppression of the signal by the stent due to its extremely low mass.

Companion Case 5: Artifactual Signal Loss due to In-Plane Flow on 2D MRA

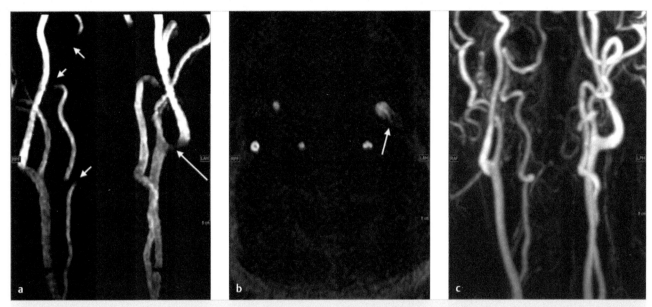

Fig. 43.18 2D time-of-flight maximum intensity projection **(a)** demonstrates signal loss secondary to in-plane flow in the horizontal portions of the internal carotid artery origin (*long arrow*) and right vertebral artery (*short arrows*). Axial images **(b)** demonstrate typical signal loss related to in-plane or turbulent flow on axial images. Contrast-enhanced MR angiography **(c)** demonstrates normal appearance of all vessels.

Companion Case 6: Motion Artifact due to Swallowing or Vascular Pulsation

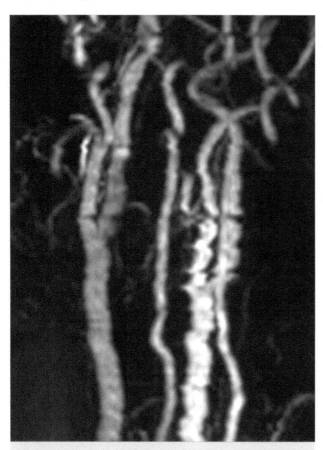

Fig. 43.19 2D time-of-flight MRA maximum intensity projection is degraded by typical motion artifact due to swallowing and/or vascular pulsation, which results in horizontal areas of irregularity and signal loss in the carotid arteries. Note that the vertebral arteries are not as affected, as their motion is restricted by the transverse foramina.

Reference

[1] Questions and Answers in MRI. Available at: https://mriquestions.com/index.html

44 MRI Technical and Sequence-Specific Artifacts

Alexander B. Simonetta, Seferino Romo, and Kaye D. Westmark

44.1 Pulse Sequence–Specific Artifacts: FLAIR

44.1.1 Case 1 Presentation

Lack of cerebrospinal fluid (CSF) suppression on fluid-attenuated inversion recovery (FLAIR) mimicking subarachnoid space abnormality (hemorrhage, meningitis, mass).

44.1.2 Imaging Findings

Axial FLAIR image (▶ Fig. 44.1a) through the posterior fossa reveals increased signal in the CSF of the prepontine cistern, anterior to the cerebellar hemispheres bilaterally and within the fourth ventricle. This CSF hyperintensity results from the incomplete suppression of signal due to the presence of a metallic pellet within the left ethmoid air cells (▶ Fig. 44.1b). Marked signal loss is seen in the immediate vicinity of the pellet due to magnetic susceptibility artifact. The artifact persists well superior to the inciting metallic object and mimics subarachnoid hemorrhage

(SAH) in the region of the frontal lobes at the vertex (▶ Fig. 44.1c). Additional images from the patient's brain MRI are shown in ▶ Fig. 44.2.

Impression: Normal brain MRI. The hyperintense CSF on FLAIR imaging is an artifact created by the presence of a metallic foreign body in the ethmoid sinus.

44.1.3 Differential Diagnosis of Subarachnoid FLAIR Hyperintensity

- **Artifactual hyperintensity:**
  - Magnetic susceptibility artifact.
  - Vascular pulsation or CSF flow artifact: Although this can occur on any pulse sequence, the FLAIR sequence is markedly affected by this artifact especially in the region of the foramen of Monro and in the posterior fossa.
  - Gadolinium: In renal dysfunction or in cases of delayed imaging after contrast administration in patients who have blood–brain barrier disruption, gadolinium may leak into the CSF space and simulate SAH or meningitis.

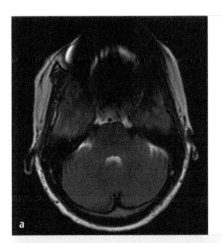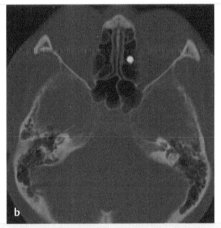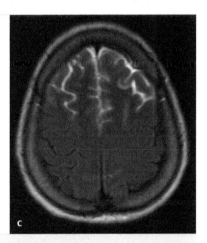

Fig. 44.1 (a–c) A 30-year-old woman with brain MRI performed for new onset of headaches. Axial FLAIR images are shown.

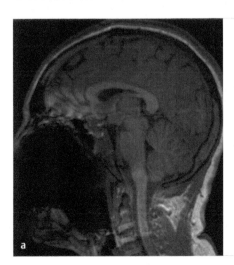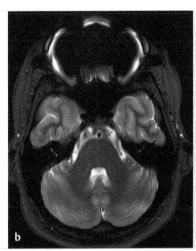

Fig. 44.2 Sagittal T1WI **(a)** shows signal loss from the metallic pellet is creating artifactual T1 shortening, which extends up into the region of the frontal lobes. Axial FSE-T2WI **(b)** reveals the metal pellet is causing local frequency alterations that lead to signal loss centrally from T2 shortening (dephasing) and piling up of signal (bright ring) as the signal is misplaced peripherally.[1] The FSE-T2 W sequence typically shows the least distortion of all the pulse sequences due to its multiple 180-degree refocusing pulses that help correct local magnetic field heterogeneity.

– One-hundred percent oxygen inhalation, but not found in those receiving 50% oxygen.[2]

– Moderate to severe motion artifact.

- True pathologic causes:
  – SAH.
  – Meningitis.
  – Meningeal carcinomatosis.
  – Melanocytosis; melanomatosis.
  – Ruptured dermoid.
  – Moyamoya disease—"ivy sign."[3]
  – Acute stroke—pathologic vascular prominence on FLAIR.

44.1.4 Pearls and Pitfalls of FLAIR Imaging

- An increase in signal on FLAIR sequences, which is artifactual, will often cross normal anatomic boundaries and fail to have expected associated findings on other sequences.
- Increased signal of the CSF on FLAIR that is due to SAH or meningitis is typically very subtle. When it is due to lack of CSF nulling from metal artifact, the signal is most often very hyperintense and involves the entirety of the region affected in a very "nonanatomic" manner.
- Examine the entire study for the presence of metallic artifact to see if the increased in CSF signal may be related.
- Clinical correlation is very important. Always consider the possibility of a true pathological condition, such as SAH or meningitis, in a patient with a metallic foreign body that may falsely lead one to assume the increased signal on FLAIR imaging is artifactual. Artifacts may conceal real pathology!
- Increased signal of the CSF due to inhalation of 100% oxygen, as often occurs in patients under general anesthesia (GA) for MRI, may result in diffuse increase in CSF signal on FLAIR that is indistinguishable from that due to meningitis or very diffuse SAH. Focal enhancing areas of the leptomeninges or dura and/or loculated CSF collections, cortical edema, and mass effect would obviously suggest an infectious etiology although their absence does not exclude it. Clinical correlation must be made.
- Normal pulsatile CSF motion results in lack of its suppression on FLAIR images and resulting areas of increased signal within the CSF. Typical areas affected include the lateral and third ventricles adjacent to the foramen of Monro and the prepontine and ambient cisterns as well as the fourth ventricle.

44.1.5 Essential Facts about FLAIR Imaging

- The FLAIR sequence is a heavily T2WI that has an initial inversion recovery pulse to null the CSF signal.[1]
- Nulling of CSF signal results in increased sensitivity for edema or increased water content in the brain, particularly at CSF interfaces such as the periventricular region and cortex.
- However, FLAIR is not used in spine imaging due to excessive CSF pulsatility artifacts.
- The inversion time (TI) is defined as the time between the initial 180-degree inversion pulse and the time of the 90-degree RF pulse, which converts any existing longitudinal magnetization into transverse magnetization.
- In inversion recovery sequences, the TI is chosen in such a way that any tissue whose longitudinal magnetization is at the null point at the time of the 90-degree RF pulse will not generate any signal, hence fluid signal suppression in FLAIR or fat signal suppression in STIR sequences.
- Factors that alter the T1 recovery time of CSF result in lack of its suppression:
  – Increased protein content in the CSF due to SAH or meningitis, whether carcinomatous or infectious, may decrease the T1 recovery time and result in increased signal on FLAIR.
  – Substances with a short T1 appear bright on FLAIR, that is, fat and gadolinium enhancement.
  – Gadolinium results in a shift to the left of the T1 recovery curve for water protons so affected by its presence and therefore generates higher signal on FLAIR images.
  – Postgadolinium, FLAIR imaging is superior for the detection of meningitis compared with conventional postcontrast T1WIs as there is very little, if any, normal cortical venous enhancement on FLAIR images, which improves confidence that leptomeningeal enhancement is abnormal.
  – Oxygen is weakly paramagnetic and, therefore, when in high concentration in the subarachnoid space, it may result in shortening of the CSF T1 recovery curve.
- The initial inversion pulse is slice selective and therefore frequency specific:
  – Patient motion or CSF pulsatility between the time of the inversion pulse and the echo acquisition may result in lack of complete CSF suppression.
  – Magnetic susceptibility artifact creating local magnetic field inhomogeneity results in differences in frequency, which often results in lack of CSF suppression.

44.1.6 Companion Cases

Companion Case 1: Confirmed Case of Meningitis with Abnormalities on the FLAIR Imaging Sequence

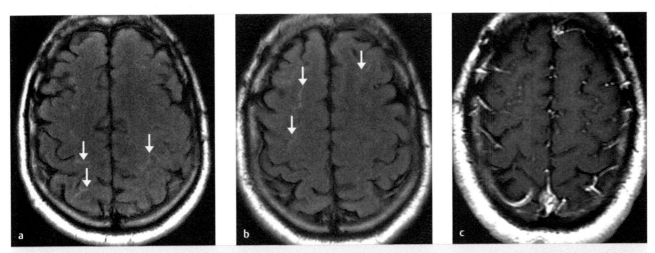

Fig. 44.3 Axial FLAIR images of the brain at the high convexities **(a, b)** reveal very focal areas of increased signal in the sulci in this patient with recent *Staphylococcus* sepsis and meningitis. Routine postcontrast T1WI **(c)** reveals very subtle enhancement that could easily be overlooked and attributed to the enhancement of normal cortical veins. Close correlation with the location of the more obvious FLAIR hyperintensity increases confidence that the enhancement is pathological and due to meningitis.

Companion Case 2: Additional Confirmed Case of Meningitis on the FLAIR Imaging Sequence

Companion Case 3: 100% O₂ Inhalation

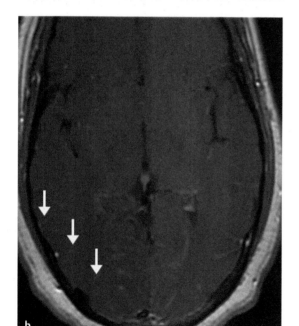

Fig. 44.4 Axial FLAIR image of the brain **(a)** reveals hyperintense signal within the sulci predominantly in the occipital regions in this patient recently diagnosed with pneumococcal meningitis. Subtle enhancement of the leptomeninges is also present on the postcontrast T1WI **(b)**. The areas affected are not at the skull base, near an aerated sinus, or a metal foreign body, which could generate magnetic susceptibility artifact.

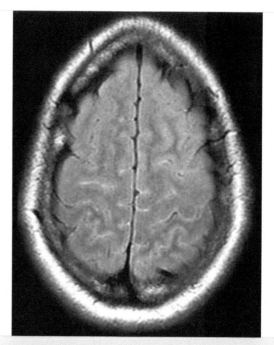

Fig. 44.5 Axial FLAIR image of a claustrophobic patient under heavy sedation for MRI. The patient had a history of cluster-type headaches for several years but was currently asymptomatic and without clinical evidence of meningitis. FLAIR images show increased signal intensity of the CSF diffusely, but particularly evidence over the convexities rather than in the basilar region.

Companion Case 4: CSF Pulsation on FLAIR Results in the Artifactual Appearance of a Lesion or Hemorrhage in the Posterior Fossa Subarachnoid Space

Companion Case 5: CSF Motion in the Lateral Ventricles on FLAIR Causes Artifactual Appearance of a Mass in the Frontal Horns Near the Foramen of Monro

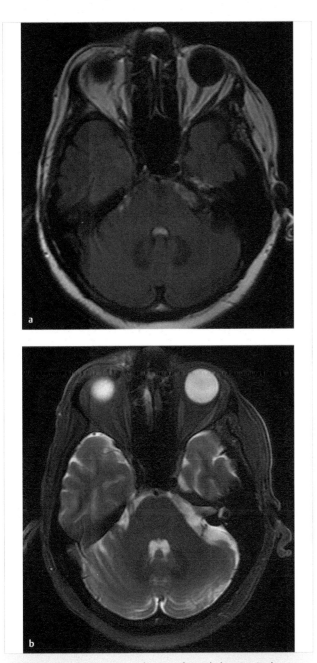

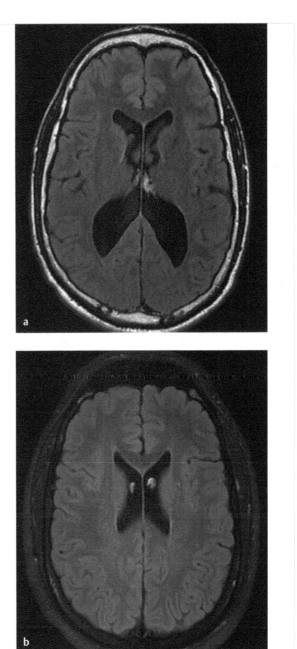

Fig. 44.6 Axial FLAIR image with areas of signal elevation in the prepontine cistern surrounding the cisternal segments of the fifth cranial nerve and extending inferiorly **(a)**. Axial FSE-T2WI **(b)** demonstrates no mass lesion of the visualized right fifth cranial nerve or mass in the contralateral cistern. The typical location for CSF flow artifacts on FLAIR should be noted. Also, lack of any mass effect upon surrounding structures helps confirm the artifactual nature of this finding. Diffusion-weighted images can also confirm the absence of a potential lesion (epidermoid) in this location.

Fig. 44.7 **(a, b)** Axial FLAIR images reveal typical areas of increased signal that appear to float within the lateral ventricles arise within areas adjacent to the foramen of Monro where CSF motion is accentuated.

44.1.7 Case 2 Presentation

FLAIR: The "bounce point artifact" mimicking superficial CNS siderosis.

44.1.8 Imaging Findings

The FLAIR T1 images (▶ Fig. 44.8a–c) all show a single pixel-thin black line at the boundary of the brain and the CSF and at the water–fat interfaces. Had this finding been present on the T2WIs, especially gradient recalled echo (GRE) T2WIs

(▶ Fig. 44.9b,c), concern would have been raised regarding the possibility of superficial CNS siderosis. However, the T2WIs (▶ Fig. 44.9a–c) are normal. Furthermore, noninversion recovery T1WI is completely normal (▶ Fig. 44.9d). Note the improved gray–white matter contrast on the FLAIR T1 sequence (▶ Fig. 44.8c) in comparison to the routine T1WI (▶ Fig. 44.9d).

Impression: Markedly low signal intensity at the interface of CSF and the brain is only present on the FLAIR T1WIs and is therefore proven to be an artifact of this inversion recovery, magnitude reconstruction-type sequence.[1]

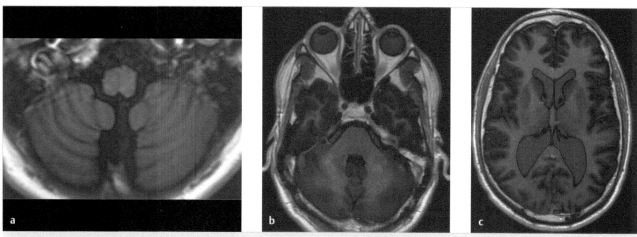

Fig. 44.8 Brain MRI performed on 3-T magnet in a patient with a headache and remote history of nonaneurysmal subarachnoid hemorrhage in the perimesencephalic cistern. Axial T1WIs are shown through the posterior fossa **(a, b)** and at the level of the lateral ventricles **(c)**.

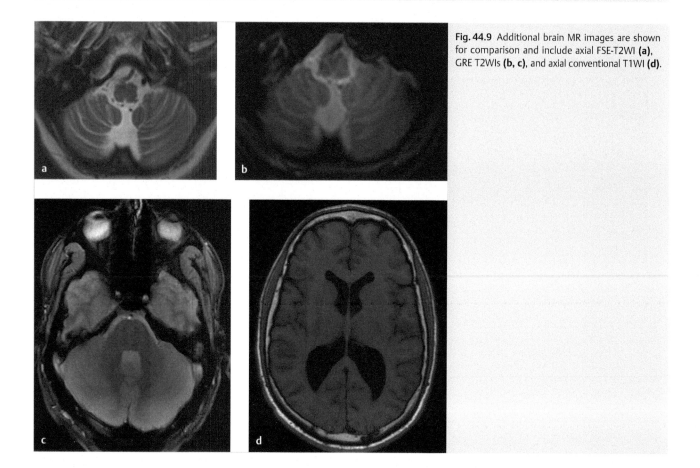

Fig. 44.9 Additional brain MR images are shown for comparison and include axial FSE-T2WI **(a)**, GRE T2WIs **(b, c)**, and axial conventional T1WI **(d)**.

44.1.9 Differential Diagnosis

- Bounce point–type artifact:
  - A thin black line artifact that exists only at the interface of tissues with very different T1 s (i.e., the brain and CSF).
  - It occurs only with inversion recovery–type sequences.
  - Absence on T2WIs, especially the GRE-type sequence, confirms the finding is artifactual.
- Superficial CNS siderosis—chronic, recurrent SAH:
  - Finding of hemosiderin deposition in the leptomeninges.
  - Most apparent on the T2WIs, especially GRE- or susceptibility weighted imaging type sequences that accentuate signal loss secondary to magnetic susceptibility artifact.
  - The classic clinical presentation is a history of hearing loss and ataxia.
- Leptomeningeal calcification:
  - More discrete areas of involvement that are better seen on T2WIs.

44.1.10 Essential Information regarding the T1W-FLAIR Sequence

- Inversion recovery sequences begin with a 180-degree RF pulse, as opposed to a 90-degree RF pulse typically used in a routine conventional T1WIs.
- As longitudinal magnetization recovers by T1 relaxation, different tissues will pass through the null point at varying times. If an echo is acquired at the time a tissue is passing through zero, or the null point (bounce point), no signal will be generated.[1]
- In magnitude reconstructed images, if a voxel contains tissues with very different T1 s, signal may cancel out and result in a black line.

- FLAIR T1 imaging sequence is routinely used on higher, 3-T, magnet systems because the T1 of tissues is prolonged at higher field strengths. This results in the CSF signal not being as dark as typically seen on T1WIs on 1.5-T and lower magnet systems.
- FLAIR T1 imaging is becoming a routine sequence for spine imaging even on 1.5-T and lower field strength systems because it has been shown to demonstrate increased conspicuity between the CSF, spinal cord, and cervical disk herniations in comparison to TSE-T1 images.[4]
- FLAIR T1 imaging also provides greater tissue contrast between normal gray and white matter on 3-T magnets.
- FLAIR T1 imaging "dark rim" effect has been reported to have diagnostic utility with high sensitivity and specificity for multiple sclerosis demyelinating lesions on double inversion recovery sequences designed to suppress CSF and gray matter signal (GM-DIR).[5]

44.1.11 Companion Case

A 55-year-old woman presents with sensorineural hearing loss, auditory hallucinations, and vertigo with a past medical history of traumatic brachial plexus injury 10 years prior to presentation.

A total spine MRI was performed and excluded an ependymoma or other hemorrhagic neoplasm. A CT angiogram was performed, which did not reveal an aneurysm or other vascular malformation. She did have a history of traumatic brachial plexus injury in the past, which was considered to be the source of the hemorrhage as no other cause was found. Brachial plexus injury and traumatic pseudomeningoceles have been previously reported to cause this condition.[6]

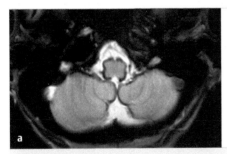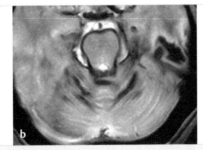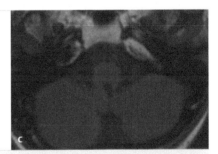

Fig. 44.10 Axial GRE T2WIs in the region of the posterior fossa **(a, b)** reveal diffuse decrease in signal of the pial surface of the brain consistent with leptomeningeal staining with hemosiderin. The axial T1WI **(c)**, however, is normal.

44.2 Hardware/Room-Related MR Artifacts

44.2.1 Case 1 Presentation

44.2.2 Imaging Findings

Sagittal T1-weighted image (T2WI; ▶ Fig. 44.11a) and fast spin echo (FSE) T2-weighted image (T2WI; ▶ Fig. 44.11b) reveal a linear area of alternating high- and low-signal bands that involve the lower cervical spine and upper thoracic levels (*arrows*). This finding was present in the same location on multiple sequences and all images within the sequence.

Note that the abnormality extends outside of the patient anteriorly and crosses normal anatomic boundaries, typical of an artifact. There is no differential diagnosis for this finding as it does not mimic pathology. It is an artifact that needs to be recognized and cause identified in order to correct the problem as the zipper artifacts degrade image quality and may obscure important anatomic detail.

Impression: Zipper artifact.

Cause: Technical equipment–related artifact that may be caused by an opening into the magnet room that is allowing penetration by outside, omnipresent radiofrequency (RF) range electromagnetic energy. The magnet room is specially constructed with copper panels, penetration seals, and an airtight, sealed door so that it acts as a Faraday cage. When correctly sealed, its most important function is to keep unwanted RF transmissions out of the room, which would be picked up by the extremely sensitive RF receivers. The artifact runs in the phase-encoding direction because it is occurring over a narrow range of contaminated RFs. Faulty light bulbs or unshielded anesthetic equipment may also generate an electromagnetic signal, which would appear identical.

Solution: The door to the magnet room should be checked for a proper seal. If new equipment has entered the room, such as new lighting fixture or pulse oximeter, it should be checked to be sure it is not generating an electromagnetic signal that is not shielded (see ▶ Fig. 44.12).

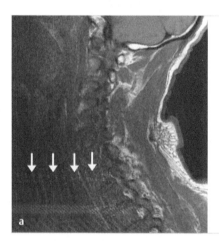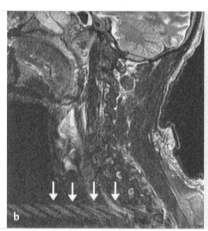

Fig. 44.11 (a, b) MRI of the cervical spine was performed for neck pain.

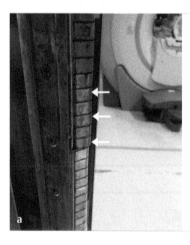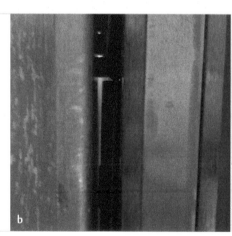

Fig. 44.12 (a) Inspection of the door to the magnet room reveals the copper clips have been damaged and are bent *(arrows)*, preventing complete closure. **(b)** The "flashlight test" shows light leakage in the area of the clip damage.

44.2.3 Companion Case 1

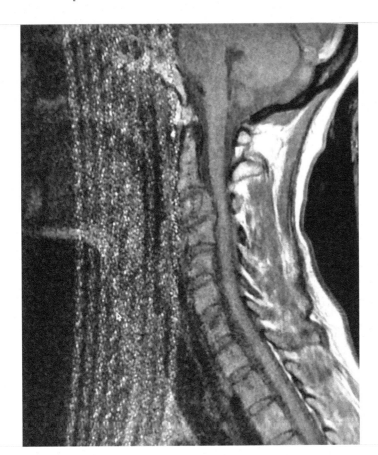

Fig. 44.13 Sagittal T1WI of a different patient's cervical spine shows extensive zipper type artifacts, which obscure the skull base and prevertebral soft tissues. This artifact was found to be due to a damaged door, which was sealing incompletely.

44.2.4 Companion Case 2

44.2.5 Imaging Findings

The sagittal T2WIs (▶ Fig. 44.14a,b) reveal a ribbon of alternating high and low signal extending superior to inferior, which in these examinations was the phase-encoding direction. Unlike the "zipper" artifact previously shown, this artifact is not uniform in appearance across the image but rather tapers in a featherlike manner. Similar to the zipper artifact, however, it does not mimic pathology as it does not respect normal anatomic boundaries. Note how the artifact obscures visualization of portions of the posterior fossa (▶ Fig. 44.14a) and limits evaluation of the paraspinous soft tissues (▶ Fig. 44.14b).

Impression: Annefact, or cusp, artifact. This artifact is seen especially in sagittal plane imaging of spines that have been performed on a C,T,L (cervical-thoracic-lumbar) phased array coil (see ▶ Fig. 44.15).

Cause: It is caused by the improper technical activation of adjacent, unneeded coil elements that are detecting signal from stimulated echoes that are outside of the intended field of view (FOV).

Solution: This is a technical error that should be corrected by the proper selection of coil elements corresponding to the region being imaged.

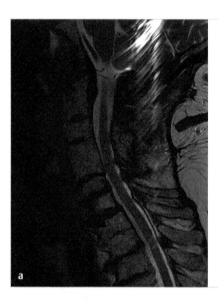 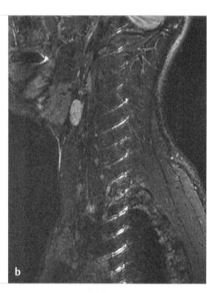

Fig. 44.14 (a, b) MR images of the cervical spine from two different patients with a similar technical artifact.

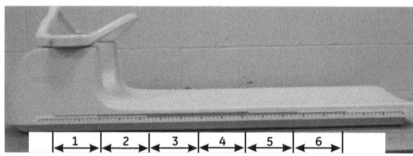

Fig. 44.15 Image of a standard C,T,L (cervical-thoracic-lumbar) phased array coil. The patient lies on this receiver coil for routine spine imaging. This coil has two elements per section and is divided into six sections. Depending upon which coil elements are activated, the field of view may be altered.

44.3 Nonspecific Pulse Sequence Technical Artifacts: Wraparound Artifact with and without the Use of Parallel Imaging Techniques

44.3.1 Case 1 Presentation

44.3.2 Imaging Findings

Axial FSE-T2WI (▶ Fig. 44.16) shows arc-shaped bands of alternating high and low signal in the region of the genu and splenium of the corpus callosum. Close inspection shows that these curvilinear bands extend laterally not only into adjacent frontal and occipital lobes but also, in the frontal region, into the skull and beyond the patient's head. The morphology of this abnormality precisely matches the frontal and occipital regions of the head that have been excluded from the image due to the small FOV.

Repeat image obtained with the same small FOV but with "no phase wrap" option selected reveals these areas are now normal (▶ Fig. 44.17).

Impression: Wraparound artifact (i.e., aliasing in the phase-encoding direction).

Cause: FOV too small for body part being imaged and no oversampling in the phase-encoding direction to remedy this problem.

Solution: There are many possible solutions, which include the following: using a larger FOV, oversampling in the phase-encoding direction and then simply eliminating the periphery of the image into which the phase wrap is occurring, using saturation bands to eliminate signal arising from the undesired body part, swapping the direction of the phase and frequency encoding so that phase encoding runs in the short axis of the body part, and use of a surface coil for signal detection so that signal from the body part outside of the region of interest is not detected.

44.3.3 Essential Information regarding Wraparound Artifact

- Spatial localization in a 2D MR image depends upon a linear relationship between frequency in one direction and differences in phase in the other as created by the magnet's gradient coils.
- As a complex echo, or signal, emitted from the patient is being converted from a continuous analog signal to a digital one, it must be sampled at a certain sampling rate that defines the FOV.
- This sampling rate must be twice the rate of the highest frequency component of the signal in order for it to be correctly distinguished from the lowest frequency components.
- If this condition is not met, and the sampling rate is too low, the highest frequency component of the signal, or highest degree of phase change, will be incorrectly interpreted as a very low frequency, or low degree of phase change, and will be misplaced to the exact opposite side of the image. This is called aliasing or wraparound artifact.

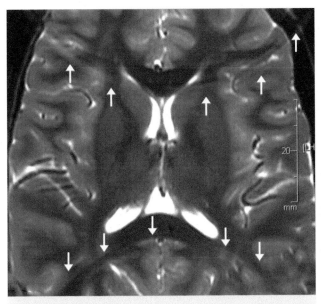

Fig. 44.16 Axial FSE-T2WI of the brain of a patient being evaluated for syncope.

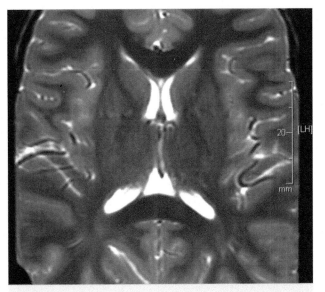

Fig. 44.17

44.3.4 Companion Case

Case 2 Presentation

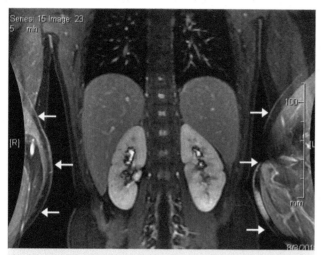

Fig. 44.18 Body coil image of the upper abdomen with arms lying to the side of the patient, just outside the prescribed FOV showing wraparound artifact.

44.3.5 Imaging Findings

FLAIR images (▶ Fig. 44.19) reveal a linear area of hyperintensity in the midline of the pontomedullary junction that was not confirmed on the FSE-T2WIs and has no evidence of associated mass effect. Importantly, the area of abnormal signal extends posterior to the dorsal aspect of the midbrain in ▶ Fig. 44.19a. Note how the left ear pinna is in the same anteroposterior plane and has the same morphology as the abnormality.

When abnormalities do not respect normal anatomic boundaries, are not confirmed in additional planes or on alterative sequences, and do not have expected associated mass effect, an artifact should be suspected and the sequence repeated for confirmation if possible.

Impression: SENSE (SENSitivity Encoding) reconstruction artifact.

Cause: The FOV for this brain MRI excluded the pinna of the left ear, which, due to its small size, would not have been detected by the body coil in the preliminary calibration scan to determine individual coil sensitivity. Signal from the ear is still detected by the head coil's individual coil element that is closest to the ear, but it cannot place the signal properly as the calibration scan determined that signal coming from this area should be set to zero. Therefore, the ear appears in the center of the image. The center of the image corresponds to the medial aspect of that imaging coil's reduced FOV.

Solution: Do not use small FOVs when utilizing SENSE as wraparound, or aliasing, type artifacts occur more readily and may be difficult to sort out as they do not have the typical appearance of wraparound artifacts as on imaging without parallel imaging techniques.

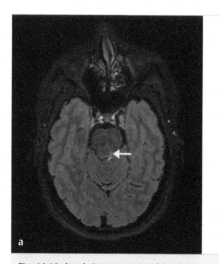
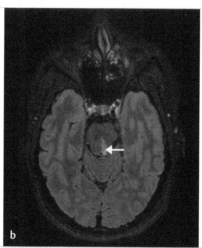
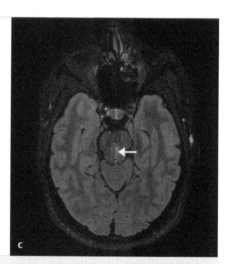

Fig. 44.19 (a–c) Contiguous axial FLAIR images of the brain obtained through the upper pons and pontomedullary junction in a woman with a diagnosis of multiple sclerosis.

44.3.6 Essential Information about Parallel Imaging and Reconstruction Artifacts

- Parallel MR imaging technology dramatically decreases the time needed to acquire an image by reducing the total number of phase-encoding steps.
- The decrease in imaging time is referred to as the acceleration factor.
- Time is decreased by having multiple coils working in parallel, each acquiring only a portion of the data required for a full image, and then recombining their data to create an "unwrapped image."
- Prior to scanning, a calibration scan is performed that uses a full FOV image obtained by the body coil to determine the sensitivity of each of the individual coils that comprise the head imaging coil.
- In routine MR imaging, without the use of parallel imaging techniques, incomplete filling of k-space (due to collecting only every other line of the phase-encoding steps) results in a "wraparound" type artifact where objects just outside the FOV would appear on the opposite (or right side) of the image.

- Aliasing with parallel imaging occurs more readily and often has an unusual appearance.
- Frequently the aliased anatomy appears in the center of the image.
- If an object lies outside the prescribed FOV and is small, and therefore not detected on the body coil calibration step, signal that arises from this small "bright object" may be displaced within the final "unwrapped image."

44.3.7 Companion Case 1

Imaging Findings

A tubular area of high signal appears in the medial right temporal lobe and extends across the tentorium into the right side of the cerebellum. There is no evidence of mass effect. The finding was not present in additional imaging planes on other sequences. Note how the morphology of this high signal area precisely corresponds to the lateral most aspect of the patient's left ear, which has decreased signal as it is just outside the intended FOV.

Impression: SENSE reconstruction artifact.

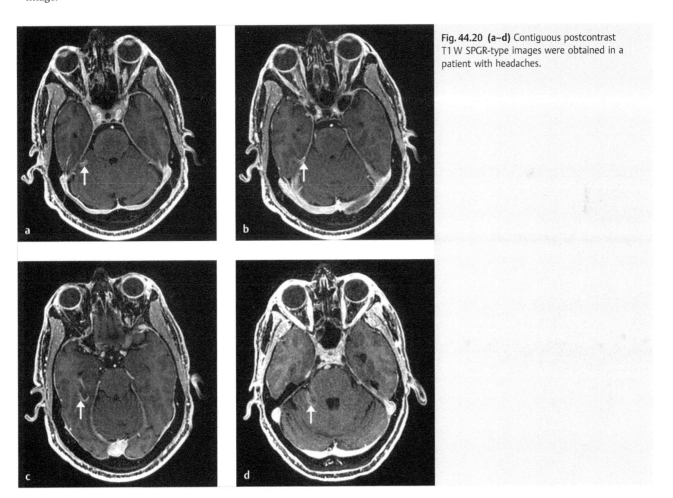

Fig. 44.20 (a–d) Contiguous postcontrast T1 W SPGR-type images were obtained in a patient with headaches.

44.3.8 Companion Case 2

Imaging Findings

Curvilinear areas of high signal that appear to be enhancement on this T1 postcontrast image are seen within the superior aspect of the brainstem extending posteriorly into the cerebellum and anteriorly into the ambient cistern in this patient with marked dilation of the temporal horns of the lateral ventricles. The fact that these structures cross normal anatomic boundaries and do not have any associated mass effect should raise suspicion that they are artifactual. The morphology of these unusual appearing "lesions" precisely matches the contralateral earlobe, which is almost excluded from the FOV but still generating high signal (*arrows* in ▶ Fig. 44.22). Small, bright objects that are just outside or nearly outside of the FOV create unusual wraparound artifacts where they commonly appear displaced toward the center of the image.

Impression: SENSE wraparound artifact.

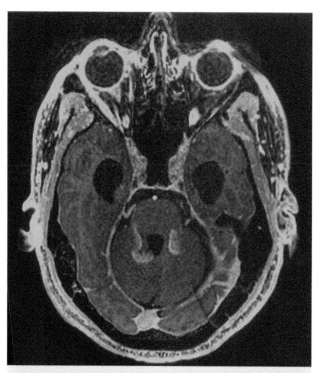

Fig. 44.21 Axial postcontrast T1WI in a patient with hydrocephalus reveals unusual appearing areas of enhancement in the posterior fossa, which raised concern for a large draining vein associated with a possible vascular malformation.

References

[1] Questions and Answers in MRI. Available at: https://mriquestions.com/index.html

[2] Frigon C, Shaw DW, Heckbert SR, Weinberger E, Jardine DS. Supplemental oxygen causes increased signal intensity in subarachnoid cerebrospinal fluid on brain FLAIR MR images obtained in children during general anesthesia. Radiology. 2004; 233(1):51–55

[3] Mori N, Mugikura S, Higano S, et al. The leptomeningeal "ivy sign" on fluid-attenuated inversion recovery MR imaging in moyamoya disease: a sign of decreased cerebral vascular reserve? AJNR Am J Neuroradiol. 2009; 30(5): 930–935

[4] Ganesan K, Bydder GM. A prospective comparison study of fast T1 weighted fluid attenuation inversion recovery and T1 weighted turbo spin echo sequence at 3 T in degenerative disease of the cervical spine. Br J Radiol. 2014; 87(1041):20140091

[5] Tillema JM, Weigand SD, Dayan M, et al. Dark rims: novel sequence enhances diagnostic specificity in multiple sclerosis. AJNR Am J Neuroradiol. 2018; 39(6): 1052–1058

[6] Bonito V, Agostinis C, Ferraresi S, Defanti CA. Superficial siderosis of the central nervous system after brachial plexus injury. Case report. J Neurosurg. 1994; 80(5):931–934

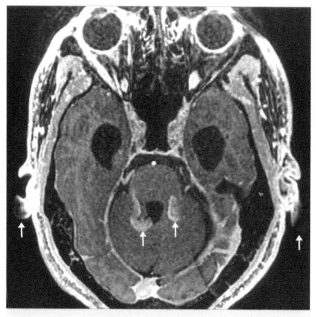

Fig. 44.22

Index